AF182058

Springer Series in Neuropsychology

Harry A. Whitaker, Series Editor

Springer Series in Neuropsychology

Harry A. Whitaker, Series Editor

Phonological Processes and Brain Mechanisms
H.A. Whitaker (Ed.)

Contemporary Reviews in Neuropsychology
H.A. Whitaker (Ed.)

Neuropsychological Studies of Nonfocal Brain Damage: Dementia and Trauma
H.A. Whitaker (Ed.)

Harry A. Whitaker
Editor

Neuropsychological Studies of Nonfocal Brain Damage

Dementia and Trauma

With 33 Illustrations

Springer-Verlag
New York Berlin Heidelberg
London Paris Tokyo

Harry A. Whitaker
Professor of Neurology
Department of Neuroscience
University of North Dakota School of Medicine
Fargo, North Dakota 58102, USA
and
Director, Cognitive Neuroscience Research Program
The Neuropsychiatric Institute
Fargo, North Dakota 58103, USA

Library of Congress Cataloging-in-Publication Data
Neuropsychological studies of non-focal brain damage.
(Springer series in neuropsychology)
Includes bibliographies and index.
1. Neuropsychological tests. 2. Dementia—Diagnosis.
3. Alzheimer's disease—Diagnosis. 4. Brain damage—
Diagnosis. I. Whitaker, Harry A. II. Series.
(DNLM: 1. Brain Injuries—psychology. 2. Dementia—
psychology. 3. Neuropsychology. WL 354 N4944]
RC386.6.N48N48 1988 617'.481 87-23509

© 1988 by Springer-Verlag New York Inc.
Softcover reprint of the hardcover 1st edition 1988

All rights reserved. This work may not be translated or copied in whole or in part without the written permission of the publisher (Springer-Verlag, 175 Fifth Avenue, New York, New York 10010, USA), except for brief excerpts in connection with reviews or scholarly analysis. Use in connection with any form of information storage and retrieval, electronic adaptation, computer software, or by similar or dissimilar methodology now known or hereafter developed is forbidden.
The use of general descriptive names, trade names, trademarks, etc. in this publication, even if the former are not especially identified, is not to be taken as a sign that such names, as understood by the Trade Marks and Merchandise Marks Act, may accordingly be used freely by anyone.
While the advice and information in this book are believed to be true and accurate at the date of going to press, neither the authors nor the editors nor the publisher can accept any legal responsibility for any errors or omissions that may be made. The publisher makes no warranty, express or implied, with respect to the material contained herein.

Typeset by Publishers Service, Bozeman, Montana.

9 8 7 6 5 4 3 2 1

ISBN-13:978-1-4613-8753-4 e-ISBN-13:978-1-4613-8751-0
DOI: 10.1007/978-1-4613-8751-0

Preface: Clinical Research in Neuropsychology

Two general research models in behavioral neurology and neuropsychology have emerged since the latter part of the 19th century; both are so-called "medical models." In the first model, the relation between a focal lesion and a specific functional impairment is observed. This relationship becomes the basis, in contemporary terms, for drawing an inference about the functional architecture of a cognitive system. From virtually the beginning of contemporary behavioral neurology and neuropsychology, this relationship has been challenged. Hughlings-Jackson argued that there was no direct or simple connection between the locus of a lesion and an element of functional architecture. Von Monakow's concept of diaschisis has been for years a theoretical concept invoked to explain away puzzling deficits associated with localized lesions. In recent research, positron emission tomography (PET) scans have shown that areas of hypometabolism occur distant from focal lesions. This fact suggests that the specific functional impairments that we observe may arise from both the locally damaged brain and the distant brain region, in spite of the fact that it is uncertain to what degree hypometabolism results in impaired function.

In the other model, patients with lesions in a similar area, or of a similar type, are assessed for a list of functional impairments. A group of patients with a similar type of lesion (e.g., stroke, tumor, closed head injury) or a similar disease (e.g., multiple sclerosis, Parkinson's disease, senile dementia of the Alzheimer type) are observed to see if they exhibit similar impairments or, in traditional terms, a syndrome. The inference about the way in which disease or lesion type affects behavior will be couched in terms of how the particular disease affects a specific brain system (e.g., myelin), chemistry (e.g., dopamine system), or region (e.g., frontal lobe).

The second model is the appropriate one for investigating nonfocal brain damage. "Nonfocal" is being used here in the conventional sense to contrast with "focal." In point of fact, both the notions of focal lesion and nonfocal lesion are misleading. As just noted above, focal lesions are typically associated with areas of hypometabolism (and, inferentially, functional changes) in other parts of the brain. Likewise, the notion of nonfocal lesion is misleading if one logically means diffusely located in all brain structures or systems. Such is not the case.

Although a particular structure, such as myelin, may be widely affected in the brain, other structures and systems remain unaffected. The so-called nonfocal or diffuse brain diseases, including closed head injury, do not result in lesions that are spread uniformly throughout the brain.

This volume does not address the neuropsychology of all nonfocal diseases; for example, multiple sclerosis is not discussed, and Parkinson's disease is not discussed in depth. However, the principles of assessment and modeling that are discussed in the following chapters also apply to other disease entities, *mutatis mutandis*. The 10 chapters are equally divided between discussions of dementia and discussions of closed head injury. A précis of each chapter follows.

Swihart and Pirozzolo compare the status of sensory, motor, cognitive, and behavioral functions in the normal aged with those of several dementias. Vision, audition, olfaction, gustation, and somesthesis all decline with age. The same is true of motor functions: Simple and complex reaction time, fine motor coordination, and postural reflexes exhibit decreased performance with age. The so-called classic aging pattern of intellectual function is marked by a relative preservation of verbal skills accompanied by a decline in nonverbal or performance skills. Some age-related language changes are actually improvements rather than decrements, such as an increased quantity and complexity of narrative discourse style. Age-declines in memory are generally acknowledged, but are problematic to interpret within a cognitive model of memory. One view is that the ability to spontaneously process to-be-remembered material—i.e., to use optimal encoding processes at a deep level—declines with age. Some research has associated this decline with age-related impaired cognitive and attentional resources. Age-related declines in visuospatial skills have been documented using standard neuropsychological tests of parietal lobe functioning. Personality, emotionality, and mood state do not decline systematically with age, but depression is a common affective disturbance in the elderly. A variety of changes in the brain's morphology, physiology, and chemistry have been associated with advancing age; correlating these with neuropsychological changes has been problematic. Swihart and Pirozzolo next review a number of disease processes that have been associated with dementia: Alzheimer's disease (DAT), multi-infarct dementia, Parkinson's disease (PD), Huntington's disease (HD), progressive supranuclear palsy, normal pressure hydrocephalus, Pick's disease, and pseudodementia. Where the information is known, Swihart and Pirozzolo discuss the clinical course, the neuropsychological functioning, and the problems in differential diagnosis associated with these dementias, comparing and contrasting normal age changes and various neuropathological changes associated with each disease entity.

Bigler compares the findings on computed tomography (CT) scans with the neuropsychological findings associated with DAT, specifically considering cortical atrophy and ventricular enlargement, based on a study of 42 patients. The neuropsychological data were taken from the Wechsler Adult Intelligence Scale (WAIS) and the Wechsler Memory Scale (WMS). No significant correlations were found between neuropsychological performance and ventricular enlargement; however, correlations were found between some neuropsychological measures of the WAIS and WMS and with the measurements of cortical atrophy. The second issue raised by Bigler is the correlation between neuropsychological performance and dementia type. In a study of 138 patients with presumptive dementia, a cluster analysis grouped them into five different types of dementia in terms of verbal and visuospatial functioning. Neither ventricular enlargement nor cortical atrophy correlated systematically with any of the dementia clusters. He concludes that neuropsychological measures are better than CT analysis at estimating as well as predicting the degree of deterioration in demented patients.

Cummings begins with an historical sketch of the issues in the clinical diagnosis of Alzheimer's disease, beginning with Alois Alzheimer's initial report in 1907. Of particular interest in this discussion is the alternating prominence of neuropathological diagnoses and clinical-behavioral diagnoses. He goes on to outline a set of clinical features that distinguish dementia of the Alzheimer type (DAT) from the other dementias, considering memory, language, visuospatial, cognitive, personality, affect, and motor systems. On clinical grounds, the most difficult differential diagnosis is between DAT and either Pick's disease or vascular dementia.

As part of a general interest in the language impairments associated with dementia of the Alzheimer type, Ulatowska, Allard, Donnell, Bristow, Haynes, Flower, and North investigated discourse performance in 10 patients diagnosed with DAT. The experimental narrative and procedural discourse tasks included a self-generated story, a story elicited by pictures, the retelling of a story, the providing of a summary and a moral for a story, and the providing of a written version of a story presented in pictures. Five types of analysis were performed: sentence structure, narrative content, discourse structure, reference, and a rating of content and clarity. The DAT subjects were impaired on some tasks, but not on others. Sentence-level and discourse-level linguistic structures were preserved, but they showed substantial deficits in both content and reference and in their ability to produce summaries and morals to stories. The most obvious disruption of discourse performance by these DAT subjects was at the level of content; they produced a greater amount of irrelevant and/or incorrect information. DAT subjects also produced many more reference errors than normal controls; not only did they use more pronouns, but they used them incorrectly more often. Measures of syntactic structure and discourse structure did not differ between the DAT subjects and normal controls. One of the interesting conclusions reached by Ulatowska et al. is that the language impairments in DAT are not best described as a form of aphasia. These impairments do seem to be similar to certain characteristics of the language of the elderly, albeit to a greater degree, which of course raises the question of whether some of the impairments in DAT are in part the effects of aging per se.

Long and Williams address some of the problems of the patient with mild to moderate closed head injury. They begin with a brief review of the physical aspects of closed head injury (CHI) and the general clinical characteristics for estimating outcome. Their recovery model emphasizes six factors: preinjury status, extent of brain damage, impairments of cognitive function, emotional adjustment, sociological-environmental factors, and vocational ability. Each of these factors is discussed in detail in subsequent sections of the chapter. They conclude with a discussion of neuropsychological rehabilitation of the CHI patient that emphasizes planning, patient and family education, stress reactions, and family support.

Goldstein and Levin correlate the distinction between automatic and volitional cognitive operations to neurological conditions that affect attention. Sources of capacity reduction—such as stress or depression, aging, or brain disease—will affect volitional, effortful, and problem-solving processes more than automatic processes. Some diseases, such as Parkinson's, produce a selective deficit of effortful/volitional but not automatic processing. Goldstein and Levin extend the application of this theoretical framework to survivors of CHI. To study the possible effects of CHI on automatic processing, they gave a group of 15 nonaphasic, long-term survivors of severe CHI, using a taped word list in which some words were repeated up to 7 times. To study the effects on effortful processing, they gave the same subjects a free-recall test, with memory for words assessed after each trial. A clear difference emerged between CHI subjects and controls on effortful processing abilities, but not on automatic processing abilities. In a second experiment to further explore the hypothesis that frequency of occurrence processing (an automatic process) is preserved after CHI, Goldstein and Levin tested a new group of 16 chronic survivors of CHI on their ability to estimate the number of times a given word had been presented. In this experiment, a difference between the experimental and control groups in the area of automatic processing was shown, although the groups did not differ in a cognitive estimation task. Goldstein and Levin conclude by comparing the current theories that amnesia represents in part a loss of automatic processing abilities to the data showing an impaired sensitivity to frequency information in CHI patients.

Wiig, Alexander, and Secord evaluated the relationships between ratings of levels of cognitive functioning (LOCF) and measures of linguistic and metalinguistic abilities in patients who had sustained closed head injury. Three groups of patients were identified according to the criteria of the Rancho Level of Cognitive Functioning Scales: VI, confused but appropriate; VII: automatic and appropriate; and VIII; purposeful and appropriate. Measures of interpreting and matching metaphors, interpreting sentence ambiguities, making inferences, and recreating sentences differentiated reliably between the confused and the automatic LOCF levels. The findings support the hypothesis that post-CHI language and cognitive dysfunctions are related to each other and involve both linguistic and metalinguistic abilities.

Mateer and Moore Sohlberg note that a reduction in memory capacity is a frequent complaint of individuals who have suffered closed head injury. Traditional approaches to memory rehabilitation have emphasized either the restoration of memory or the development of compensatory strategies. Setting these aside, Mateer and Moore Sohlberg address the question of an ecologically valid memory rehabilitation approach that considers memory mechanisms as they operate in natural contexts. An example is prospective memory, or the ability to remember to perform future acts. Prospective memory, along with five other classes of memory (retrograde, anterograde, episodic, semantic, and working), were used as the basis for a questionnaire that was sent to a randomly selected group of 178 head-injured patients and 157 control subjects. Analysis of the survey data showed that 47% of the variance in responses to the questionnaire was accounted for by items that loaded on the Attention/Prospective Memory factor, suggesting that the ability to carry out planned actions in the future depends a great deal on attention. Both brain-injured and control individuals ranked the failures of prospective memory as occurring most often. In other words, most people are concerned with their ability to remember to perform some action and with attention-based memory processes, such as keeping a number in your head while dialing; yet there are currently no established assessment or treatment tools available with which to rehabilitate Prospective Memory. Mateer and Moore Sohlberg outline three treatment programs for memory rehabilitation: attention process training, prospective memory training, and memory notebook training. Patient data providing some evidence for the efficacy of these training programs are discussed.

Cytowic, Stump, and Larned address the problem of the head-injured patient who, though not overtly impaired, nevertheless sustains a variety of symptoms that affect work and personal activities. This is the patient who is often neglected by primary care personnel, the patient who has sustained a shaking injury of the brain. The authors evaluated 178 patients with closed head injury for the incidence and follow-up prevalence of 20 different self-assessed symptoms and 7 different formal behavioral neurology tests. A number of the findings are of interest. There were high incidences of neck pain, dizziness, nonvascular headache, and memory and thought changes, as well as a wide range of subjective visual symptoms, in spite of normal acuity and normal oculomotor function on standard testing. Patient outcome—clinically defined as the point at which the patient was discharged from active medical care—was assigned to one of three groups: normal, symptomatic, or impaired. About half of the patients were discharged as normal; they were able to return to work or the home without medication and with no evident need for follow-up medical care or medications, although they were not all symptom-free on careful testing. About 30% remained symptomatic; these subjects had identifiable complaints that they felt were tolerable or acceptable and that were relieved by medication. About 20% remained impaired with an unsatisfactory outcome. Subjective visual function impairments were found in a majority of the patients in the study, including nearly a third of the patients in the normal outcome group. These impairments do not show up on routine ophthalmic examination, but must be tested for specifically. Since one question raised by Cytowic, Stump, and Larned was the efficacy of treatment, they conducted an alprazolan study on 40 patients in the group; 20 patients were given alprazolan, and 20 comprised the control group. The alprazolan-treated group had a more rapid recovery in terms of the number of treatment days from injury to discharge (a mean of 93 days compared to a mean of 155 days), although injuries prevented all 40 patients in this study from returning to work. A different study on a new group of CHI patients was undertaken to assess how well magnetic resonance imaging (MRI) scans revealed structural lesions in this patient population. Gross lesions usually were not seen, but there was an increased prevalence of unidentified bright objects (UBOs) in white matter. The location of UBOs did correspond to predicted location based on neuropsychological examination. Based on a study of 25 patients, the MRI scan showed abnormalities in less than half of those who had abnormal neuropsychological test results, but when the MRI did show abnormalities, it agreed with the neuropsychological results over 80% of the time. The data suggest that UBOs appear sometime after CHI, and they may ultimately disappear; this is based on the observation that the patients in this study who had normal MRIs (no UBOs) tended to have been scanned either very early or very late after their head injury. Cytowic, Stump, and Larned conclude with discussions of the criterion of returning to work as an indicator of persisting brain damage, as well as a discussion of neck injuries associated with CHI. The overall message of this chapter is quite clear: Shaking injuries to the brain produce real injuries and deficits, in spite of the failure of superficial clinical examination or gross brain scanning to reveal them.

Smith, Butters, and Granholm address the different nature of the semantic memory disorder in two types of dementing illnesses – DAT, which has primarily cortical involvement, and Huntington's disease (HD), which has primarily subcortical involvement. Using the network model of semantic memory, they show that DAT involves a disruption of spreading activation among nodes, leading to a breakdown in the structure and usage of semantic knowledge. However, orthographic and phonological processing abilities remain largely intact from the early to the middle stages of the disease. In contrast, HD spares language abilities for the most part, although recent studies of HD patients suggest impairments in tasks that require lexical access or that require specific knowledge about semantic relations between lexical items. Focusing on their own research, Smith, Butters, and Granholm completed several studies on the organization of semantic memory in DAT and HD. In the first study, control and HD patients were compared on a word-pair priming task, where the word pairs were strong or moderate associates. Control subjects and mild and moderate HD subjects all exhibited positive priming effects, regardless of the strength of association or type of relationship between the word pairs. However, with progression of HD, there was a trend of decreasing priming effects for strongly associated word pairs and increasing priming effects for moderately associated word pairs, thus suggesting an overall decline in the degree of associative strengths of word pairs. When considered in the light of other language tests, it is suggested that HD does in fact break down some aspects of lexical-semantic organization. In a second study comparing DAT and HD patients, a stem-completion priming task was employed. Somewhat unexpectedly, DAT patients were severely impaired on this priming task; HD patients were somewhat impaired. In a third study, semantic priming of word pairs was compared between DAT and HD patients. DAT patients exhibited no priming effects at all, whereas this new group of HD patients performed like the HD group in the first study, exhibiting priming comparable to that of control subjects. Smith, Butters, and Granholm conclude that a levels-of-processing model of semantic memory accounts for the impairments seen in DAT patients: DAT involves a breakdown in activation (or loss of representation) of attributes and features that relate and differentiate concepts in a semantic network. HD involves a degeneration in the system of spreading activation in semantic networks. Smith, Butters, and Granholm suggest that the progression of HD may involve subtle changes in the organization of activation in semantic networks; in contrast, DAT may involve an actual shrinkage of semantic networks, resulting in an incomplete representation of concepts and their relationships in semantic memory.

A proper and careful neuropsychological analysis is the cornerstone of medical management of dementing illnesses and closed head injury and, in fact, of any disease of the central nervous system. Neuropsychological evaluation is the basis for deciding both the degree of impairment and the degree of recovery; it is the basis for assessment and rehabilitation.

HARRY A. WHITAKER

Contents

Contributors

ELIZABETH W. ALEXANDER 191 Old Post Road, Box 185, Centerville, Massachusetts 02632, USA.

LEE ALLARD University of Texas at Dallas, Callier Center for Communication Disorders, Dallas, Texas 75235-7298, USA.

ERIN D. BIGLER Austin Neurological Clinic and Department of Psychology, University of Texas at Austin, Austin, Texas 78705, USA.

JEAN BRISTOW University of Texas at Dallas, Callier Center for Communication Disorders, Dallas, Texas 75235-7298, USA.

NELSON BUTTERS Psychology Service, V.A. Medical Center, San Diego, California 92161, USA.

JEFFREY L. CUMMINGS Director, Neurobehavior Unit, West Los Angeles V.A. Medical Center (Brentwood Division), Los Angeles, California 90073, USA.

RICHARD E. CYTOWIC President, Capitol Neurology and Associated Specialties, Bethesda, Maryland 20814-4810, USA.

ADRIENNE DONNELL University of Texas at Dallas, Callier Center for Communication Disorders, Dallas, Texas 75235-7298, USA.

ADELAIDE FLOWER University of Texas at Dallas, Callier Center for Communication Disorders, Dallas, Texas 75235-7298, USA.

ERIC GRANHOLM Department of Psychology, University of California at Los Angeles, Los Angeles, California 90024, USA.

FELICIA C. GOLDSTEIN Department of Neurology, The University of Texas Medical Branch, Galveston, Texas 77550, USA.

SARA M. HAYNES University of Texas at Dallas, Callier Center for Communication Disorders, Dallas, Texas 75235-7298, USA.

DAVID C. LARNED Capitol Neurology and Associated Specialties, Bethesda, Maryland 20814-4810, USA.

HARVEY S. LEVIN Division of Neurosurgery, The University of Texas Medical Branch, Galveston, Texas 77550, USA.

CHARLES J. LONG Department of Psychology, Memphis State University, Memphis, Tennessee 38152, USA.

CATHERINE A. MATEER Neuropsychological Services, Good Samaritan Rehabilitation Center, Puyallup, Washington 98371, USA.

MCKAY MOORE SOHLBERG Center for Cognitive Rehabilitation, Good Samaritan Rehabilitation Center, Puyallup, Washington 98371, USA.

ALVIN J. NORTH Department of Psychology, University of Texas Health Science Center at Dallas, Dallas, Texas 75245, USA.

FRANCIS J. PIROZZOLO Department of Neurology, Baylor College of Medicine, Houston, Texas 77030, USA.

WAYNE SECORD Department of Human Services Education, The Ohio State University, Columbus, Ohio 43210-1172, USA.

STAN SMITH Division of Neuropsychology and Behavioral Neurology, Good Samaritan Hospital and Medical Center, Portland, Oregon 97210, USA.

DAVID A. STUMP Department of Neurology, Bowman Gray School of Medicine, Wake Forest University, Winston-Salem, North Carolina 27103, USA.

ANDREW A. SWIHART Departments of Psychiatry and Neurology, University of Pittsburgh School of Medicine, Pittsburgh, Pennsylvania 15213, USA.

HANNA K. ULATOWSKA University of Texas at Dallas, Callier Center for Communication Disorders, Dallas, Texas 75235-7298, USA.

ELISABETH H. WIIG 7107 Lake Powell Drive, Arlington, Texas 76016, USA.

J. MICHAEL WILLIAMS Neuropsychology Laboratory, Memphis State University Memphis, Tennessee 38103, USA.

1
The Neuropsychology of Aging and Dementia: Clinical Issues

ANDREW A. SWIHART and FRANCIS J. PIROZZOLO

The major disorders of aging that are of most direct relevance to the neuropsychologist are the dementias. Although significant interstudy variations exist, the prevalence of severe dementia can reasonably be estimated as approximately 4% in persons over age 65 (Mortimer, Schuman, & French, 1981). Estimates of the prevalence of mild and moderately severe dementia are unreliable, but their prevalence may conservatively be expected to approximately double that of severe dementia. That a problem of such magnitude engenders enormous personal suffering, family trauma, and personal and public economic burden is obvious. The attainment of knowledge concerning the epidemiology, etiology, clinical course, and possible amelioration, treatment, or prevention of dementia, is, consequently, of great importance.

As dementia is primarily a disorder of the aged, a knowledge of normal aging, upon which dementia is superimposed, must be obtained. The changes experienced during normal aging are numerous and varied. Functional decrements commonly occur in sensory systems, motor abilities, and cognitive functions; changes also can occur in emotional functioning, personality, and behavior. The term *normal aging*, therefore, must not be understood as implying an absence of change in any factor other than chronological age, but rather, as encompassing a wide variety of relatively frequent or characteristic, but nonpathological, changes with increasing age.

This chapter, then, reviews the status of sensory, motor, cognitive, and psychological functioning in aged individuals without evidence of neurological or other physical or psychological pathology; neurophysiological and neuromorphological changes concomitant with normal aging also are briefly discussed. This picture of "successful aging" is then contrasted with the changes that occur in various dementias.

Normal Aging

SENSORY FUNCTIONS

In summarizing the research to date, Botwinick (1984) states, "Probably in no other area of psychological investigation are the findings as clear-cut as they are in sensory age changes. Old people do not see or hear as well as young people do, and decline in sensitivity is present also in taste, smell, touch, and possibly pain" (p. 203). Such sensory system functional declines can have potentially significant implications for neuropsychological test performance and interpretation, and the neuropsychologist must take care in distinguishing performance deficits secondary to age-related sensory changes from true neuropsychological impairment stemming from central processing deficiencies per se.

Vision

Studies of specific visual subsystems are numerous and, invariably, functional declines are found with advancing age. Visual acuity undergoes little change up to age 40–50, but exhibits a marked decline after this time, even in the absence of identifiable eye disease (Cohen & Lessell, 1984). By age 70 poor visual acuity is the rule rather than the exception, and by age 80 only one in five individuals will have corrected visual acuity of 20/20 or better (Botwinick, 1984; Cohen & Lessell, 1984). Contrast sensitivity declines with age, but the question of whether low or high spatial frequencies are differentially affected remains unresolved (Hutman & Sekuler, 1980; Kline, 1984; Sekuler & Hutman, 1980). The sensitivity of the eye to low levels of illumination also decreases with age (Fozard, Wolf, Bell, McFarland, & Podolsky, 1977; Ordy, Brizzee, & Beavers, 1980). Accompanying these declines in acuity, contrast sensitivity, and visual threshold is a decrease in the size of the visual field (Fozard et al., 1977; Harrington, 1976). Maximum visual sensitivity following dark adaption decreases with age (Botwinick, 1984). Finally, there are losses in sensitivity and discrimination ability in color vision by the fourth decade of life, with a more prominent decline in blue-green than in red-yellow sensitivity and discrimination (Cohen & Lessell, 1984; Ordy et al., 1980).

These visual sensory changes are accompanied by changes in ocular motor functions, which in turn produce additional age-related visual sensory changes. Such ocular motor decrements include decreased accommodative convergence, restriction of upgaze, and reduced efficiency of smooth pursuit and saccadic eye movement systems (Chamberlain, 1970; Cohen & Lessell, 1984). The accommodative convergence changes, combined with presbyopia (a hyperopia, or farsightedness, associated with old age), frequently produce a marked change in acuity of near-object perception by the sixth decade of life (Botwinick, 1984). Decrements in depth perception are frequently observed beginning at approximately age 45 (Bell, Wolf, & Bernholz, 1972; Jani, 1966; Ordy et al., 1980).

Changes in visual sensory-perceptual processes with aging also have been well documented. These include the observations that the fusing point in critical flicker fusion paradigms decreases with advancing age, the critical interstimulus interval in backward masking procedures increases with age, and components of the visual evoked response demonstrate age-related latency increases (Cohen & Lessell, 1984; Kline, 1984). Together, these findings suggest that aged subjects do not process visual information as rapidly or as efficiently as younger subjects.

Audition

Over 13% of all individuals age 65 or older experience significant bilateral hearing loss (Hayes & Jerger, 1984). Presbycusis (a progressive, bilaterally symmetrical hearing loss with age, particularly for the higher frequencies) and difficulty in speech perception are the most important of these age-related auditory function declines. The age of onset and rate of decline for presbycusis, although varying with sex, noise exposure, and genetic background, can generally be stated as post-age 40, with quite accelerated decline for the 4,000 to 8,000 Hz range between ages 50 and 80 (Corso, 1963, 1977; Glorig, 1977). Pitch discrimination also declines with age, with a marked functional decline post-age 55, especially for frequencies greater than 1,000 Hz (Botwinick, 1984).

Speech perception declines with age, with the difficulty in perception roughly proportional to the extent of presbycusis and pitch discrimination disability (Botwinick, 1984). The decline for perception in the "speech" region (500 to 4,000 Hz) is most evident post-age 60 (Hayes & Jerger, 1984). Jerger and Hayes (1977) report that both word recognition and sentence identification abilities decline with age, but that sentence identification abilities show a decline of significantly greater magnitude. Furthermore, this speech perception decline is exacerbated under difficult listening conditions (Corso, 1977; Hayes & Jerger, 1984). For example, declines in the ability to use interaural time delay cues in the localization of sound can produce functional deficits in speech comprehension under noisy ("real world") listening conditions (Herman, Warren, & Wagener, 1977).

Olfaction and Gustation

Multiple dimensions of olfactory sensibility clearly decline with age. Olfactory detection and recognition thresholds are elevated in the aged (Schiffman & Covey, 1984). Smell identification abilities exhibit performance peaks between ages 20 and 40, and decline markedly post-age 60 (Doty et al., 1984). By age 65, more than 60% of all individuals experience major olfactory impairment (Doty et al., 1984).

It is often stated that gustatory sensibilities decline with advancing age. It does appear that threshold sensitivity declines slightly with age (Cowart, 1981), but much of the reported gustatory decline with aging may, in fact, be secondary to olfactory declines (Murphy, 1983). However, given the frequency of decline in olfactory function with advancing age, a decline in gustatory sensory parameters (whether they be primary or secondary phenomena) would appear to be the rule rather than the exception.

Somesthesis

Decrements in tactile sensitivity are seen in approximately 25% of the aged, but such a decline may be specific to glabrous skin (e.g., palm) (Kenshalo, 1977; Thornbury & Mistretta, 1981). Vibratory sensitivity, specifically for the higher frequencies, decreases with age (Verrillo, 1980), but again, such a decline is not universal (Drachman & Long, 1984; Kenshalo, 1977). Clark and Mehl (1971), utilizing a signal detection paradigm, demonstrated a loss in cutaneous pain sensitivity with age, but this effect was observed only in females. Harkins and Chapman (1976, 1977) report a decrease in ability to discriminate between painful stimuli of differing intensity with advancing age. Performance in double simultaneous stimulation and stereognosis procedures also is observed to decline with age (Kenshalo, 1977).

Implications

Reduced sensory acuity can significantly confound the neuropsychological differentiation of normal and impaired cognitive functioning. For example, decrements in hearing acuity have been shown to adversely affect measures of mental status in otherwise healthy elderly individuals (Thomas et al., 1983), and an association between hearing loss and reduced intellectual functioning has been reported (Granick, Kleban, & Weiss, 1976). Hearing loss also has been reported to be associated with depression (Botwinick, 1984; Corso, 1981), and depression, in turn, can have a major impact on cognitive functioning in the elderly (Caine, 1981). The implications are apparent: The clinician must take care to discriminate between true neuropsychological impairment and spuriously reduced neuropsychological performance secondary to uncorrected, age-related sensory declines.

Motor Functions

Mortimer, Pirozzolo, and Maletta (1982) enumerate multiple changes in the motor system that can be considered virtually universal concomitants of aging: (a) significant dendritic, synaptic, and neuronal density declines in brain regions crucial for motor function; (b) decrease in number and percentage of fast-twitch muscle fiber and associated motor neurons; (c) decline in dopaminergic function in the basal ganglia; (d) sensory decrements (e.g., decreased stereopsis function) which, in turn, limit motor performance in complex tasks; (e) disturbances in the temporal organization of motor synergies mediated by the long latency postural reflex system; (f) decline in the maximum rate of sequential repetitive movements; and (g) functional performance decline in tasks requiring complex programming or transformations (e.g., choice reaction time tasks requiring symbolic or spatial transformations).

These age-related changes and declines in the motor system may manifest themselves as decrements in a variety of tasks that include significant motor function or motor skill components. For example, maximum strength of handgrip muscles, although relatively well maintained into the fifth decade, undergoes an accelerating decline thereafter (Larsson, 1982). Other muscle groups show varying rates of strength decline, with the proximal muscles of the lower extremities undergoing the most marked decline (44%, ages 20 to 80), and shoulder strength undergoing significant declines (26% and 32%, respectively, ages 20 to 80) (Larsson, 1982; Potvin et al., 1981). Maximum speed of movement of various muscle groups also declines with age (Larsson, Grimby, & Karlsson, 1979; Welford, 1977). Such speed decrements for simple movements are generally of a 30% magnitude; more complex movements (e.g., timed digit copying) display up to 100% increases in time necessary for completion of task (Welford, 1977). Such complex tasks, of course, also depend upon nonmotor factors such as visual sensory processing, response biases, and self-monitoring time, all of which may change with age and contribute to this slowing of performance.

Both simple and complex reaction times show age-related performance decrements, with the magnitude of such decline reported at 19% for simple reaction time between ages 20 and 80 (Potvin et al., 1981). Choice reaction times show greater decrements (Welford, 1977). Again, however, perceptual and central processing components are important factors in such slowing, and contribute to this decline in at least as significant a fashion as do motor components of reaction time.

Fine motor coordination and related activities of daily living display age-related declines. Potvin and associates (1981) have documented a number of such changes. For example, Purdue Pegboard speed has been shown to decline 16% to 18% from ages 20 to 80, implicating decreased upper extremity coordination and dexterity. Documented declines in speed for such skills as managing small and large buttons, bow-tying, and manipulating a safety pin or zipper serve as examples of daily life consequences of these fine motor coordination decrements.

Changes in long-latency postural reflex system motor synergies with aging can produce greater postural instability and an increased tendency to fall. Age-related visual and vestibular system changes exacerbate this problem (Woollacott, Shumway-Cook, & Nasher, 1982). Decrease in walking speed and stride length, as well as broader gait and toeing-out are all seen with increasing frequency in the aged, and may be compensatory consequences of these postural reflex system changes (Woollacott et al., 1982).

Contrary to the stereotype of aged individuals as stooped in posture, tremorous, and shuffling in gait, such extrapyramidal motor signs do not generally increase with age in otherwise healthy persons (Mortimer & Webster, 1982). There is some evidence that experimental indicators of bradykinesia (e.g., pursuit of a moving target with the hand, number of steps required to negotiate a 30-foot course) do correlate with age, but tremor and rigidity display no such relationship (Mortimer & Webster, 1982).

Cognitive Functions

Intelligence

It is now generally agreed that many intellectual functions begin to decline between ages 50 and 60, with a much more pronounced decline beginning between ages 70 and 80 (Bank & Jarvik, 1978; Botwinick, 1977, 1984; Hochanadel & Kaplan, 1984; Schaie & Labouvie-Vief, 1974). However, broad generalizations such as "performance on a variety of psychometric tests declines with advancing age" are of little usefulness in such broad brush terms. A more precise understanding of which specific intellectual measures do and do not decline, when such declines begin, and of the magnitude of such performance declines is needed.

It appears that some indicators of intellectual ability remain stable, or even show slight improvement with advancing age. Horn (1982) reviews multiple studies that document improving performance, up to approximately age 65, on measures of facility in recalling and expressing connotations from semantic memory (e.g., recalling words that are similar in meaning to the word *warm* within a 3-minute test period), or measures of "cleverness or creativity" (i.e., specifying different ways in which an object might be used), and other measures. Several of the Wechsler Adult Intelligence Scale–Revised (WAIS-R) verbal subtests (particularly Information, Vocabulary, and Comprehension) hold up very well with advancing age (Sattler, 1982).

Other intellectual performance measures decline with age. Speeded psychomotor tasks, such as the WAIS Digit Symbol subtest, virtually always display significant decrements with advancing age (Botwinick, 1984; Storandt, 1976). Performance on the Block Design and Picture Arrangement subtests of the WAIS also declines markedly with age (Botwinick, 1984; Sattler, 1982).

This pattern of intellectual performance in the aged (i.e., verbal intellectual measures remaining relatively stable with concurrent decline in so-called "nonverbal" or performance measures) has come to be known as the "classic aging pattern." A compelling theoretical interpretation of this pattern arises from the work of Cattell, Horn, and associates, who postulate that it reflects fundamental developmental changes in fluid and crystallized intellectual abilities (Horn, 1982; Horn & Cattell, 1967; Horn, Donaldson, & Engstrom, 1981). Crystallized intelligence is reflected in an individual's ability to manipulate relatively familiar material in familiar ways; it is associated with overlearned material involving educational and cultural knowledge. Fluid intelligence, on the other hand, involves problem solving with novel, unfamiliar material in tasks requiring the apprehension of more complex relations and, frequently, perceptual-integrative and manipulative skill (Baltes & Willis, 1982; Botwinick, 1984). Generally speaking then, the classic aging pattern is one of relatively well preserved (or even improving) crystallized intellectual abilities and a slow decline in fluid intellectual skills.

Horn (1982) ascribes the decline in fluid intelligence between ages 20 and 60 to functional decrements in short-term memory and performance speed that, in turn, decline due to more fundamental age-related decrements in capacities for maintaining spontaneous alertness and focused intensive concentration, and in the ability to effectively organize and encode otherwise unorganized material. Concurrent with this age-related loss in fluid intelligence, Horn reports a *rise* of crystallized intelligence of approximately equal absolute magnitude.

Further support for Horn's explanation of this fluid intellectual decline arises from several studies. Storandt (1977) found that the decrement in WAIS performance subtest scores for the elderly remained when the effect of bonus points for speedy performance was removed, suggesting that more than just response speed underlies such decrements. Furthermore, Storandt and associates parceled out the effects of both copying speed and memorization of digit-symbol associations on the WAIS Digit Symbol subtest, and still obtained unexplained performance slowing, suggesting that other, unidentified factors significantly contribute to the decline (Erber, Botwinick, & Storandt, 1981; Storandt, 1976).

In summary, then, healthy individuals do undergo changes in intellectual performance with advancing age. The magnitude and pattern of such changes must be carefully considered in all questions of differential neuropsychological diagnosis in the elderly.

Memory

The observation that memory function, in general, declines with advancing age is a well-accepted banality. The more fruitful and important questions have narrowed in focus: which specific memory processes do and do not decline; under what environmental and task conditions, with what type of information, and with which subject characteristics is stability or decline in function noted; what is the nature of the change in cognitive processing underlying such declines? Research on these questions has produced a body of literature too enormous and complex to properly review here. Instead, a brief overview of the major issues in this literature is presented. The reader is referred to Burke and Light (1981), Craik (1977), Craik and Rabinowitz (1984), Craik and Trehub (1982), and Poon (1985) for more complete reviews of current theoretical and empirical approaches to these questions.

Age-related decrements in memory functioning do occur, but are much more apparent in some tasks than in others (Craik, 1984). Waugh and Norman (1965) draw a distinction between primary and secondary memory (PM and SM, respectively). Primary memory is conceptualized as a "temporary holding and organizing *process*," not a structured memory store (Craik, 1977, p. 387). Items in PM are those that are still in conscious awareness, still being rehearsed, still the focus of attention. Secondary memory, on the other hand, subsumes all other information in memory not currently being processed in PM. When to-be-remembered items are fully perceived and require no reorganization, age differences in PM are found to be minimal or nonexistent (Craik, 1977; Wright, 1982). Measures of immediate memory span (e.g., digits forward) typically exhibit no significant age difference (e.g., Drachman & Leavitt, 1972), or only slight but reliable declines with age (e.g., Parkinson, Lindholm, & Inman, 1982). Craik (1977) describes such declines as representing the combined functioning of an intact PM and a small, less efficient, SM component. Others (Parkinson et al., 1982; Parkinson & Perey, 1980) argue that the decrements represent impairments in both PM and SM.

Age differences in SM processes are universally acknowledged, but debate continues as to the underlying cognitive changes responsible for these deficits. Age-related declines in free recall of word lists (when the subject is simply instructed to learn the words) are undeniable. When gist recall of more ecologically valid material (newspaper articles) is required, memory decrements remain (Dixon, Simon, Nowak, & Hultsch, 1982). Standard neuropsychological tests reveal consistent declines in verbal memory for both word associates and meaningful text (Bak & Greene, 1980, 1981; Cauthen, 1977; Haaland, Linn, Hunt, & Goodwin, 1983; McCarty, Siegler, & Logue, 1982; Siegler, McCarty, & Logue, 1982). Recall of episodic material over longer time periods (e.g., memory for news events occurring 1 month to 2 years distant) decreases with advancing age (Warrington & Silberstein, 1970). Recall for more remote sociohistoric events and entertainment world events (drawn from the 60-year period prior to assessment), on the other hand, exhibits little decline in some studies (Botwinick & Storandt, 1974, 1980; Storandt, Grant, & Gordon, 1978), while other studies suggest a deficit with advancing age (Squire, 1974; Warrington & Sanders, 1971). Recall and recognition of remote material, such as names of school teachers and classmates, also decline (Bahrick, Bahrick, & Wittlinger, 1975; Schonfield, 1969), although the confounding of age of subject and age of memory in such studies makes straightforward interpretation of these results problematic. A temporal gradient in remote memory (i.e., better memory for more remote events than more recent events) also has been observed in normal aged individuals (Moscovitch, 1982).

Age-related declines in memory for nonverbal materials also have been noted. Visual nonverbal memory has been observed to decline, with the slope of the decline for the nonverbal material being indistinguishable from that for verbal material, suggesting that the rates of decline for verbal and nonverbal material do not differ (Winograd, Smith, & Simon, 1982). The types of visually presented nonverbal materials used to document such declines have included geometric designs from the Memory-for-Designs test (Davies, 1967; Kendall, 1962; Shelton, Parsons, & Leber, 1982), the Benton Visual Retention Test (Arenberg, 1978, 1982), black-and-white line drawings of common objects (Winograd et al., 1982), and faces from the Memory for Faces Test (Ferris, Crook, Clark, McCarthy, and Rae, 1981). Memory for nonverbal auditory and tactile materials also may decline with advancing age (Riege & Inman, 1981).

Attempts to interpret and understand these declines have been made within the context of several differing models of memory. The "levels-of-processing" approach (Craik & Lockhart, 1972), in particular, has been extremely influential over the past decade. In brief, this approach suggests that memory is a product of information extraction and elaboration processes carried out for the purposes of perception and comprehension of environmental information and events. Such extraction and elaboration analyses occur upon a continuum of differing "levels" or "depths" of information processing, with the depth (i.e., the quality and extent) of the processing determining the nature and durability of the information in memory. At one extreme of the continuum, information is processed in a relatively shallow or surface level, that is, at a level concerned primarily with the physical features of the stimuli (e.g., "How many times does the letter *e* occur in the following list of words?"). At the other extreme is relatively deep processing of information, involving more elaborate semantic, associative, or inferential analyses of the stimuli (e.g., "For each of the words in the following list, decide whether a pleasant or unpleasant association is evoked for you."). Deeper levels of processing (or encoding), in general, are thought to produce better retention and subsequent recall of the relevant information.

Craik (1977, 1984), in reviewing the experimental literature on aging and memory, attributes much of the age-related decrement in memory to a failure of older people to *spontaneously* process the to-be-remembered material at an adequate, deep level. He states that if "effective encoding operations are induced by means of a semantic orienting task . . . and this encoding task is coupled with a retrieval test in which processes are again guided—for example, cued recall or recognition . . . age differences are slight or non-existent" (Craik, 1984, p. 10). On the other hand, if encoding and retrieval processes are not guided, as in free recall of a list of words studied simply with an intent to memorize, age decrements are large.

There is considerable evidence in support of Craik's interpretation of the data. For example, Sanders, Murphy, Schmitt, and Walsh (1980) studied the rehearsal strategies of young and older adults during word list learning. They found that the older subjects were less likely to use clustering strategies, frequently using single-item naming (the repetition of each of the to-be-remembered words once to oneself), and that, in general, the older subjects' rehearsal was "best characterized as inactive and essentially nonstrategic" (p. 556). Hence, deficiencies in the spontaneous use of deeper encoding processes may have produced the age-related memory decrement.

Other investigators (e.g., Erber, 1984; Puglisi, 1980; Rabinowitz & Ackerman, 1982), utilizing differing methodological approaches (e.g., encoding congruence effects, release from proactive interference phenomena, manipulation of semantic encoding along a prototypic-unique dimension), have achieved experimental results congruent with the hypothesis that older and younger subjects differ in their spontaneous use of optimal encoding processes, but not in their ability to process deeply per se.

It is often observed that age decrements are greater in tasks requiring free recall relative to simple recognition (Craik, 1977). This observation has led many investigators (e.g., Burke & Light, 1981; Buschke, 1974; Perlmutter & Mitchell, 1982; Till, 1985) to conclude that age differences in retrieval processes exist and that these differences also contribute to age-related memory declines.

Recently, attempts have been made to understand age-related differences in spontaneous use of optimal encoding strategies (and some aspects of the age-related retrieval deficiency) in terms of a more fundamental decline in mental "processing resources," processing capacity, or pool of attentional resources (e.g., Craik, 1984; Craik & Byrd, 1982; Macht & Buschke, 1983; Rabinowitz & Ackerman, 1982; Wright, 1981). In brief, these investigators suggest that the failure of older subjects to spontaneously encode material deeply is due to the fact that such encoding placed heavy demands upon age-depleted cognitive or attentional resources.

The theoretical model proposed by Hasher and Zachs (1979), which distinguishes between "automatic" and "effortful" processes, also has been invoked to explain decrements in memory with advancing age (e.g., Craik & Byrd, 1982; Perlmutter & Mitchell, 1982; Rabinowitz & Ackerman, 1982). Automatic processes are those that "drain minimal energy from the limited-capacity attention mechanism and do not interfere with ongoing cognitive capacity" (Perlmutter & Mitchell, 1982, p. 136). Effortful processes, on the other hand, require considerable attentional capacity and interfere with other cognitive activities. It has been postulated that aspects of memory performance dependent primarily upon automatic processes are preserved with advancing age (e.g., memory for frequency of occurrence, memory for temporal information, spread of semantic activation during memory encoding, well overlearned encoding strategies), but that memory functions requiring significant levels of effortful processing display greater declines with age (e.g., deeper semantic encoding, difficult or novel operations, manipulation or reorganization of the to-be-remembered information) (Attig & Hasher, 1980; Craik, 1984; Howard, Lasaga, & McAndrews, 1980; McCormack, 1981; Rabinowitz & Ackerman, 1982; Zacks, 1982).

Language

The common wisdom purports that language functions show little, if any, decrements with advancing age. Results of recent research, however, challenge this notion. Albert (1980, 1981) reports that the elderly have greater linguistic variability than younger adults, and that impairments in language functions, such as active naming and comprehension, are more common with advancing age. Other investigators have produced similar results.

Schaie (1980) has documented increases in passive recognition vocabulary up to age 60, with a modest performance decrement thereafter. Albert (1981) confirms this finding, but further reports that older individuals use a wider range of vocabulary when in natural (i.e., not under laboratory or experimental conditions) settings. Confrontation naming ability also may increase up through age 60, but some investigators report that significant decrements are characteristic of age groups post-age 60 (Goodglass, 1980; Obler & Albert, 1984; Schaie, 1980). More recently, other investigators have reported little or no significant decrement in confrontation naming with advancing age (e.g., LaBarge, Edwards, & Knesevich, 1986). In general, it appears that older individuals (post-age 60) typically have preserved passive lexicon use, but may have mild decrements in active lexicon use.

Changes in narrative discourse style with advancing age have been documented. Albert and associates (Albert, 1981; Obler, 1980; Obler & Albert, 1984) describe an increased elaborateness of speech and written language beginning in the sixth decade. Production of spoken language is characterized by more total words, more words per theme, more details, greater syntactic complexity, and more frequent use of modifiers in this older group. Verbal fluency, under *untimed* conditions, reportedly shows no significant change with advancing age. Verbal fluency under timed conditions (e.g., naming as many words as possible from a given semantic category within 60 seconds) does decline with advancing age (Bayles, Tomoeda, & Boone, 1985).

Verbal comprehension decrements with advancing age also have been demonstrated, but such change is usually small, and hence may produce no noticeable disruption in real-life verbal communication (Brookshire & Manthie, 1980). Albert (1980) reports that both speech discrimination and comprehension decline with advancing age. Feier and Gertsman (1980) have demonstrated decreased comprehension of spoken sentences containing relative clauses beginning at approximately age 60. Decreased performance levels with advancing age have been reported for the more syntactically complex portions of the Token Test (Brookshire & Manthie, 1980). Albert (1981) states that these declines in auditory verbal comprehension cannot be explained by peripheral hearing loss alone, and that older individuals depend more upon contextual and nonverbal cues for comprehension of interpersonal communications.

In summary, changes in language production and comprehension do occur in aged individuals. When combined with the effects of presbycusis, such decrements in language abilities may affect the older individual's ability to consistently and completely comprehend spoken task instructions and interpersonal communications. The otherwise neuropsychologically intact elderly person may be unaware of, or deny, faltering comprehension abilities and attempt to feign full comprehension of what is said. Responses may therefore appear confused or unrelated to the task at hand, leading the clinician to falsely suspect a central cognitive dysfunction. Consequently, great care must be taken to discriminate between the aged individual with unusual performance decrements secondary to these multiple age-related changes, and the individual manifesting a true dementing disorder.

Visuoperceptual, Visuospatial, Visuoconstructive, and Related Abilities

Age-related declines in the ability to perform both spatial and nonspatial visuoperceptual tasks rapidly and accurately are well documented. Benton and associates have demonstrated moderate but steady declines (approximately ½ *SD* per decade post-age 65) in the discrimination and matching of unfamiliar faces and in the identification of the spatial orientation of lines in relation to a standard (Benton, Eslinger, & Damasio, 1981; Eslinger & Benton, 1983). However, complex visual form discrimination abilities per se appear to undergo no significant change with advancing age (Benton, Hamsher, Varney, & Spreen, 1983).

Older adults have been demonstrated to be generally slower and less efficient in mental rotation abilities (Cerella, Poon, & Fozard, 1981). Such declines in the solving of problems involving spatially rotated figures are not due to differing problem-solving strategies, but represent true slowing in the rate of mental rotation abilities per se (Cohen & Faulkner, 1983).

Research using the Parietal Lobe Tests of the Boston Diagnostic Aphasia Examination has demonstrated age-related performance declines on several visuoperceptual and visuoconstructive tasks (Farver & Farver, 1982). These decrements are found in drawing to command of such items as clocks, daisies, and houses; construction of match-stick geometric figures; and three-dimensional block construction of photographically presented models. Farver and Farver also documented the type of errors made on these tasks, and noted frequent reduction or enlargement of drawn figures; poor reduction of angles, loss of perspective, rotations, and errors of spatial relations in drawings; and disorganization of shape, rotation, and perseveration in the stick constructions. They also observed that the performance of aging individuals declined on the Hooper Visual Organization Test (which requires identification of pictures of cut-up objects) and the Poppelreuter Superimposed Figures Test (a figure-ground task).

Finally, tactile perception of two-dimensional geometric figures made of fine-grade sandpaper declines slightly with advancing age (Benton et al., 1983). Hence, spatial perception and recognition ability declines are not confined solely to the visual modality.

In summary, it is important to note that healthy older adults display decrements in performance that, when present in younger adults, are considered to reflect central nervous system dysfunction. Simple application of "cut-off" scores or "impairment indices" in the diagnostic discrimination of normal and demented individuals, therefore, may well result in a false determination of impairment in otherwise normal aged adults.

Speed of Cognitive Processing

Behavioral and cognitive slowing are universal accompaniments of advancing age. The literature on this topic is extensive, and several excellent syntheses and critiques exist (e.g., Cerella, 1985; Salthouse, 1985). Consequently, a detailed summary and evaluation will not be given here; the reader is referred to the above-cited literature for a more complete discussion.

Multiple explanations for the decreased speed of behavior and cognition with aging have been advanced. Salthouse (1985) reviews the most prominent hypotheses and their underlying empirical support. A slowing secondary to peripheral sensory and/or motor changes, in the *absence* of changes in central processing speed, is perhaps the oldest hypothesis. However, this explanation has been convincingly demonstrated to be at odds with the available data, and is now universally rejected. A difference in cognitive strategies between young and old subjects, rather than a difference in processing speed per se, has been proposed as an explanatory factor. Investigations of this hypothesis have produced results that are either in conflict with, or inconsistent in their support for, this claim. A difference in working memory capacity between young and old adults has been proferred as the underlying factor. However, even tasks placing minimal demands upon working memory capacity show age-related performance speed declines, a phenomenon inconsistent with the strong form of this hypothesis. Differences in the allocation of available mental resources (i.e., submaximal allocation by older subjects) has been proposed as responsible for the performance slowing in the elderly. Salthouse concludes that the currently available data are insufficient for acceptance or rejection of this proposal. Finally, the so-called "Birren hypothesis," postulating a generalized slowing that affects all components of performance (sensory input, cognitive processing, and motor output), has been tendered, and appears to be the most viable explanation to date.

Cerella (1985) reviews various mathematical functions that may serve to model the Birren hypothesis. He concludes that "two slowing factors are adequate to account for changes in the information-processing latencies of elderly adults" (p. 82). The first is a slowing in sensorimotor processes; the second is a slowing in a central, computational, higher order factor. The degree of slowing in the elderly on any given task is predicted by the additive effects of a central factor and a peripheral factor, with each factor attenuated by the proportion of the task dependent upon that factor. Furthermore, Cerella finds that the degree of slowing in the sensorimotor component is less severe than that in the higher order (computational) factor.

Psychological Functions

Only those aspects of personality, emotionality, and mood state most relevant to the neuropsychologist are discussed here. For a review of the theoretical and methodological issues involved in this area, the reader is referred to Botwinick (1984), Neugarten (1977), and Schulz (1982a).

Botwinick (1984), in reviewing the literature to date, concludes that personality is generally stable with advancing age, and that findings to the contrary are artifacts of cohort differences in cross-sectional studies rather than reflections of maturational changes per se. McCrae, Costa, and Arenberg (1980) provide both cross-sectional and longitudinal data supporting Botwinick's conclusion.

Cameron (1975) and Malatesta and Kalnok (1984) provide strong evidence that emotionality and mood state show no significant age changes. Cameron, in a relatively large study (n = 6,452), found no significant differences in the frequency of happy, sad, or neutral mood states from childhood to old age. Malatesta and Kalnok found no change in negative or positive affect frequency with advancing age.

Depression is the most common affective disturbance of late life (Schulz, 1982b), and is of considerable significance in the process of differential neuropsychological diagnosis in the aged. The rate of clinically significant depression in the general elderly population has been estimated as 10% to 15% (Gurland & Toner, 1982). Given the experience of increasingly frequent and severe ill health, the losses through death of spouse and/or close friends, and decreased earning capacity and frequent decline in standard of living, such a significant frequency of depression is not surprising.

Depression can produce cognitive changes closely resembling those observed in the true dementias (Caine, 1981; Folstein & McHugh, 1978; Kiloh, 1961; Wells, 1979). Pirozzolo (1982), in a study of geriatric outpatients referred for evaluation of suspected dementia, reports that 24% were eventually given the diagnosis of major depressive disorder. Because of their age and the current lack of effective treatment for the dementing disorders, patients with a diagnosis of dementia are frequently simply maintained in an institution or nursing care facility. Consequently, the misdiagnosis of depression (a treatable disorder) as a dementia represents a catastrophic error for the depressed individual, and a painstakingly careful approach to this differential diagnosis must be adopted.

Neuromorphology and Neurophysiology

Neuromorphological and neurophysiological changes in the healthy aged have been well documented (for more comprehensive reviews, see Brizzee, Ordy, Knox, & Jirge, 1980; Cote & Kremzner, 1983; Freedman, Knoefel, Naeser, & Levine, 1984; Katz & Harner, 1984; Kemper, 1984; Meyer & Shaw, 1984; Pedley & Miller, 1983; and Polich & Starr, 1984). On first impression, much of the evidence appears to suggest that the differences in brain morphology of healthy aged and demented persons are quantitative only. However, such an impression is erroneous (with the possible, still controversial, exception of Alzheimer's disease), and it will be seen that the changes occurring in the various dementias are not mere accentuations of normal age-related changes, but rather, represent qualitatively distinct neuropathological phenomena unique to the dementing process itself.

A number of gross morphological central nervous system changes occur reliably with advancing age. Brain weight decreases by approximately 7% to 8% beginning at approximately age 60 (Brizzee et al., 1980). Brain volume decreases of from 5% to 15%, indicating brain atrophy, occur most strikingly post-age 60 (Curcio, Buell, & Coleman, 1982; Kemper, 1984). Ventricular volume increases, cortical sulci widen and deepen, and the mass and width of gyri decrease with advancing years (Kemper, 1984).

The changes described above, initially noted through autopsy study, have more recently been confirmed in computed tomography (CT) scan studies of living healthy elderly. Gyral atrophy, beginning at approximately age 40, is observable (Freedman et al., 1984). Although enlargement of the left Sylvian fissure has been reported to correlate with decline in intellectual function in the otherwise healthy elderly (Soininen, Puranen, & Riekkinen, 1982), no relationship between sulcal widening in general and neuropsychological test performance is evident (Earnest, Heaton, Wilkinson, & Manke, 1979; Soininen et al., 1982).

Changes at the microscopic level include increased lipofuscin deposition with age, the appearance of amyloid and senile (neuritic) plaques, the development of neurofibrillary tangles, observable granulovacuolar degeneration, the appearance of Hirano bodies, and loss or distortion of axonal and dendritic processes (Brizzee et al., 1980; Kemper, 1984). Senile plaques are most frequently observed in the healthy elderly beginning in the fifth decade and increasing with advancing age. Neurofibrillary tangles often make their first appearance by the fourth decade of life. Granulovacuolar degeneration is uncommon before age 60, but occurs in approximately 20% of healthy elderly after that age, increasing to 75% of all individuals age 80 or greater (Kemper, 1984). Hirano bodies usually occur after age 60.

The region of brain observed and the neurohistological technique employed determine, in large measure, whether neuron loss with advancing age will be observed (Curcio et al., 1982). Research to date suggests that diffuse cortical and hippocampal neuron loss may be a veridical age change, but that age-related neuron loss occurs only on a selective basis in all other brain areas (Kemper, 1984). In general, higher order association cortex appears to experience greater cell loss than the primary projection areas (Kemper, 1984). The cerebellum, anterior thalamic nucleus, striatum, substantia nigra, locus ceruleus, and selected amygdaloid nuclei also display neuronal depopulation (Brizzee et al., 1980; Curcio et al., 1982). Other subcortical regions, however, undergo no such changes, hence, it is important to avoid the tempting but overly simplistic impression of an unvarying and general central nervous system (CNS) cell loss with advancing age.

Neurotransmitter systems also undergo age-related change. Selective declines in the activity of tyrosine hydroxylase and dopa decarboxylase (necessary for the synthesis of dopamine), glutamic acid decarboxylase (essential for γ-aminobutyric acid [GABA] synthesis), and choline acetyltransferase (necessary for acetylcholine synthesis) are often observed in selected brain regions (Bartus, Dean, Beer, & Lippa, 1982; Cote & Kremzner, 1983). Neurotransmitter receptor sites also may undergo age-related changes. Positron emission tomography (PET) studies of dopamine and serotonin receptors in living human brain have demonstrated a receptor decrease in the caudate, putamen, and frontal cortex (Wong et al., 1984). Despite this impressive array of demonstrated changes, the functional significance of such declines remains uncertain, and the implications of these changes for the cognitive and behavioral functioning of the elderly continue to be unclear.

Various neurophysiological changes with advancing age have been documented. The local cerebral metabolic rate for glucose has been reported to decline in some studies, but others have failed to replicate this finding (de Leon et al., 1983; Kuhl, Metter, Riege, & Phelps, 1982; Rapoport et al., 1983). Cerebral blood flow does decline with normal aging (Meyer & Shaw, 1984; Naritomi, Meyer, Sakai, Yamaguchi, & Shaw, 1979; Tachibana et al., 1984), but this decline may be specific for the regions of the frontal lobe and central Rolandic fissure (Warren, Butler, Katholi, & Halsey, 1985).

The most frequent concomitants of advancing age observed during electroencephalographic study are a slowing of the alpha frequency and intermittent temporal slow wave activity, particularly on the left (Katz & Harner, 1984). Event-related potentials display well-documented changes with advancing age, indicating possible changes in both objective neurological function and cognition. There is evidence that both peripheral and central transmission time latencies for the auditory brainstem response increase with age (Patterson, Michalewski, Thompson, Bowman, & Litzelman, 1981; Polich & Starr, 1984).

The visual evoked response exhibits a similar increased latency, particularly in P100 (the prominent positive going peak occurring approximately 100 msec after stimulus presentation). Increased latencies also are observed in recordings of somatosensory evoked potentials (Polich & Starr, 1984). Evoked potentials more closely associated with cognitive functions also have been studied in the aged. The P300 event-related potential, thought to reflect perception of novelty, surprise, or decision making, shows an increase in latency with both auditory and visual stimulus presentations (Pfefferbaum, Ford, Roth, & Kopell, 1980; Polich & Starr, 1984). The contingent negative variation (CNV), postulated to indicate expectation, preparation, attentional changes, or arousal, displays a decreasing amplitude, especially over frontal sites (Michalewski et al., 1980).

In summary, numerous neuromorphological and neurophysiological changes occur with normal aging. Kemper (1984) points out that decreased brain weight, gyral atrophy, ventricular dilatation, neuronal cell loss, and the presence of amyloid are prominent age-related changes that also occur, sometimes indistinguishably, in Alzheimer's disease. However, clear differences between normal aging and this form of dementia occur in the frequency and distribution of neurofibrillary tangles and granulovacuolar degeneration; the frequency and distribution of these changes display little overlap between normal aging and Alzheimer's. The presence and extent of neuritic plaques and Hirano bodies in normal elderly persons occupy an area of intermediate overlap with this dementia. Kemper concludes that no simple quantitative neuromorphological continuum exists to connect normal aging and Alzheimer's disease; even Alzheimer's must be considered a qualitatively distinct disease process.

Summary

It is clear that there is a wide range of sensory, motor, cognitive, psychological, neuromorphological, and neurophysiological changes in normal elderly persons. At times, the convergence of these biological, cognitive, and psychological declines within a given elderly individual may produce a clinical presentation strongly resembling that of a dementia. The clinician must be able to differentiate neuropsychological and behavioral changes secondary to age-related sensory and motor decrements, age-related cognitive changes, and/or affective disturbance in the elderly from neuropsychological impairment secondary to a true dementia.

The Dementias

Definition

Dementia is a general clinical term lacking a precise definition. It does *not* refer to a specific disease entity, but rather, identifies a general clinical symptom complex characterized by a progressive deterioration of intellectual and other cognitive capacities secondary to known or suspected brain dysfunction. It is a *nonspecific* diagnosis of diffuse mental deterioration and does not imply an invariant etiology. Dementia implies a *global* deterioration or decline in virtually all aspects of higher cognitive function, and not an isolated or circumscribed neuropsychological deficit (e.g., amnesia, aphasia). Dementia is typically characterized as a *progressing* deterioration, in this manner differentiating itself from other acquired clinical syndromes with nonprogressing, diffuse mental dysfunction, such as severe closed head injury and impairment secondary to significant anoxic episodes. Furthermore, dementia is frequently referred to as an *irreversible* process, hence distinguishing itself from delirium, a potentially reversible syndrome of acute confusion and diffuse decline in neuropsychological abilities.

In practice, the characteristics of *global* decline, *progressive* course, and *irreversibility* must all be qualified to some degree. Defining dementia as a generalized mental decline does not imply temporally concurrent onset and decline in each individual neuropsychological ability. It merely implies that, *at some point* in the disease process, all cognitive abilities will be affected. The progressive nature of a dementing disorder may be difficult to discern over the course of many months, or even several years; it is presumed, however, that the course will *eventually* progress despite such apparently prolonged plateaus. And finally, the irreversibility of dementia most imperatively must not imply the irrelevance of treatment attempts. It is certainly hoped that all of the dementias will eventually yield to attempts at treatment, despite our current lack of effective treatment approaches.

The individual dementias, then, will be considered as qualitatively differing and distinct disease entities that can be conveniently, if loosely, grouped together as disorders producing the general symptom complex of dementia. Each has its own known (or presumed) unique etiology, and neuropathology, specific clinical presentation, and eventually, treatment approach. One point, though, repeatedly emphasized in the first half of this chapter, must be kept in mind. Before any change in intellectual or cognitive functioning is attributed to a specific dementing disorder, one must first know, recall, and rule out of consideration those changes considered "normal" in an otherwise healthy elderly person. Any changes suspected of occurring secondary to a specific dementia must first be compared to a baseline established for normally functioning persons of the same age.

Alzheimer's Disease

Alzheimer's disease (AD) is the most common cause of serious cognitive decline in the elderly, accounting for up to 55% of patients referred for evaluation of suspected dementia (Rocca, Amaducci, & Schoenberg, 1986). The incidence of AD rises throughout the life span, with the earliest onset of the disease virtually always being post-age 40. Multiple investigators report a higher prevalence ratio of AD among women than in men, but this finding is not universally accepted (Katzman, 1986; Rocca et al., 1986). The time course of the disease is quite variable. Early age at onset is associated with shortened survival and greater severity of illness, until approximately age 65 when the greater likelihood of death from competing causes turns the curve back toward shorter survival with advancing age (Heston, 1983). Clinical progression of symptom severity is not uniform and some patients have been reported to remain in the mildly demented stage for up to 7 years duration (Botwinick, Storandt, & Berg, 1986).

Traditionally, only those patients whose illness began before age 65 were given the diagnosis of AD, while those whose illness began after 65 were diagnosed as experiencing senile dementia of the Alzheimer's type (SDAT). This distinction, based solely upon age at onset, has been largely abandoned due to the demonstrated histopathological unity of these two groups, and in this discussion we shall group all patients together under the single nosological rubric of Alzheimer's disease.

Clinical Course

The clinical course of AD is frequently divided into three relatively distinct phases (e.g., Schneck, Reisberg, & Ferris, 1982). The first phase (the *forgetfulness phase*) is characterized by subtle decrements in memory functioning (e.g., misplacing objects, difficulty remembering names and appointments, etc.) and affective or behavioral changes such as decreased spontaneity and initiative, social withdrawal, and perhaps anxiety secondary to subjective awareness of failing abilities. Language disturbances, such as anomia, verbal paraphasias, mild comprehension deficits, perseverations, and halting speech also have been noted, with somewhat less frequency, as initial symptoms of degenerative dementia (Kirshner, Webb, Kelly, & Wells, 1984). Topographic disorientation and constructional apraxia also may be evident. Formal neuropsychological testing is usually necessary to firmly demonstrate the presence of such mild cognitive dysfunction at this stage.

During the second phase (the *confusional phase*), the cognitive deficits characteristic of dementia become manifestly apparent. These include clearly deteriorating memory functions, temporal and/or spatial disorientation, poor judgment, and the classical signs of cortical dysfunction, including frequent aphasic symptomatology, apraxia, impaired visuospatial abilities, and possibly agnosia. Definite deterioration in activities of daily living and further affective and/or personality changes also are readily apparent at this time.

The final phase (the *dementia phase*) is characterized by profound disturbances in orientation and memory, global and severe intellectual decline, frequent inability to recognize persons significant within the patient's life (e.g., spouse, children), motor restlessness, and psychotic symptomatology. This picture soon progresses to one of a bedridden state, limb rigidity and flexion posture, incontinence of urine and feces, and ultimately, death.

Neuropsychological Functions

Fuld (1982, 1984) and Brinkman and Braun (1984) describe a WAIS subtest profile "typical of patients with Alzheimer's disease" (Fuld, 1982, p. 193). The profile, computed using age-corrected scaled scores, is as follows: ½ (Information + Vocabulary) > ½ (Similarities + Digit Span) > ½ (Block Design + Digit Symbol) ≤ Object Assembly, and ½ (Information + Vocabulary) > Object Assembly. Roughly one half of the patients examined in these studies were correctly classified by this profile as experiencing AD. However, other investigators (Feher, Swihart, & Largen, 1987) have failed to validate this profile (only 2 of 15 patients manifested this pattern in the Feher study). Other patterns of so-called "hold" and "don't hold" WAIS subtest profiles have been found equally wanting (Larrabee, Largen, & Levin, 1985). On the basis of purely theoretical grounds, the existence of a diagnostically useful WAIS profile would appear quite unlikely. The symptoms of AD can be quite variable (e.g., some patients present with early constructional apraxia, others with late apraxia; language disturbances are present early in some patients and late in others, etc.); premorbid differences in ability have significant effects on WAIS scores and Verbal IQ-Performance IQ (VIQ-PIQ) relationships; and the individual WAIS subtests tend to have relatively low reliability. Hence, it appears unlikely that any diagnostically useful unitary pattern of intellectual function, as assessed by currently available psychometric instruments, will be demonstrated in AD.

Memory dysfunction is typically identified as the earliest symptom of AD, and is perhaps the best investigated of all neuropsychological deficits in this disorder. Deficits have been documented in primary memory, secondary memory, verbal learning and memory, nonverbal learning and memory, episodic memory for remote events, and semantic memory (Miller, 1971; Muramoto, 1984; Ober, Dronkers, Koss, Delis, & Friedland, 1986; Weingartner et al., 1981; Weingartner, Grafman, Boutelle, Kaye, & Martin, 1983; Wilson, Bacon, Kramer, Fox, & Kaszniak, 1983; Wilson, Kaszniak, Bacon, Fox, & Kelly, 1982; Wilson, Kaszniak, & Fox, 1981).

Miller (1971) demonstrated impaired free recall of previously learned word lists in AD patients relative to age-matched controls, and attributed the deficit to "an abnormally rapid loss of material from short-term storage and a difficulty in transfer between short-term and long-term storage" (p. 80). The question of whether rates of forgetting are abnormally rapid in AD remains an open one (Becker, Boller, Saxton, & McGonigle-Gibson, 1987; Hart, Kwentus, Taylor, & Harkins, 1987; Kopelman, 1985; Morris, 1986), with evidence available to support either side of the debate. However, more recent investigations (e.g., Weingartner et al., 1981, 1983) tend to attribute these failures in the ability to retain verbal material to a deficit in encoding processes, rather than impaired memory "stores" or "transfer." Weingartner and associates postulate that AD patients are unable to adequately access their own semantic memory structures, and hence are impaired in their ability to organize and encode the to-be-remembered material or events in a manner facilitating later recall. Deficits in accessing semantic memory are reflected in the AD patients' poor performance in the generation of words for a given semantic category (e.g., "In the next 60 seconds name aloud all the different vegetables you can think of . . ."), in their difficulty in completing highly structured sentences (e.g., "The wet clothes were hung out to ______"), and in their frequent errors in judging the correct sequence of common, verbally described activities (e.g., "If you were eating in a restaurant is this the correct sequence? First eat your food and then read the menu?"). This failure to access semantic memory, then, prohibits the AD subject from successfully encoding new episodic events in a semantically organized, readily memorable, and/or readily retrievable manner. Recent research has also focused on the issue of whether disruption in the *structure* of semantic memory (as distinguished from impaired *access* to semantic memory) may also contribute to the memory deficit in AD (e.g., Martin and Fedio, 1983; Nebes, Boller, & Holland, 1986; Nebes, Martin, & Horn, 1984).

Memory for nonverbal, visually presented material (e.g., spatial location of objects, recognition of previously presented unfamiliar faces) also has been shown to decline in AD, with such a decline not simply reducible to a more fundamental failure of visuoperceptual mechanisms (Muramoto, 1984; Wilson et al., 1982). The question of whether memory for verbal material declines relatively more or less rapidly than that for nonverbal material remains unresolved, however. Remote memory is impaired in AD, with a relatively "flat" recall deficit observed across all time periods examined (Wilson et al., 1981).

The status of visuoperceptual and visuospatial abilities in AD has not been well studied. Eye movement impairments are present in AD, and the severity of this impairment has been shown to correlate with the severity of dementia (Pirozzolo & Hansch, 1981). A loss of sensitivity to spatial contrast of all spatial frequencies has been reported in AD subjects, and such a deficit could produce decrements in normal spatial vision (Nissen et al., 1985). Such a spatial vision deficit may not, however, be present in AD patients with normal visual acuity (Schlotterer, Moscovitch, & Crapper-McLachlan, 1983). Visuoperceptual discrimination abilities for both nonmeaningful (e.g., mosaic designs) and meaningful (e.g., faces) material has been shown to decline in AD patients relative to age-matched normal controls (Brouwers, Cox, Martin, Chase, & Fedio, 1984; Eslinger & Benton, 1983), and the identification of the spatial orientation of lines in relation to a standard shows a similar decline in 80% of demented subjects (Eslinger & Benton, 1983).

Language dysfunction is a universal concomitant of AD, and can occur as the initial symptom of this disorder (Bayles, 1984; Kirshner et al., 1984). Despite significant intersubject variability, several general features of the dysphasia in AD are apparent. In the early phases of the dementia, object-naming and word-finding difficulties are the most apparent deficits (Appell, Kertesz, & Fisman, 1982). These problems manifest themselves as anomia, circuitous and circumstantial speech, semantic paraphasias, and verbal perseverations (Bayles, 1984). Articulation, phonology, syntax, fluency of speech, repetition, and oral reading are well preserved relative to semantic aspects of speech; comprehension difficulties may or may not be apparent (Appell et al., 1982; Bayles, 1984; Cummings, Benson, Hill, & Read, 1985). As the dementia progresses, speech becomes vague or empty, with indefinite or generic terms (e.g., "this one," "thing") substituted for substantive nouns, an increase in semantic paraphasias and verbal perseverations occurs, and comprehension abilities deteriorate (affecting both auditory and written materials) (Bayles, 1984; Cummings et al., 1985). Verbal fluency, as measured by the ability to retrieve words belonging to a specific semantic or alphabetic category within a limited time period, declines significantly despite relatively fluent, if empty, spontaneous verbal output (Rosen, 1980). Late stages of the disease see the appearance of echolalia, palilalia, nonsensical or jargon speech, syntactic and phonological disturbances, and a frequent late-stage mutism (Bayles, 1984).

Diagnostic Consideration

There is currently no known, unique behavioral or biological marker for AD (see Hollander, Mohs, & Davis, 1986, and the concurrently published commentaries for an excellent review). Definitive diagnosis is possible only at autopsy or via biopsy, based upon the finding of neurofibrillary tangles and senile plaques in the cerebral cortex of clinically demented individuals (Khachaturian, 1985). Recent research (Wolozin & Davies, 1986; Wolozin, Pruchnicki, Dickson, & Davies, 1986) has suggested that an abnormal protein (A68) may be characteristic of AD and detectible in the cerebrospinal fluid (CSF) using an antibody (Alz-50) that binds to it. Although refinement of the CSF assay procedure is not complete, and large-scale study of diagnostic sensitivity and specificity have yet to be conducted, this test represents the best current hope for a diagnostic test for AD. Clinical diagnosis of AD, lacking brain specimen or a proven diagnostic test, is an exclusionary process of ruling out all other possible causes for the observed cognitive and behavioral decline. The importance of a meticulous search for reversible or treatable causes of the dementing process cannot be over emphasized; the consequences of missing such a cause and falsely diagnosing the patient as experiencing AD are tragic.

The procedures necessary for this diagnostic process have recently been enumerated by an NINCDS-ADRDA Work Group on clinical diagnosis of AD (McKhann et al., 1984). A careful clinical history must be obtained to establish an insidious onset and progressive, deteriorating course for the cognitive decline. A neurological examination is necessary to demonstrate the absence of focal neurological signs and symptoms. Neuropsychological evaluation is necessary to verify and document deficits in memory and at least one additional area of cognition, and to rule out depression as a causative agent. Laboratory studies must include blood and urine studies, with care taken to rule out diseases producing reversible or treatable cognitive decline (e.g., pernicious anemia, syphilis, hepatic failure, renal failure, thyroid dysfunction, folate or B_{12} deficiency, heavy metal toxicity, etc.). Examination of cerebrospinal fluid may be helpful in excluding inflammatory or infectious etiologies (the CSF is typically normal in AD). CT scanning and magnetic resonance imaging are necessary to eliminate focal lesions as possible sources of the dementia (slow-growing tumor, subdural hematoma, and hydrocephalus are perhaps the most important such etiologies). Electroencephalographic study is frequently normal or characterized by nonspecific changes (e.g., diffuse slow wave activity) in AD. Only upon the completion of this broad array of procedures can other possible causes of the cognitive decline be eliminated and a diagnosis of probable AD be made (McKhann et al., 1984).

Misdiagnosis is, unfortunately, a much too frequent occurrence. Some studies have revealed that up to 20% of cases given an initial diagnosis of AD prove, at autopsy, to have been inaccurately diagnosed, with conditions other than AD having been responsible for the cognitive decline (e.g., McKhann et al., 1984; Sulkava, Haltia, Paetau, Wikstrom, & Palo, 1983). Long-term follow-up studies (e.g., Ron, Toone, Garralda, & Lishman, 1979) indicate an initial misdiagnosis rate of up to 31%. Approximately one half of those misdiagnosed as having AD later proved to have been experiencing an affective disorder that produced symptoms strongly resembling those seen in dementia. A number of clinical features can differentiate such pseudodementia (the mimicking of dementia by a functional psychiatric illness, usually depression) from dementia, and careful consideration of these features may assist in decreasing this unacceptable rate of misdiagnosis (the reader is encouraged to consult Wells, 1979, for a review of such features). The use of Hachinski's Ischemic Score will, in similar fashion, assist in the differential diagnosis of multi-infarct dementia from AD (Hachinski et al., 1975; Rosen, Terry, Fuld, Katzman, & Peck, 1980).

Neuromorphology and Neurophysiology

It can be persuasively argued that the neuromorphological changes observed to occur in AD represent only quantitative accentuations of normal age-related brain changes. Decrease in brain weight, gyral atrophy, ventricular dilatation, neuronal cell loss, and amyloid accumulation all occur with normal aging, are accentuated relative to the normal aged in AD patients, and show significant quantitative overlap between normal aging and AD (Kemper, 1984). The frequency and extent of occurrence of neuritic plaques and Hirano bodies show somewhat less quantitative overlap between AD and normal aging, but do occur with regularity in both. It is only when one observes the extent and location of neurofibrillary tangles and granulovacuolar degeneration that minimal overlap between the two groups is observed. Neurofibrillary tangles and granulovacuolar degeneration occur in small numbers and relatively restricted locations in the normal aged; they display striking increases in density and extent in AD (Kemper, 1984).

Terry (1983) reports that the neuron loss in AD is confined primarily to large neurons; small neurons are relatively unaffected. The cause of this cell death remains unknown. Marked subcortical neuronal losses are observed in all areas of the amygdala, the locus ceruleus, and the nucleus basalis of Meynert (Kemper, 1983; Mann, Yates, & Marcyniuk, 1984). Nucleus basalis neuron loss of approximately 75%, relative to normal aged subjects, has been reported in AD patients in studies from several laboratories (e.g., Mann et al., 1984; Whitehouse et al., 1982). The hippocampus and subiculum undergo similar significant depopulation (approximately 50%) (Kemper, 1984). Neuronal loss in the substantia nigra (with additional findings of Lewy bodies and neurofibrillary tangles) is also frequently observed in patients with AD, suggesting an association between AD and Parkinson's disease (Leverenz & Sumi, 1986).

Cerebrovascular amyloidosis occurs in over 90% of AD patients (Glenner, 1983). Neuritic plaques occur most frequently in the cortex of the temporal lobe, and preponderantly in the association cortex of this lobe. The amygdala is the subcortical site most prominently affected by these plaques. Neurofibrillary tangles occur in association cortex, limbic cortex, hippocampus, amydgala, thalamus, hypothalamus, and mammillary bodies, a range of locations never observed in nondementing aged controls (Kemper, 1984; McDuff & Sumi, 1985). Granulovacuolar degeneration (observed virtually exclusively in Sommer's sector of the hippocampus in the normal aged, and never affecting more than 10% of those cells) is found in multiple hippocampal areas and affects up to 60% of all cells observed (Kemper, 1984). Finally, a white matter disorder has been described in up to 60% of AD patients (Brun & Englund, 1986).

The neuromorphology of AD, as revealed via CT scanning, has received considerable study. There is currently general agreement that ventricular size and severity of dementia correlate positively, and that significant group differences on measures of ventricular enlargement between AD and normal aged do exist (Albert, Naeser, Levine, & Garvey, 1984a). In the individual case, however, CT scan results cannot be used alone diagnostically, given the significant degree of overlap between normal aged and demented individuals (Freedman et al., 1984). In the near future, though, the use of CT density numbers may make such a case-by-case diagnostic differentiation possible (Albert, Naeser, Levine, & Garvey, 1984b). Additionally, rate of change in various CT parameters over time may prove much more valuable in diagnosis than findings obtained from a single CT scan (Bird, Levy, & Jacoby, 1986; Brinkman & Largen, 1984). Unlike the relationship between ventricular enlargement and degree of dementia, no consensus has been reached on the relationship between sulcal prominence and severity of cognitive decline. Finally, white matter lucencies have been observed in both CT and MRI study of normal aging persons and in studies of AD patients, and a relationship of these changes to presence and severity of cognitive decline has been suggested (George, de Leon, Gentes, et al., 1986; George, de Leon, Kalnin, et al., 1986; Steingart, Hachinski, Lau, Fox, Diaz, et al., 1987; Steingart, Hachinski, Lau, Fox, Fox, et al., 1987). The clinical significance of these findings, however, is unclear in the individual case.

There is general agreement that numerous indicators of neurophysiological status differentiate AD patients from healthy aged controls. Cerebral blood flow is significantly and diffusely decreased in AD, and this decrease is secondary to, rather than causative of, a primary hypometabolism (Tachibana et al., 1984). The regional cerebral metabolic rate for glucose (rCMRglu) displays a mild, generalized decrease relative to controls, with frontal and parietotemporal association cortex relatively more affected than primary cortex, a finding congruent with the known distribution of neuromorphological pathology (Benson, 1983; Benson et al., 1983; de Leon et al., 1983). Furthermore, the cerebral localization of the diminished rCMRglu corresponds well with the pattern of cognitive failure (e.g., subjects with disproportionate language dysfunction show markedly greater diminution of rCMRglu in left hemispheric regions; subjects with disproportionate visuospatial dysfunction show the opposite lateralization) (Foster et al., 1983). The most common EEG findings in AD include diffuse alpha slowing (or a complete absence of alpha activity) and diminished bilateral coherence of electrical activity in the central-temporal regions (Hansch et al., 1980; Katz & Harner, 1984). The degree of EEG abnormality has been shown to correlate with the degree of dementia in multiple studies (e.g., Kaszniak, Garron, Fox, Bergen, & Huckman, 1979; Pedley & Miller, 1983), although in individual cases progression of the dementia may not be accompanied by an increasingly abnormal EEG (Rae-Grant et al., 1987). Significant changes in various evoked potential measures also have been demonstrated in AD, including increased latency and amplitude in P300 (Goodin, Squires, & Starr, 1978; Hansch et al., 1980).

Etiology

Despite the existence of numerous promising hypotheses and significant research effort, the etiological basis of AD remains unknown. A complete review of the relevant data and proposals is beyond the scope of this chapter; a brief review of the more important points is presented in its stead (see Wurtman, 1985, for a more complete review).

A genetic basis is often postulated for at least a subset of AD cases. Estimates of the number of cases that are familial in nature vary from 10% to over 50% (Breitner & Folstein, 1984; Drachman, 1983; Heston, 1983; Prusiner, 1984a). Heston and associates (Heston, Mastri, Anderson, & White, 1981) review the evidence implicating a genetic basis for AD, citing several quite suggestive phenomena: (a) the well-documented existence of single families with multiple cases of AD, generally characterized by relatively early age at onset, rapid progression, and apparently autosomal dominant transmission; (b) increased risk to first- and second-degree relatives in such families; (c) an excessive incidence of Down syndrome in the relatives of AD patients in such families; (d) an increased incidence of lymphoma in these relatives; and (e) the increased frequency of putative immune system disorders in such families (e.g., rheumatoid arthritis, rheumatic valvular disease, multiple sclerosis, diabetes mellitus). Furthermore, it is an oft-cited finding that virtually all Down syndrome patients surviving to age 35 will develop the pathological brain lesions characteristic of Alzheimer's disease (Epstein, 1983).

The genetic defect that produces the familial form of AD has recently been localized to a restricted region of chromosome 21 (St. George-Hyslop et al., 1987). Furthermore, the gene responsible for the production of amyloid in both AD and Down syndrome has also been isolated and localized in the same region of chromosome 21 (Goldgaber, Lerman, McBride, Saffiotti, and Gajdusek, 1987; Robakis et al., 1987: Tanzi et al.. 1987). At the time of this writing, it is uncertain whether the gene(s) responsible for the genetic defect in familial AD and the gene for amyloid protein are the same, or different but localized closely to one another on chromosome 21. Delabar and colleagues (1987) have also demonstrated that in both AD and Down syndrome three copies (rather than the normal two) of the gene for brain amyloid protein are present, and suggest that this duplication of the gene may be the underlying defect responsible for AD. Whether this defect alone is, in fact, necessary and sufficient for the development of AD is currently unknown.

The development and accumulation of abnormal protein structure had been proposed as a proximal causative factor in AD prior to these recent genetic findings (e.g., Glenner, 1983; Schlaepfer, 1983). Amyloid, senile plaques, and neurofibrillary tangles are all examples of abnormal protein structure, and charcteristic of AD. The number of senile plaques has been shown to correlate with severity of impairment of competence in personal, domestic, and social activities (Blessed, Tomlinson, & Roth, 1968), and hence the formation of such plaques might suggest itself as a fundamental pathogenic process in AD (Wisniewski & Merz, 1983). It has been proposed that neurofibrillary tangles, which upon electromicrographic examination appear to be composed of paired helical filaments, are abnormally transformed neurofilaments, a normally occurring neuronal fibrous protein (Schlaepfer, 1983). The abnormal transformation of neurofilaments into paired helical filaments and then into neurofibrillary tangles, and the subsequent abnormal accumulation of the latter within the neuron, is thought to disrupt normal cytoplasmic transport, subsequently resulting in reduced synaptic activity and, ultimately, neuronal degeneration (Crapper-McLachlan and De Boni, 1980). The primary cause of such postulated neurofilament transformation is unknown. Finally, Glenner (1983) proposes the process of cerebrovascular amyloidosis as the initial step in a cascade of changes leading to neurofibrillary tangles; this proposal, as with others, lacks an initial causative factor.

Infectious agents have been proposed as the etiological basis producing AD. Both scrapie (a slow, progressive, neurological disease of sheep and goats) and Creutzfeldt-Jakob disease (a rare degenerative dementia producing death within approximately 1 year of symptom onset) have been shown to be transmissible disorders, hence implicating the existence of an infectious agent. The infectious agent in these disorders remains poorly understood, but is thought to be an "unconventional virus," perhaps the scrapie-associated fibril or "prion" (these two entities may, in fact, be one-and-the-same phenomenon) (Gajdusek, 1986; Prusiner, 1984b). Prions form dense, rodlike collections that, in aggregate, resemble amyloid plaques, suggesting that the plaques in AD are in fact prion rods. Consequently, it has been suggested that prions are the causative, infectious agent producing AD (Prusiner, 1984a, 1984b). However, recent work has demonstrated that although amyloid plaque from scrapie and Creutzfeldt-Jakob disease brain show prion-protein immunoreactivity, no such reactivity is observed in amyloid plaque, vascular amyloid, or neurofibrillary tangles from AD brain (Roberts et al., 1986). Furthermore, the gene responsible for producing the human prion-protein has been localized to chromosome 20 (Liao, Lebo,

Clawson, & Smuckler, 1986). Hence, a causative link between the prion-protein and AD (and Down syndrome) appears unlikely at this time. Additionally, attempts to demonstrate the transmissibility of AD have been unsuccessful to date (e.g., Goudsmit et al., 1980).

Environmental toxins, such as aluminum, have received attention as potential etiological factors in AD (e.g., Crapper, Krishman, & Quittkat, 1976). Neurofibrillary degeneration can be produced in rabbits by exposing the CNS to aluminum, and increased amounts of aluminum have been reported in the brains of AD patients (Perl, 1983). However, the ultrastructural details of the tangles produced in rabbits differ from those seen in AD, and the association between tangles and aluminum may merely represent an increased affinity for aluminum and not a causative relationship at all (Wurtman, 1985).

The major etiological hypothesis of the past decade has been the so-called cholinergic hypothesis. Specific dysfunction in cholinergic neurons and neurotransmitter activity has been demonstrated in AD (Coyle, Price, & DeLong, 1983); the severity of this disruption correlates with the severity of the dementia in AD patients (Francis et al., 1985), and artificial disruption of cholinergic activity in young people produces AD-like cognitive dysfunction (Bartus et al., 1982). Together, these findings have suggested to many that AD is caused by a specific cholinergic system dysfunction.

Despite this empirical support, recent work has cast doubt upon the validity of this hypothesis. First, if AD is caused by a loss of cortical cholinergic innervation, it would be expected that enhancing central cholinergic activity in AD patients would result in significantly reduced cognitive deficits. To date, however, results of the numerous studies attempting such an intervention have indicated no replicable clinical benefit from such treatment approaches (Bartus et al., 1982). One exception might be the recent study of the efficacy of oral tetrahydroamino acridine (THA) by Summers, Majovski, Marsh, Tachiki and Kling (1986), which, however, still awaits replication. Previous use of the same drug by another group of investigators (Kaye et al., 1982) did not show encouraging results. Second, evidence has accumulated that strongly indicates that deficiencies in cholinergic system markers are not the only deficits seen in AD patients. It remains true that reductions in cholinergic system activity are the most consistent findings, and the findings of greatest magnitude, across various studies of the neurochemistry of the disorder. However, significant losses in norepinephrine, serotonin, somatostatin, substance P, and cholecystokinin octapeptide indicators are also found to accompany such cholinergic declines in numerous individual studies (e.g., Crystal & Davies, 1982; Davies & Terry, 1981; Francis et al., 1985; Perry, Blessed, et al., 1981; Perry & Perry, 1985a; Perry, Tomlinson, et al., 1981). Additionally, the cholinergic hypothesis postulates a primary degeneration of neurons in the nucleus basalis of Meynert (NBM, the primary source of cortical cholinergic innervation), which in turn produces neocortical plaques composed of degenerating NBM neurites and neocortical decreases in choline acetyltransferase (ChAT) (Coyle et al., 1983; Struble, Cork, Whitehouse, & Price, 1982). However, it is now clear that severe degeneration of the NBM can occur without concomitant neocortical senile plaque formation, that neocortical ChAT activity does not invariably correlate with NBM neuron counts in AD, that significant cell loss in the NBM does not always accompany AD, and that cellular changes in the NBM (when they do occur) are also consistent with a process of retrograde degeneration following damage to the cortex, rather than necessarily prior to and causative of cortical changes per se (Pearson, Sofroniew, et al., 1983; Perry, et al., 1985; Perry & Perry, 1985b). Hence, although reductions in cholinergic system activity may be characteristic of AD, it now appears doubtful that such dysfunction represents the primary or sole causative mechanism underlying the dementia occurring in AD.

The last several years have witnessed a shift in thinking concerning the pathophysiological mechanisms underlying AD. Although a number of investigators continue to assert that subcortical (NBM) dysfunction precedes and produces cortical pathology, others have reaffirmed their long-standing conviction that the cortical lesions per se are primary. Perry and Perry (1985a), for example, assert that the subcortical degeneration in AD is a consequence of retrograde axonal degeneration that, in turn, results from primary cortical pathology. Numerous lines of evidence suggest and support this hypothesis (Pearson, Gatter, & Powell, 1983; Pearson, Sofroniew, et al., 1983; Perry & Perry, 1985a; Perry et al., 1985). Furthermore, the severity of the cortical histopathological lesions of AD has repeatedly been shown to correlate with various measures of the severity of dementia (e.g., Blessed et al., 1968; Wilcock & Esiri, 1982). Reductions in cortical somatostatin (SS) are a consistent finding in AD, both in advanced and early-to-middle disease stages (Beal & Martin, 1986). Destruction of the NBM, however, produces decreases in cortical ChAT activity but not in cortical SS concentrations (McKinney, Davies, & Coyle, 1982). Hence, primary cortical lesions are again suggested.

Recent work has suggested that a deficit in the cortico-cortical association system may be fundamental in producing the dementia in AD. Multiple laboratories have demonstrated reduced concentrations of cortical SS in AD (Arai, Moroji, & Kosaka, 1984; Beal, Mazurek, Svendsen, Bird, & Martin, 1986; Davies & Terry, 1981; Ferrier et al., 1983; Rosser, Emson, Mountjoy, Roth, & Iverson, 1980). Morphological changes consistent with neuronal degeneration have been shown to occur in SS containing neurons in the cerebral cortex of AD patients (Joynt & McNeill, 1984; Morrison, Rogers, Scherr, Benoit, & Bloom, 1985; Roberts, Crow, & Polak, 1985). Somatostatin immunoreactivity (SRIF) has been demonstrated in senile plaques in AD patients, and neurofibrillary tangles have been shown to be localized in SS containing neurons in AD (Armstrong, LeRoy, Shields, & Terry, 1985; Morrison et al., 1985; Roberts et al., 1985). The regional cortical and cortical laminar distributions of somatostatin have been demonstrated to show a striking similarity to the regional cortical and cortical laminar distributions of both cell loss and senile plaques in AD (Morrison et al., 1985). Additionally, the cortical laminar localization of somatostatin-containing neurons coincides with the origin of most of the projection neurons comprising the cortico-cortical association system (Morrison et al., 1985).

Together, these data have been interpreted as supporting the hypothesis that the profound cognitive loss characteristic of AD arises, in part, from the disconnection of cortical association regions with one another, secondary to this breakdown in the cortico-cortical association system (Morrison et al., 1985). The primary cause of this cortical pathological process remains unknown. Recent work has demonstrated that CSF levels of SRIF correlate with cognitive functioning in AD (Tamminga, Foster, Fedio, Bird, & Chase, 1987). Furthermore, close associations between SRIF measured in cortical biopsy samples and concurrently measured neuropsychological functions have been demonstrated.

Multi-Infarct Dementia

Next to AD, multi-infarct dementia (MID) is the most frequent dementing disorder in the aged. MID is brought about by the occurrence of multiple vascular occlusions that collectively produce a stuttering course of intellectual and other cognitive loss. MID is characterized by dementia (which may be its earliest symptom), focal and/or asymmetric neurological deficits, and evidence of probable arteriosclerosis outside of the CNS (e.g., systolic hypertension, cardiac enlargement, electrocardiographic abnormalities). Elicitation of a detailed clinical history, thorough physical, neurological, and laboratory evaluation, and CT study are usually sufficient for the differential diagnosis of this disorder in life. CT scanning can be confirmatory by demonstrating multiple focal areas of infarction and/or patchy cerebral atrophy (in contrast to the diffuse atrophy often seen in AD), but the CT scan also can appear normal when the dementia is produced by small, widely distributed occlusions. Cerebral blood flow studies and positron emission tomography studies also have been shown to discriminate between MID and AD, with MID patients displaying the expected focal or patchy reductions in contrast to the more diffuse dysfunction observed in AD (Benson et al., 1983; Tachibana et al., 1984). Careful history taking will benefit from the utilization of Hachinski's Ischemic Score, which has been shown to differentiate MID and AD, but will not distinguish a mixed etiology group from either "pure" disorder (Hachinski et al., 1975; Rosen et al., 1980).

The etiological and pathological subtypes of MID are legion, and have been reviewed elsewhere (see Cummings & Benson, 1983). Appropriate management and treatment of the disorder are dependent upon careful differentiation of the subtype involved in the individual case, but such a differentiation is not within the province of the neuropsychologist.

Neuropsychological Functions

The differentiation of MID and AD through neuropsychological assessment can be a difficult if not, at times, impossible task. The characteristics of the dementia produced by a multi-infarct process are determined by both the location of the individual infarctions and the total amount of brain tissue compromised by the multiple infarctions (Cummings & Benson, 1983). Consequently, there will exist individual cases of MID that are utterly indistinguishable from AD in terms of their neuropsychological presentation, a fact that further emphasizes the importance of eliciting a careful and detailed clinical history from the patient's family.

Multi-infarct processes with primarily a neocortical focus will produce the classical neuropsychological indicators of higher cortical dysfunction, such as dysphasia, apraxia, memory disturbance, and visuoperceptual and/or visuospatial dysfunction. A primarily subcortical focus for the pathology will more likely produce a generalized psychomotor slowing, disturbances in memory, language, and visuospatial abilities secondary to these more fundamental deficits. Obviously, many cases of MID will be characterized by concurrent cortical and subcortical infarctions, and the neuropsychological presentation will reflect this mixture. When MID is neuropsychologically distinguishable from AD, it is its presentation of select neuropsychological deficits reflecting focal lesions (rather than a generalized cognitive decline indicative of diffuse cerebral dysfunction) that makes the differentiation possible.

Parkinson's Disease

Parkinson's disease (PD) is a relatively common degenerative neurological disorder of the aged, affecting 1% of the population at age 50 and increasing to 2% of the population by age 75 (Alexander & Geschwind, 1984; Gilroy & Meyer, 1979). The mean age of onset has been variously reported as occurring in the mid-50s (e.g., Zetusky, Jankovic, & Pirozzolo, 1985) and mid-60s (e.g., Appel, 1981). In any case, onset of the disease prior to age 40 is unusual (such cases accounted for 6.7% of the sample in the Zetusky study, for instance). Onset of the disease is insidious, the course of the disorder is extremely variable, and the nature of the change in neuropsychological functioning with this disease remains an issue of considerable contention.

Although the label "Parkinson's disease" is widely used and generally accepted, such use is, in the strictest sense, erroneous. Parkinson's disease is, in fact, not a unitary disease entity at all, but rather, a syndrome that can result from numerous differing etiologies. Verified causes of Parkinsonism are encephalitis lethargica (producing postencephalitic Parkinsonism) and occlusive cerebrovascular disease (producing arteriosclerotic Parkinsonism). Parkinsonism also is thought to result from various toxicities (e.g., manganese poisoning) and adverse reactions to pharmacological agents (e.g., the phenothiazines). However, the vast majority of Parkinsonism cases are of unknown etiology, and such "idiopathic Parkinsonism" is the disorder usually referred to by the nosological label "Parkinson's disease."

Clinically, PD is characterized by tremor at rest, muscular rigidity, and bradykinesia. Multiple other signs and symptoms can accompany this "cardinal triad," the most common being postural changes, slowed and shuffling gait, masked facies, and dysarthric speech. Few patients show all such symptoms, and when symptoms do occur, they are usually bilateral but not necessarily symmetrical. The prevalence of dementia in PD has not been clearly defined, but there is now little debate that cognitive and intellectual dysfunction are a frequent and significant consequence of the disease.

Neuropathologically, PD is characterized by neuronal degeneration in the substantia nigra, and to a somewhat lesser extent, the locus ceruleus, raphe nuclei, and motor nucleus of vagus. Lewy bodies (relatively dense, spheroidal intracytoplasmic inclusion bodies) are diagnostic of idiopathic PD when occurring in large numbers in the neurons of the substantia nigra, and also have been frequently observed in locus ceruleus and substantia innominata (Kemper, 1984). Recently, significant neuronal depopulation in the NBM has been reported in the brains of demented PD patients, but such depopulation is not significant in nondemented PD patients (Perry et al., 1985; Whitehouse, Hedreen, White, & Price, 1983). Diffuse cortical atrophy (greater than normal for age) is a frequent finding in PD, occurring in approximately 60% of PD patients (Alvord et al., 1974; Becker, Grau, Schneider, Fischer, & Hacker, 1976; Selby, 1968). In addition, abnormal ventricular enlargement has been noted in up to 30% of PD patients (Selby, 1968; Sroka, Elizan, Yahr, Burger, & Mendoza, 1981). Further indication of cortical dysfunction in PD stems from investigations of regional cerebral blood flow, which have demonstrated significant reductions in nondemented PD subjects (Lavy, Melamed, Cooper, Bentin, & Rinot, 1979).

Parkinson's Disease and Dementia

As previously stated, the prevalence of dementia in PD has not been well defined. Estimates range from approximately 20% to 80%, with most estimates in the 40% to 60% range (Alexander & Geschwind, 1984; Boller, 1980; Boller, Mizutani, Roessmann, & Gambetti, 1980; Hakim & Mathieson, 1979; Lieberman et al., 1979; Martin, Loewenson, Resch, & Baker, 1973; Wells, 1982). This wide range of prevalence estimates is attributable to differences in the patient populations studied (e.g., autopsy cases, inpatients only, outpatients only) and to differences in criteria for inclusion under the classification of dementia. Furthermore, Pirozzolo has stressed that cognitive dysfunction in PD occurs along a continuum of impairment (rather than occurring in a clearly bimodal distribution of *unimpaired* versus *impaired* patients), that 93% of PD patients experience some level of such impairment, and that consequently any attempt to estimate the prevalence of dementia in PD must of necessity employ an arbitrary cutoff point between demented and nondemented cases (Pirozzolo, Hansch, Mortimer, Webster, & Kuskowski, 1982). Whatever the true frequency of significant cognitive dysfunction in PD may be, it is clearly much higher than the frequency of such dysfunction in the population at large (by a factor of 6 to 10 according to recent reports), and hence a real and significant association of dementia and PD does exist (Boller et al., 1980; Lieberman et al., 1979).

The neuropathological mechanism responsible for the dementia in PD is presently unknown. Two major hypotheses are currently extant: the first attributes the cognitive decline to cortical dysfunction secondary to co-occurring

Alzheimer's disease; the second ascribes major importance to basal ganglia dysfunction in producing the known cognitive decline. Hakim and Mathieson (1979), in an autopsy study of 19 demented PD patients, report neuropathological changes consistent with co-occurring AD in 17 of the 19 patients. Boller and associates (Boller et al., 1980) found significantly increased numbers of senile plaques and neurofibrillary tangles in 75% of their demented PD patients at autopsy, and 100% of their severely demented PD subjects had this distinctive, AD-like neuropathology. Significant levels of cortical atrophy are known to exist in PD, although a direct correlation of such atrophy with cognitive decline is lacking to date (Boller, 1980; Selby, 1968). Furthermore, decreases in cortical ChAT activity have been reported in some demented PD patients (Perry et al., 1985), and significant, AD-like cell loss in the NBM has been documented in demented PD subjects (Perry et al., 1985; Whitehouse et al., 1983). Other investigators, however, report an absence of significant AD-like neuropathology in PD patients (e.g., Heston, 1980). Neocortical plaques and tangles were at normal levels in the demented patients studied by Perry and associates (Perry et al., 1985). Heilig, Knopman, Mastri, and Frey (1985) report on five demented PD patients who lacked significant neocortical or hippocampal plaques, tangles, or granulovacuolar degeneration and additionally failed to show significant NBM cell loss. Given these findings, it appears that some demented PD patients may well be experiencing cognitive decline secondary to co-occurring AD, but many other PD patients can and do experience dementia in the absence of AD. Hence, the co-occurring AD hypothesis may explain some, but certainly not all, cases of dementia in PD.

Multiple other investigators have emphasized the role of basal ganglia dysfunction in producing the cognitive decline in PD. Specifically, basal ganglia degeneration is purportedly responsible for the visuoperceptual, visuospatial, and perceptual motor deficits commonly occurring in PD as well as the frequent and well-documented deficits in performance of tasks requiring shifting of set and complex, predictive, sequential voluntary motor movements (Boller et al., 1984; Cools, van den Bercken, Horstink, van Spaendonck, & Berger, 1984; Danta & Hilton, 1975; Lees & Smith, 1983; Mayeux & Stern, 1983; Mortimer, Pirozzolo, Hansch, & Webster, 1982; Pirozzolo et al., 1982; Stern, 1983; Stern, Mayeux, Rosen, & Ilson, 1983). Basic behavioral studies in animals, utilizing both ablation and stimulation of the basal ganglia, have amply demonstrated the critical role of these structures in these functions (see Stern, 1983, for a review). Significant correlations between the various motor symptoms of PD and concomitant cognitive dysfunction have been reported, again suggesting a role for the basal ganglia in the production of this cognitive decline in PD (e.g., Garron, Klawans, & Narin, 1972; Marttila & Rinne, 1976; Mortimer, Pirozzolo, Hansch, et al., 1982; Zetusky et al., 1985). Given the available evidence then, it appears that basal ganglia dysfunction may be responsible for selected aspects of the cognitive decline observed in many PD patients. However, there is no evidence to suggest that basal ganglia degeneration alone can explain the generalized dementia observed in so many of these patients.

Neuropsychological Functions

The neuropsychological characteristics of PD are a matter of considerable contention. For example, Boller (1980) and Pirozzolo (1982) claim that the dementias accompanying AD and PD are essentially the same in their qualitative aspects and difficult, if not often impossible, to distinguish neuropsychologically. Alexander and Geschwind (1984) and Albert (1978), on the other hand, state that the dementias occurring with AD and PD are qualitatively different, and in fact, exemplify the contrasting characteristics of cortical versus subcortical dementias, respectively. In the brief review that follows, we do not claim to resolve this area of contention. However, multiple specific neuropsychological characteristics are reported with notable frequency in studies of demented PD patients, and we suggest that these findings may serve as a basis for common agreement and provide a perspective from which remaining areas of contention may begin to be resolved.

As alluded to in the previous section, complex abstract reasoning, conceptual flexibility, and set-shifting ability are functions frequently disrupted in PD. Lees and Smith (1983) report evidence that decreased conceptual shifting ability and an increase in perseverative errors are common cognitive deficits in the early stages of PD, and that these deficits are not due to concomitant depression or generalized intellectual impairment. Albert (1978) and Bowen (1976) also have previously emphasized declines in written concept formulation, diminished conceptual flexibility, and deficits in set-shifting performance in PD. In a more recent study, Cools and associates (1984) demonstrate an impairment in set shifting at both motor and cognitive levels (e.g., finger-pressing sequences, verbal fluency, sorting of blocks and animal names into multiple categories) even in the presence of intact concept formation (i.e., WAIS Similarities subtest performance). They conclude that PD is characterized by diminished "shifting aptitude" at both motor and cognitive levels of behavioral organization, and cite the abundant available animal literature in support of the postulate that basal ganglia dysfunction underlies this deficit.

Memory dysfunction is a second frequently noted characteristic of PD. Alexander and Geschwind (1984) and Boller (1980) state that memory impairment may be the single most-frequent cognitive deficit in PD. Furthermore, El-Awar, Becker, Hammond, Nebes, and Boller (1987) point out that the memory deficit may be severe even in the absence of a generalized dementia. Deficits have been documented in visual memory (Albert, 1978), verbal memory (Pirozzolo et al., 1982), speed of scanning in short-term memory (Wilson, Kaszniak, Klawans, & Garron, 1980), and remote memory (Huber, Shuttleworth, & Paulson, 1986).

The nature of this memory dysfunction in PD has not, however, been well investigated. Tweedy, Langer, & McDowell (1982) demonstrate verbal memory impairments for both recall and recognition performance in PD patients. They found no decrease in the semantic organization of the to-be-remembered material, but the PD subjects did show less benefit from semantic cueing relative to age- and education-matched controls. Additionally, the PD subjects' performance on a Brown-Peterson task indicated an abnormally rapid loss of information from memory. Flowers, Pearce, and Pearce (1984) failed to demonstrate a decline in recognition memory performance for visually presented verbal and nonverbal material at either immediate or 45-minute delayed recall intervals. Consequently, they suggest that the PD memory impairment involves retrieval stage mechanisms, and not dysfunction during initial encoding or subsequent retention. In summary, memory functioning in PD patients may be characterized by slowed scanning of short-term memory, performance impairments with both verbal and nonverbal material, possible impairments in the use of semantic information in facilitating verbal recall, and abnormally rapid forgetting. The status of recognition memory performance in PD remains uncertain at this time.

Changes in speech and language functions have been noted in PD patients. Matison and associates state that the speech of PD patients is frequently characterized by hypophonia, tachyphemia, palilalia, and inappropriate silent periods (Matison, Mayeux, Rosen, & Fahn, 1982). Additionally, they note that the language performance of nondemented PD patients is frequently marred by impaired confrontation naming and decreased category naming (verbal fluency). They suggest that this verbal fluency deficit is due to a difficulty in semantic (rather than phonetic) retrieval, and that the fundamental disturbance in semantic retrieval may be one of "planning". They suggest that successful category naming requires systematic lexical search within categories and the ability to shift between categories, and that impaired shifts and an inability to plan and follow a particular strategy result in decreased verbal fluency. Scott, Caird, and Williams (1984) have demonstrated a decreased ability to match facial expression with appropriate speech intonation, and an inability to produce appropriate affective intonations when speaking (particularly interrogative and angry intonations). In summary, impaired verbal fluency, and defective production and appreciation of affective aspects of language, have all been demonstrated in PD. Full-blown aphasic dysfunction in PD subjects, however, appears to be uncommon.

As mentioned in the previous section, visuoperceptual, visuospatial, and perceptual motor defects commonly occur in PD patients. Visuoperceptual and visuospatial defects documented in PD include impaired judgment of the visual vertical and horizontal (Danta & Hilton, 1975), defective recognition of complex visual stimuli after a brief delay (Delancy-Horne, 1971), and impaired, discrimination of nonmeaningful visual stimuli (Boller et al., 1984; Pirozzolo et al., 1982). Other visuospatial and perceptual motor defects found in PD patients include impaired drawing of Benton Visual Retention Test figures (Boller et al., 1984), defective WAIS Block Design and Digit Symbol subtest performance (Pirozzolo et al., 1982), and defective map- or route-walking ability (Bowen, Hoehn, & Yahr, 1972). These specific neuropsychological defects have been observed in PD patients without overt dementia and also are known to occur as recognizably severe defects within the context of a generalized cognitive impairment in demented PD patients (Hovestadt, de Jong, & Meerwaldt, 1987; Pirozzolo et al., 1982). Furthermore, severity of bradykinesia has been shown to correlate with severity of disability on visuospatial task performance (e.g., Pirozzolo et al., 1982), again suggesting a role for basal ganglia dysfunction in the production of these deficits.

As would be expected, psychomotor and motor task performances are disrupted by PD. Slowing in such tasks, although certainly explicable in part by bradykinesia, also is produced in part by central defects of motor programming, manifested specifically as deficits in sequencing and planning of voluntary motor movements (Stern et al., 1983).

Certain specific neuropsychological abilities are frequently preserved in PD. Multiple investigators have noted that the general fund of information (as manifested in performance on tests such as WAIS Vocabulary and Information) is rarely impaired in PD (e.g., Pirozzolo, 1982). Apraxia and agnosia also are rarely observed (Albert, 1978; Alexander & Geschwind, 1984). Aphasia is often cited as absent in PD (e.g., Albert, 1978; Alexander & Geschwind, 1984), although recent studies report individual cases manifesting this deficit (e.g., Perry et al., 1985).

Finally, depression is a common correlate of PD, and may contribute to the presence and/or severity of the above-described neuropsychological deficits. The prevalence of depression in PD has been variously estimated at 30% (Lieberman et al., 1979) to 76% (Alexander & Geschwind, 1984). Mayeux, Stern, Rosen, and Leventhal (1981) report that 31% of nondemented PD patients are mildly depressed, and an additional 16% are moderately-to-severely depressed. Furthermore, they find that this prevalence rate is significantly greater than that observed in patients with other progressive, crippling medical diseases.

Huntington's Disease

Huntington's disease (HD) is a hereditary condition with confirmed autosomal dominant transmission and complete penetrance. Symptoms typically first appear between the ages of 30 and 50, although a so-called "juvenile chorea," beginning prior to age 30 occurs in approximately 5% of all cases (Finch, 1980; Spokes, 1981). HD is rare, occurring in only 1 in 10,000 individuals (Spokes, 1981). Duration of the disease is typically between 10 and 15 years (Lezak, 1983).

Clinically, HD is characterized by a triad of motor, affective, and cognitive changes. Clumsiness of movement, dropping things, and slowness of finer movements are the early harbingers of the coming motor dysfunction; athetosis and chorea follow (Gilroy & Meyer, 1979). Motor dysfunction in the late stages of HD is characterized by a lessening of these involuntary movements and the appearance of upper limb flexion and lower extremity extension (Sax et al., 1983). Related neurological signs, with onset at various points in the disease course, include gait impairment, hypotonia, hyperreflexia, dysarthria, and eye movement abnormalities (Gilroy & Meyer, 1979; Sax et al., 1983).

Frequently cited affective changes in HD include depression (particularly early in the course of the disease), anxiety, irritability, emotional lability, behavioral impulsivity (frequently manifested in aggressive or sexual behaviors), apathy, and later onset of frank psychosis in approximately 50% of HD patients (Caine, Hunt, Weingartner, & Ebert, 1978; Pincus & Tucker, 1985; Sax et al., 1983). The risk of suicide is significantly greater in HD patients relative to the normal population, particularly in younger patients (Schoenfeld et al., 1984; Spokes, 1981). The question of whether these various affective changes are primary or reactive remains unresolved.

Cognitively, HD is virtually always characterized by dementia, with the pattern and severity of the cognitive impairment differing across the various stages of the disease course. Lyle and Gottesman (1977), in a prospective study of a population at risk for HD ($N = 85$), demonstrate that relatively small but significant declines in intellectual abilities frequently begin years before the onset of motor dysfunction, with scores on the various Wechsler scales decreasing as temporal proximity to the onset of overt HD motor symptomology increases. Significant deficits on selected subtests of the Wechsler intellectual scales become apparent with the onset of motor symptomology, with Digit Symbol and Picture Arrangement often cited as the first to be affected (Butters, Sax, Montgomery, & Tarlow, 1978; Caine et al., 1978; Josiassen, Curry, Roemer, DeBease, & Mancall, 1982). Josiassen and associates interpret this pattern of decline as indicative of decreases in auditory alertness, immediate memory, motor skills, and the ability to organize and sequentially arrange relevant information. In the advanced stages of HD, of course, such focal deficits give way to a more global impairment, with HD patients performing worse than normals on all subtests of the intellectual scales (Butters et al., 1978; Josiassen et al., 1982).

Memory also is adversely affected early in the disease course, with an anterograde impairment characterized by a pronounced recall deficit often cited (Butters et al., 1978; Caine et al., 1978). It also is frequently noted that performance on short-term memory tasks is not improved by manipulations of proactive interference, rehearsal time, or cues, suggesting that the locus of the memory impairment is not at the level of initial encoding or stimulus analysis, but rather, at storage or retrieval levels (Butters, 1984; Butters, Tarlow, Cermak, & Sax, 1976). The rate of forgetting of pictoral material over a 1-week period has been shown to be normal in HD, implicating deficits in retrieval, rather than storage, as the underlying mechanism. Additionally, it has been demonstrated that the recognition memory performance of HD patients may be disproportionately better than their free-recall performance, again implicating a retrieval deficit rather than an impairment of consolidation or storage mechanisms (Butters, 1984; Butters, Wolfe, Granholm, & Martone, 1986). HD patients also experience an extensive remote memory impairment, with no temporal gradient apparent either in early or advanced disease stages, again consistent with the retrieval mechanism deficit hypothesis (Albert, Butters, & Brandt, 1981a, 1981b).

Early in the disease course decreases in verbal fluency, impairment in visuospatial performance (e.g., WAIS Block Design and Object Assembly, Benton Visual Retention Test), and difficulties with constructional tasks (both two- and three-dimensional) become apparent (Butters et al., 1978; Caine et al., 1978; Josiassen, Curry, & Mancall, 1983). As the disease advances, decreases in cognitive flexibility, concept formation, and set shifting become apparent (Josiassen et al., 1983). Additional indicators of frontal lobe dysfunction occurring in this middle stage include an increasing inability to plan, organize, sequence, execute, and integrate complex activities, failure to spontaneously initiate activities (giving the perhaps erroneous appearance of apathy), and a difficulty in comprehending complex or subtle social situations (Caine et al., 1978; Sax et al., 1983). Generally, language dysfunction is not thought to be characteristic of HD (Butters et al., 1978; Josiassen et al., 1983); recent studies, however, challenge this notion (Caine, Bamford, Schiffer, Shoulson, & Levy, 1986).

It has been noted that the progression of cognitive deficits parallels the known progression of neuropathological changes in HD (Sax et al., 1983). Early in the disease course memory, visuospatial, and motor abilities are disrupted. Middle stages of the disorder are characterized by additional deficits in conceptual, executive, and specific intellectual abilities associated with frontal lobe functioning. In advanced HD, a more global intellectual and cognitive impairment occurs, supplanting these earlier focal deficits. Hence, the progression of cognitive changes is consistent with a neostriatal to frontal lobe to posterior cortex sequence of neuropathological degeneration.

Neuropathologically, HD has been characterized as a neostriatal and frontal disorder in its early stages, with additional areas of involvement appearing as the disease progresses (Sax et al., 1983). Specifically, characteristic and marked changes in the caudate and putamen include loss of small neurons, morphological changes in the dendrites of medium-sized spiny neurons, and consequent atrophy of the neostriatum to approximately 50% of its normal size (Caine et al., 1978; Finch, 1980; Graveland, Williams, & DiFiglia, 1985). Concomitant cortical degeneration occurs (spreading in an anterior to posterior manner), degeneration of the corpus callosum has been observed, changes in thalamic nuclei, hypothalamus, and brainstem structures are common, and significant ventricular dilatation has been noted (Sax et al., 1983). Neurochemically, it appears that multiple neurotransmitter systems are affected, including massive depletion of neostriatal GABA-ergic cells, some loss of cholinergic cells, decrease in number of dopamine receptors (but dopamine neurotransmitter levels per se appear unchanged), and decreased glutamate binding in the neostriatum (Finch, 1980; Greenamyre et al., 1985). Furthermore, several neuropeptides (e.g., somatostatin, neuropeptide Y) show caudate increases; the significance of this finding remains unknown (Martin & Gusella, 1986).

Progressive Supranuclear Palsy

Progressive supranuclear palsy (PSP) is a rare degenerative neurological disorder characterized clinically by supranuclear opthalmoplegia, with additionally frequent complaints of falling (typically backwards), nuchal rigidity, moderate axial dystonia, pseudobulbar palsy, difficulty swallowing, dysarthria, bradykinesia, masked facies, nonspecific changes in personality, sleep disturbance, and performance decrements on various neuropsychological tasks (Hynd, Pirozzolo, & Maletta, 1982; Steele, 1972; Steele, Richardson, & Olszewski, 1964). The symptomological overlap with Parkinson's disease is apparent; however, the supranuclear opthalmoplegia that is the hallmark of PSP is not characteristic of Parkinson's disease, and the tremor associated with Parkinson's disease is typically absent in PSP. It is on this basis that the two disorders can be clinically differentiated.

PSP usually has its onset in the sixth decade of life (Steele, 1972), although onset as early as age 16 has been reported (Hynd et al., 1982). Precise estimates of the incidence of PSP are lacking, but occurrence in less than 1% of elderly patients *presenting* with symptoms of dementia appears probable (Hynd et al., 1982). The disease is terminal in 4 to 7 years in one half of all patients (Steele, 1972), although durations of up to 24 years have been observed (Jellinger, Riederer, & Tomonasa, 1980).

At present, there is no diagnostic test specific for PSP; such diagnosis is essentially clinical in nature. Routine CSF, blood, and urine studies are typically normal; EEG findings may be normal or suggestive of diffuse slowing, and CT scan findings are often negative or characterized by nonspecific atrophic changes (Hynd et al., 1982; Jackson, Jankovic, & Ford, 1983). There is currently no effective treatment for the entire range of symptoms associated with PSP, but dopamine agonists and methysergide have proven effective in reducing the severity of selected symptoms in some PSP patients (Jackson et al., 1983; Rafal & Grimm, 1981).

Whether or not a true dementia occurs in association with PSP is a matter of significant disagreement. Albert and associates (1974) describe PSP as a prototypical "subcortical dementia," characterized by: (a) "forgetfulness" (not a true memory defect per se, but rather a difficult and slowed, but accurate retrieval); (b) slowing of thought processes; (c) personality changes (e.g., apathy, depression, irritability, and inappropriate displays of emotion); and (d) an impaired ability to manipulate acquired knowledge (as manifested by disturbances in abstraction and calculation). Furthermore, the higher cortical disorders (i.e., aphasia, apraxia, agnosia) that characterize the so-called "cortical dementias" (e.g., Alzheimer's disease) are said to be absent in the subcortical dementia of PSP. Albert and colleagues postulate an underlying disturbance of "timing and activation" as the fundamental defect responsible for the four above-described clinical characteristics of PSP. They propose that impaired functioning of the reticular activating system, or a disconnection of the reticular activating system from thalamic and subthalamic nuclei, produces this slowing of normal intellectual and memory processes.

Other investigators have, however, taken issue with this formulation, and deny that any true, progressing, diffuse cognitive decline occurs in PSP. Kimura, Barnett, and Burkhart (1981) have demonstrated that performance IQ decrements appear to be produced by poor performance only on those tasks requiring significant visual scanning (e.g., Digit Symbol); performance subtests lacking this pronounced visual search requirement (e.g., Picture Completion) were completed at a level comparable to the nondemented groups. Furthermore, PSP patients did not differ from the focal lesion groups in terms of Wechsler Memory Scale memory quotient scores. Hence, it appears that PSP is characterized by defective performance on tasks with a strong visual scanning requirement, but not by defective intellectual and memory performance per se. Finally, Hynd and colleagues (1982) note that the cognitive decline associated with PSP is non-progressing. Hence, given the lack of both a generalized and progressive cognitive decline in PSP, it appears that a classification of PSP with the dementing disorders is indefensible from a definitional standpoint alone.

Normal Pressure Hydrocephalus

Normal pressure hydrocephalus (NPH) is characterized by enlargement of the ventricular system with concomitant normal CSF pressure. Pathophysiologically, NPH is thought to begin with an initial elevation of CSF pressure, producing ventricular dilatation, and a subsequent return of pressure to normal or borderline elevated levels with persisting hydrocephalus (Adams, 1980). NPH must be differentiated from hydrocephalus *ex vacuo*, in which ventricular dilatation is secondary to atrophy of cerebral white matter.

NPH is a relatively infrequent cause of dementia, accounting for approximately 5% to 6% of final diagnoses in cases presenting with dementia (Katzman, 1978). Onset is typically in the late 50s, with a number of differing etiologies responsible for the development of NPH (Katzman, 1977). These etiologies fall into two groups: (a) idiopathic NPH, in which no causal agent is apparent; and (b) secondary NPH, in which hydrocephalus is produced by subarachnoid hemorrhage, head trauma, subdural hematoma, cerebellar hematoma, meningitis, or other insult, producing damage to the arachnoid membrane. Approximately one third of all cases of NPH are of the idiopathic variety; two thirds are of identifiable etiology, with subarachnoid hemorrhage alone accounting for 35% of all cases (Katzman, 1977).

Pathologically, NPH typically produces pronounced dilatation of the frontal horns and body of the lateral ventricles, with somewhat less pronounced enlargement of the remaining ventricles (Adams, 1980). CT scanning frequently fails to demonstrate cortical atrophy, but periventricular density decreases, having the characteristics of white matter edema, are common (Jacobs, Kinkel, Painter, Murawski, & Heffner, 1978). Multiple studies have documented decreases in cerebral blood flow relative to an aged control group (e.g., Kushner et al., 1984); the EEG is typically normal or characterized by diffuse slowing (Katzman, 1977). Radioisotopic cisternography should reveal ventricular stasis, considered by some to be the *sine qua non* for diagnosis of NPH (Katzman, 1977). Direct measurement of CSF pressure may, in fact, demonstrate either normal levels or intermittent to virtually constant mild elevations of pressure (Hartmann & Alberti, 1977).

Clinically, NPH is characterized by the classic triad of gait disturbance, urinary incontinence, and dementia. The disturbance of gait may manifest itself as unsteadiness of gait, shuffling gait, or spasticity, and is usually the first of these three symptoms to appear (Katzman, 1977). Other neurological deficits reported include snout and grasp reflexes, nystagmus, spasticity, seizures, parkinsonian features, and akinetic mutism (Katzman, 1977; Wood, Bartlet, James, & Udvarhelyi, 1974). Botez and co-workers report that headache, depression, memory difficulties, and sudden, transient decreases in muscle tone (producing "drop attacks") may precede the classic symptomological triad and associated neurological abanormalities (Botez, Ethier, L'eveille, & Botez-Maquard, 1977).

Neuropsychologically, the dementia accompanying NPH is frequently described as "mild," with a slowing of thought processes, inattention, apathy, disorientation, and motor slowing predominating (Cummings, 1983; Katzman, 1977). Adams (1980) notes that a difficulty in planning, sequencing, maintaining, and monitoring sustained activities is common, and attributes this to frontal lobe dysfunction or disconnection caused by a stretching of the long fiber tracts that connect the frontal lobes to other cortical and subcortical areas, a stretching readily produced by the known dilatation of the frontal horns. Furthermore, disruption of these long fiber tracts provides a plausible neuropathological mechanism for the production of the concomitant gait disturbance and incontinence. Collignon and associates, in a study of 10 NPH patients, report constructional apraxia in 8; memory disturbance, anosagnosia, and poor judgment and insight in 7; ideational or motor apraxia in 5; spatial disorientation in 4; and changes in mood or affective behavior in 3 (Collignon, Rectem, Laterre, & Stroobandt, 1975). Gustafson and Hagberg (1978) emphasized impaired memory functioning in their sample ($n = 23$). Multiple authors have noted the absence of language dysfunction in NPH (Adams, 1980; Cummings, 1983; Gustafson & Hagberg, 1978; Katzman, 1977).

Careful differential diagnosis in cases of suspected NPH is crucial, as NPH represents a potentially treatable disorder. NPH and AD frequently dissociate on several dimensions: in NPH, psychomotor retardation frequently precedes frank intellectual decline, the reverse usually holds true in AD; gait disturbances occur early in NPH and late (if at all) in AD; the memory difficulties in NPH may have a relatively rapid onset and may represent a slowing or inattention rather than a true memory dysfunction per se, whereas onset of memory decline in AD is less acute and represent true memory impairment; language disturbances, common in AD, are rare in NPH; and finally, abnormal CT and CSF flow findings characterize NPH but not AD (Adams, Fisher, Hakim, Ojemann, & Sweet, 1965; Lezak, 1983; Katzman, 1978).

Ventricular shunting has received much attention as a potential treatment for NPH. However, mortality with this procedure is high (6% to 9%), and postoperative morbidity is common (40%), while reports of symptom improvement or lessening, in comparison, are disappointingly low (range of 10% to 100%, with most estimates clustering around 60%) (Cummings, 1983; Hughes et al., 1978;

Katzman, 1977; Kirshner, 1986; Kushner et al., 1984; Thomsen, Borgesen, Bruhn, & Gjerris, 1986).

Pick's Disease

Pick's disease is a relatively rare form of dementia, occurring in both sporadic (80%) and familial (20%) forms, with onset most common between the ages of 40 and 60 (Alexander & Geschwind, 1984). Pathologically, Pick's disease is characterized by severe atrophy of the anterior temporal lobes and frontal lobes with relative preservation of the pre- and postcentral gyri and the posterior superior temporal gyrus (Cummings & Duchen, 1981; Wechsler, Verity, Rosenschein, Fried, & Scheibel, 1982). Atrophy is secondary to neuron cell loss, and secondary areas of such cell depopulation include the amygdala (all sections), basal ganglia, and thalamus (Cummings & Duchen, 1981; Uhl, Hilt, Hedreen, Whitehouse, & Price, 1983). Although not observed in all cases, severe degeneration of the NBM has been reported with Pick's disease (Uhl et al., 1983). The cause of Pick's disease is unknown and no treatment currently exists.

Neuropsychologically, Pick's disease can sometimes be difficult, if not impossible, to distinguish from AD. However, in many cases, multiple clinical features can make such a differentiation possible. First, language changes are usually an early feature of Pick's disease, and occur in a severity out of all proportion to losses observed in other cognitive abilities (Cummings & Duchen, 1981; Wechsler et al., 1982). Such changes first include word-finding difficulties, frequent paraphasias, and jargon, with a rapid disintegration to the use of single words or phrases, echolalia, mutism, and amimia. Language dysfunction, although common in AD, is not usually so disproportionately and acutely disrupted, and features such as echolalia and mutism typically occur only in the later disease stages. Memory dysfunction, an early indicator of AD, usually has a later onset in Pick's disease (Gustafson & Nilsson, 1982). A similar pattern of dissociation holds true for visuospatial and constructional dysfunction (Cummings & Duchen, 1981; Wechsler et al., 1982). Personality changes, including a frank Kluver-Bucy syndrome, usually occur much earlier and with greater severity in Pick's disease (Alexander & Geschwind, 1984; Cummings & Duchen, 1981). Finally, CT scanning may reveal the relatively restricted temporal and/or frontal cortical atrophy associated with Pick's disease, in contrast to the normal or diffusely atrophic changes observed in AD (Wechsler et al., 1982).

Pseudodementia

Pseudodementia is a nosological entity currently unbounded by clearly defined clinical diagnostic criteria. In general terms, pseudodementia is usually defined as: (a) an impairment of intellectual and other cognitive functioning in a patient with a primary psychiatric disorder, (b) in the absence of a primary neuropathological process responsible for the production of the cognitive decline, (c) with the neuropsychological impairment resembling, at least in part, the presentation of the cognitive decline in dementias with primary neuropathological bases, and (d) with the cognitive impairment being potentially reversible given accurate diagnosis of the psychiatric disorder and subsequent appropriate treatment (Caine, 1981). The logical and conceptual difficulties of defining pseudodementia as lacking in a primary underlying neuropathological process are self-evident; however, the point of this statement—that the neuropsychological decline in pseudodementia is secondary to a functional psychiatric illness rather than an identifiable neurological disorder—is well taken. Functional psychiatric illnesses, and the pseudodementias that arise from them, are potentially treatable; many of the "true" dementias are not. Hence accurate differential diagnosis between these two is of paramount importance.

The types of psychiatric disorders that can produce a pseudodementia are numerous, the most commonly cited are major depression, conversion and hysterical reactions, bipolar affective disorders, and various psychiatric disorders (Caine, 1981; McAllister, 1983; Wells, 1979). Although pseudodementia can occur at any point in the adult life span, onset is most often in the mid-50s and beyond (Folstein & McHugh, 1978; McAllister, 1983). Why the cognitive dysfunction should be experienced almost exclusively by these older patients is unclear. However, the combined deleterious effects of a functional disturbance of the biogenic amine pathways interacting with the well-documented age-related loss of neurons in these pathways is often cited as a plausible mechanism for this phenomenon (e.g., Folstein & McHugh, 1978).

As implied in the definition above, pseudodementia can be virtually indistinguishable from dementia in terms of its neuropsychological presentation. However, certain features of the clinical course and history, the patient's test-taking behavior, and qualitative aspects of the patient's neuropsychological performance can help in distinguishing between the two. Pseudodementia is typically associated with rapid onset and progression of the cognitive decline, short duration of symptoms before professional help is sought, history of previous psychiatric dysfunction, pervasive affective change in the patient, the complaining of cognitive loss (typically in some detail and with a marked sense of distress) by the patient, the patient's emphasis on his or her disability and highlighting of this performance failure, poor effort or low motivation on the part of the patient vis-à-vis the neuropsychological tasks required, "don't know" responses (rather than "near miss" answers), equally severe loss of recent and remote memory recall, and marked variability in the performance of tasks of similar difficulty (McAllister, 1983; Wells, 1979). Obviously, the presence of any one of these differentiating points cannot be considered diagnostically conclusive; rather, it is the general pattern of the clinical history and presentation that is of diagnostic utility (Wells, 1979).

References

Adams, R.D. (1980). Altered cerebrospinal fluid dynamics in relation to dementia and aging. In L. Amaducci, A.N. Davison, & P. Antuono (Eds.), *Aging of the brain and dementia* (pp. 217–225). New York: Raven Press.

Adams, R.D., Fisher, C.M., Hakim, S., Ojemann, R.G., & Sweet, W.H. (1965). Symptomatic occult hydrocephalus with "normal" cerebrospinal fluid pressure. *New England Journal of Medicine, 273*, 117–126.

Albert, M.L. (1978). Subcortical dementia. In R. Katzman, R.D. Terry, & K.L. Bick (Eds.), *Aging: Vol. 7. Alzheimer's disease: Senile dementia and related disorders* (pp. 173–180). New York: Raven Press.

Albert, M.L. (1980). Language in normal and dementing elder. In L.K. Obler & M.L. Albert (Eds.), *Language and communication in the elderly* (pp. 145–150). Lexington, MA: Lexington Books.

Albert, M.L. (1981). Changes in language with aging. *Seminars in Neurology, 1*, 43–46.

Albert, M.L., Feldman, R.G., & Willis, A. (1974). The "subcortical dementia" of progressive supranuclear palsy. *Journal of Neurology, Neurosurgery, and Psychiatry, 37*, 121–130.

Albert, M.S., Butters, N., & Brandt, J. (1981a). Patterns of remote memory in amnesic and demented patients. *Archives of Neurology, 38*, 495–500.

Albert, M.S., Butters, N., & Brandt, J. (1981b). Development of remote memory loss in patients with Huntington's disease. *Journal of Clinical Neuropsychology, 3*, 1–12.

Albert, M.S., Naeser, M.A., Levine, H.L., & Garvey, A.J. (1984a). Ventricular size in patients with presenile dementia of the Alzheimer's type. *Archives of Neurology, 41*, 1258–1263.

Albert, M.S., Naeser, M.A., Levine, H.L., & Garvey, A.J. (1984b). CT density numbers in patients with senile dementia of the Alzheimer's type. *Archives of Neurology, 41*, 1264–1269.

Alexander, M.P., & Geschwind, N. (1984). Dementia in the elderly. In M.L. Albert (Ed.), *Clinical neurology of aging* (pp. 254–276). New York: Oxford University Press.

Alvord, E.C., Forno, L.S., Kusske, J.A., Kauffman, R.J., Rhodes, J.S., & Goetowski, C.R. (1974). The pathology of Parkinsonism: A comparison of degenerations in cerebral cortex and brainstem. In F.H. McDowell & A. Barbeau (Eds.), *Advances in Neurology* (Vol. 5, pp. 175–193). New York: Raven Press.

Appel, S.H. (1981). A unifying hypothesis for the cause of amyotrophic lateral sclerosis, Parkinsonism, and Alzheimer's disease. *Annals of Neurology, 10*, 499–505.

Appell, J., Kertesz, A., & Fisman, M. (1982). A study of language functioning in Alzheimer patients. *Brain and Language, 17*, 73–91.

Arai, H., Moroji, T., & Kosaka, K. (1984). Somatostatin and vasoactive intestinal polypeptide in postmortem brains from patients with Alzheimer-type dementia. *Neuroscience Letters, 52*, 73–78.

Arenberg, D. (1978). Differences and changes with age in the Benton Visual Retention Test. *Journal of Gerontology, 33*, 534–540.

Arenberg, D. (1982). Estimates of age changes on the Benton Visual Retention Test. *Journal of Gerontology, 37*, 87–90.

Armstrong, D.M., LeRoy, S., Shields, D., & Terry, R.D. (1985). Somatostatin-like immunoreactivity within neuritic plaques. *Brain Research, 338*, 71–79.

Attig, M., & Hasher, L. (1980). The processing of frequency of occurrence information by adults. *Journal of Gerontology, 35*, 66–69.

Bahrick, H.P., Bahrick, P.O., & Wittlinger, R.P. (1975). Fifty years of memory for names and faces: A cross-sectional approach. *Journal of Experimental Psychology, 104*, 54–75.

Bak, J.S., & Greene, R.L. (1980). Changes in neuropsychological functioning in an aging population. *Journal of Consulting and Clinical Psychology, 48*, 395–399.

Bak, J.S., & Greene, R.L. (1981). A review of the performance of aged adults on various Wechsler Memory Scale subtests. *Journal of Clinical Psychology, 37*, 186–188.

Baltes, P.B., & Willis, S.L. (1982). Plasticity and enhancement of intellectual functioning in old age. In F.I.M. Craik & S. Trehub (Eds.), *Advances in the study of communication and affect: Vol. 8. Aging and cognitive processes* (pp. 353–389). New York: Plenum Press.

Bank, L.I., & Jarvik, L.F. (1978). A longitudinal study of aging human twins. In E.L. Schneider (Ed.), *The genetics of aging* (pp. 303–333). New York: Plenum Press.

Bartus, R.T., Dean, R.L., Beer, B., & Lippa, A.S. (1982). The cholinergic hypothesis of geriatric memory dysfunction. *Science, 217*, 408–417.

Bayles, K.A. (1984). Language and dementia. In A. Holland (Ed.), *Language disorders in adults* (pp. 209–244). San Diego: College-Hill Press.

Bayles, K.A., Tomoeda, C.K., & Boone, D.R. (1985). A view of age-related changes in language function. *Developmental Neuropsychology, 1*, 231–264.

Beal, M.F., & Martin, J.B. (1986). Neuropeptides in neurological disease. *Annals of Neurology, 20*, 547–565.

Beal, M.F., Mazurek, M.F., Svendsen, C.N., Bird, E.D., & Martin, J.B. (1986). Widespread reduction of somatostatin-like immunoreactivity in the cerebral cortex in Alzheimer's disease. *Annals of Neurology, 20*, 489–495.

Becker, H., Grau, H., Schneider, E., Fischer, P.A., & Hacker, H. (1976). CT examination series of Parkinson patients. In W. Lauksch & E. Kazner (Eds.), *Cranial computerized tomography* (pp. 249–251). New York: Springer-Verlag.

Becker, J.T., Boller, F., Saxton, J., & McGonigle-Gibson, K.L. (1987). Normal rates of forgetting of verbal and non-verbal material in Alzheimer's disease. *Cortex, 23*, 59–72.

Bell, B., Wolf, E., & Bernholz, C.D. (1972). Depth perception as a function of age. *Aging and Human Development, 3*, 77–83.

Benson, D.F. (1983). Alterations in glucose metabolism in Alzheimer's disease. In R. Katzman (Ed.), *Banbury Report 15: Biological aspects of Alzheimer's disease* (pp. 309–314). Cold Spring Harbor, NY: Cold Spring Harbor Laboratory.

Benson, D.F., Kuhl, D.E., Hawkins, R.A., Phelps, M.E., Cummings, J.E., & Tsai, S.Y. (1983). The fluordeoxyglucose ^{18}F scan in Alzheimer's disease and multi-infarct dementia. *Archives of Neurology, 40*, 711–714.

Benton, A.L., Eslinger, P.J., & Damasio, A.R. (1981). Normative observations on neuropsychological test performances in old age. *Journal of Clinical Neuropsychology, 3*, 33–42.

Benton, A.L., Hamsher, K., Varney, N.R., & Spreen, O. (1983). *Contributions to neuropsychological assessment*. New York: Oxford University Press.

Bird, J.M., Levy, R., & Jacoby, R.J. (1986). Computed tomography in the elderly: Changes over time in a normal population. *British Journal of Psychiatry, 148*, 80–85.

Blessed, G., Tomlinson, B.E., & Roth, M. (1968). The association between quantitative measures of dementia and of senile change in the cerebral grey matter of elderly subjects. *British Journal of Psychiatry, 114*, 797–811.

Boller, F. (1980). Mental status of patients with Parkinson disease. *Journal of Clinical Neuropsychology, 2*, 157–172.

Boller, F., Mizutani, T., Roessmann, U., & Gambetti, P. (1980). Parkinson disease, dementia, and Alzheimer disease: Clinicopathological correlations. *Annals of Neurology, 7*, 329-335.

Boller, F., Passafiume, D., Keefe, N.C., Rogers, K., Morrow, L., & Kim, Y. (1984). Visuospatial impairment in Parkinson's disease: Role of perceptual and motor factors. *Archives of Neurology, 41*, 485-490.

Botez, M.I., Ethier, R., L'eveille, J., & Botez-Maquard, T. (1977). A syndrome of early recognition of occult hydrocephalus and cerebral atrophy. *Quarterly Journal of Medicine, 46*, 365-380.

Botwinick, J. (1977). Intellectual abilities. In J.E. Birren & K.W. Schaie (Eds.), *Handbook of the psychology of aging* (pp. 508-605). New York: Van Nostrand Reinhold.

Botwinick, J. (1984). *Aging and behavior: A comprehensive integration of research findings* (3rd ed.). New York: Springer.

Botwinick, J., & Storandt, M. (1974). *Memory related functions and age*. Springfield, IL: Thomas.

Botwinick, J., and Storandt, M. (1980). Recall and recognition of old information in relation to age and sex. *Journal of Gerontology, 35*, 70-76.

Botwinick, J., Storandt, M., & Berg, L. (1986). A longitudinal, behavioral study of senile dementia of the Alzheimer type. *Archives of Neurology, 43*, 1124-1127.

Bowen, F.P. (1976). Behavioral alterations in patients with basal ganglia lesions. In M. Yahr (Ed.), *The basal ganglia* (pp. 169-180). New York: Raven Press.

Bowen, F.P., Hoehn, M.M., & Yahr, M.O. (1972). Parkinsonism: Alterations in spatial orientation as determined by a route-walking test. *Neuropsychologia, 10*, 355-361.

Breitner, J.C.S., & Folstein, M.F. (1984). Familial nature of Alzheimer's disease. *New England Journal of Medicine, 311*, 192.

Brinkman, S.D., & Braun, P. (1984). Classification of dementia patients by a WAIS profile related to central cholinergic deficiencies. *Journal of Clinical Neuropsychology, 6*, 393-400.

Brinkman, S.D., & Largen, J.W., Jr. (1984). Changes in brain ventricular size with repeated CAT scans in suspected Alzheimer's disease. *American Journal of Psychiatry, 141*, 81-83.

Brizzee, K.R., Ordy, J.M., Knox, C., & Jirge, S.K. (1980). Morphology and aging in the brain. In G.J. Maletta & F.J. Pirozzolo (Eds.), *The aging nervous system* (pp. 10-39). New York: Praeger.

Brookshire, R.H., & Manthie, M.A. (1980). Speech and language disturbances in the elderly. In G.J. Maletta & F.J. Pirozzolo (Eds.), *The aging nervous system* (pp. 241-263). New York: Praeger.

Brouwers, P., Cox, C., Martin, A., Chase, T., & Fedio, P. (1984). Differential perceptual-impairment in Huntington's and Alzheimer's dementias. *Archives of Neurology, 41*, 1073-1076.

Brun, A., & Englund, E. (1986). A white matter disorder in dementia of the Alzheimer type: A pathoanatomic study. *Annals of Neurology, 19*, 253-262.

Burke, D.M., & Light, L.L. (1981). Memory and aging: The role of retrieval processes. *Psychological Bulletin, 90*, 513-546.

Buschke, H. (1974). Two stages of learning by children and adults. *Bulletin of the Psychonomic Society, 2*, 392-394.

Butters, N. (1984). The clinical aspects of memory disorders: Contributions from experimental studies of amnesia and dementia. *Journal of Clinical Neuropsychology, 6*, 17-36.

Butters, N., Sax, D., Montgomery, K., & Tarlow, S. (1978). Comparison of the neuropsychological deficits associated with early and advanced Huntington's disease. *Archives of Neurology, 35*, 585–589.

Butters, N., Tarlow, S., Cermak, L.S., & Sax, D. (1976). A comparison of the information processing deficits of patients with Huntington's chorea and Korsakoff's syndrome. *Cortex, 12*, 134–144.

Butters, N., Wolfe, J., Granholm, E., & Martone, M. (1986). An assessment of verbal recall, recognition and fluency abilities in patients with Huntington's disease. *Cortex, 22*, 11–32.

Caine, E.D. (1981). Pseudodementia: Current concepts and future directions. *Archives of General Psychiatry, 38*, 1359–1364.

Caine, E.D., Bamford, K.A., Schiffer, R.B., Shoulson, I., & Levy, S. (1986). A controlled neuropsychological comparison of Huntington's disease and multiple sclerosis. *Archives of Neurology, 43*, 249–254.

Caine, E.D., Hunt, R.D., Weingartner, H., & Ebert, M.H. (1978). Huntington's dementia: Clinical and neuropsychological features. *Archives of General Psychiatry, 35*, 377–384.

Cameron, P. (1975). Mood as an indicant of happiness: Age, sex, social class, and situational differences. *Journal of Gerontology, 30*, 216–224.

Cauthen, N.R. (1977). Extension of the Wechsler Memory Scale norms to older age groups. *Journal of Clinical Psychology, 33*, 208–211.

Cerella, J. (1985). Information processing rates in the elderly. *Psychological Bulletin, 98*, 67–83.

Cerella, J., Poon, L.W., & Fozard, J.L. (1981). Mental rotation and age reconsidered. *Journal of Gerontology, 36*, 620–624.

Chamberlain, W. (1970). Restriction in upward gaze with advancing age. *Transactions of the American Ophthalmological Society, 68*, 234–244.

Clark, W.C., & Mehl, L. (1971). Thermal pain: A sensory decision theory analysis of the effect of age and sex on d', various response criteria, and 50 percent pain threshold. *Journal of Abnormal Psychology, 78*, 202–212.

Cohen, G., & Faulkner, D. (1983). Age differences in performance on two information-processing tasks: Strategy selection and processing efficiency. *Journal of Gerontology, 38*, 447–454.

Cohen, M.M., & Lessell, S. (1984). Neuro-ophthalmology of aging. In M.L. Albert (Ed.), *Clinical neurology of aging* (pp. 313–344). New York: Oxford University Press.

Collignon, R., Rectem, D., Laterre, E.C., & Stroobandt, G. (1975). Aspect neuropsychologique de l'hydrocephalie normopressive. *Acta Neurologica Belgica, 76*, 74–82.

Cools, A.R., van den Bercken, J.H.L., Horstink, M.W.I., van Spaendonck, K.P.M., & Berger, H.J.C. (1984). Cognitive and motor shifting aptitude disorder in Parkinson's disease. *Journal of Neurology, Neurosurgery, and Psychiatry, 47*, 443–453.

Corso, J.F. (1963). Age and sex differences in pure-tone thresholds. *Archives of Otolaryngology, 77*, 385–405.

Corso, J.F. (1977). Auditory perception and communication. In J.E. Birren & K.W. Schaie (Eds.), *Handbook of the psychology of aging* (pp. 535–553). New York: Van Nostrand Reinhold.

Corso, J.F. (1981). *Aging sensory systems and perception* (p. 218). New York: Praeger.

Cote, L.J., & Kremzner, L.T. (1983). Biochemical changes in normal aging in human brain. In R. Mayeux & W.G. Rosen (Eds.), *The dementias* (pp. 19–30). New York: Raven Press.

Cowart, B.J. (1981). Development of taste perception in humans: Sensitivity and preference throughout the life span. *Psychological Bulletin, 90*, 43–73.
Coyle, J.T., Price, D.L., & DeLong, M.R. (1983). Alzheimer's disease: A disorder of cortical cholinergic innervation. *Science, 219*, 1184–1190.
Craik, F.I.M. (1977). Age differences in human memory. In J.E. Birren & K.W. Schaie (Eds.), *Handbook of the psychology of aging* (pp. 384–420). New York: Van Nostrand Reinhold.
Craik, F.I.M. (1984). Age differences in remembering. In. L.R. Squire & N. Butters (Eds.), *Neuropsychology of memory* (pp. 3–12). New York: Guilford Press.
Craik, F.I.M., & Byrd, M. (1982). Aging and cognitive deficits: The role of attentional resources. In F.I.M. Craik & S. Trehub (Eds.), *Advances in the study of communication and affect: Vol. 8. Aging and cognitive processes* (pp. 191–211). New York: Plenum Press.
Craik, F.I.M., & Lockhart, R.S. (1972). Levels of processing: A framework for memory research. *Journal of Verbal Learning and Verbal Behavior, 11*, 671–684.
Craik, F.I.M., & Rabinowitz, J.C. (1984). Age differences in the acquisition and use of verbal information. In H. Bouma & D.G. Bouwhuis (Eds.), *Attention and performance X* (pp. 471–499). Hillsdale, NJ: Erlbaum.
Craik, F.I.M., & Trehub, S. (Eds.). (1982). *Advances in the study of communication and affect: Vol. 8. Aging and cognitive processes*. New York: Plenum Press.
Crapper, D.R., Krishman, S.S., & Quittkat, S. (1976). Aluminum neurofibrillary degeneration and Alzheimer's disease. *Brain, 99*, 67–80.
Crapper-McLachlan, D.R., & De Boni, U. (1980). Etiologic factors in senile dementia of the Alzheimer type. In L. Amaducci, A.N. Davison, & P. Antuono (Eds.), *Aging of the brain and dementia* (pp. 173–181). New York: Raven Press.
Crystal, H.A., & Davies, P. (1982). Cortical substance P like-immunoreactivity in cases of Alzheimer's disease and senile dementia of the Alzheimer's type. *Journal of Neurochemistry, 38*, 1781–1784.
Cummings, J.L. (1983). Treatable dementias. In R. Mayeux & W.G. Rosen (Eds.), *The dementias* (pp. 165–183). New York: Raven Press.
Cummings, J.L., & Benson, D.F. (1983). *Dementia: A clinical approach*. Boston: Butterworth.
Cummings, J.L., Benson, D.F., Hill, M.A., & Read, S. (1985). Aphasia in dementia of the Alzheimer type. *Neurology, 35*, 394–397.
Cummings, J.L., & Duchen, L.W. (1981). Kluver-Bucy syndrome in Pick disease: Clinical and pathologic correlations. *Neurology, 31*, 1415–1422.
Curcio, C.A., Buell, S.J., & Coleman, P.D. (1982). Morphology of the aging central nervous system: Not all downhill. In J.A. Mortimer, F.J. Pirozzolo, & G.J. Maletta (Eds.), *The aging motor system* (pp. 7–35). New York: Praeger.
Danta, G., & Hilton, R.C. (1975). Judgment of the visual vertical and horizontal in patients with Parkinsonism. *Neurology, 25*, 43–47.
Davies, A.D. (1967). Age and the Memory-for-Designs test. *British Journal of Social and Clinical Pathology, 6*, 228–233.
Davies, P., & Terry, R.D. (1981). Cortical somatostatin-like immunoreactivity in cases of Alzheimer's disease and senile dementia of the Alzheimer-type. *Neurobiology of Aging, 2*, 9–14.
Delabar, J-M., Goldgaber, D., Lamour, Y., Nicole, A., Huret, J-L., de Grouchy, J., Brown, P., Gajdusek, D.C., & Sinet, P-M. (1987). Beta-amyloid gene duplication in Alzheimer's disease and karyotypically normal Down syndrome. *Science, 235*, 1390–1392.

DeLancy-Horne, D.J. (1971). Performance on delayed response tasks by patients with Parkinsonism. *Journal of Neurology, Neurosurgery, and Psychiatry, 34*, 192–194.

de Leon, M.J., Ferris, S.H., George, A.E., Reisberg, B., Christman, D.R., Kricheff, I.I., & Wolf, A.P. (1983). Computed tomography and positron emission transaxial tomography evaluations of normal aging and Alzheimer's disease. *Journal of Cerebral Blood Flow and Metabolism, 3*, 391–394.

Dixon, R.A., Simon, E.W., Nowak, C.A., & Hultsch, D.F. (1982). Text recall in adulthood as a function of level of information, input modality, and delay interval. *Journal of Gerontology, 37*, 358-364.

Doty, R.L., Shaman, P., Appelbaum, S.L., Giberson, R., Siksorski, L., & Rosenberg, L. (1984). Smell identification ability: Changes with age. *Science, 226*, 1441–1443.

Drachman, D.A. (1983). In R. Katzman (Ed.), *Banbury Report 15: Biological aspects of Alzheimer's disease* (p. 15). Cold Spring Harbor, NY: Cold Spring Harbor Laboratory.

Drachman, D.A., & Leavitt, J. (1972). Memory impairment in the aged: Storage versus retrieval deficit. *Journal of Experimental Psychology, 93*, 302–308.

Drachman, D.A., & Long, R.R. (1984). Neurological evaluation of the elderly patient. In M.L. Albert (Ed.), *Clinical neurology of aging* (pp. 97–113). New York: Oxford University Press.

Earnest, M.P., Heaton, R.K., Wilkinson, W.E., & Manke, W.F. (1979). Cortical atrophy, ventricular enlargement and intellectual impairment in the aged. *Neurology, 29*, 1138–1143.

El-Awar, M., Becker, J.T., Hammond, K.M., Nebes, R.D., & Boller, F. (1987). Learning deficit in Parkinson's disease: Comparison with Alzheimer's disease and normal aging. *Archives of Neurology, 44*, 180–184.

Epstein, C.J. (1983). Down's syndrome and Alzheimer's disease: Implications and approaches. In R. Katzman (Ed.), *Banbury Report 15: Biological aspects of Alzheimer's disease* (pp. 169–182). Cold Spring Harbor, NY: Cold Spring Harbor Laboratory.

Erber, J.T. (1984). Age differences in the effect of encoding congruence on incidental free and cued recall. *Experimental Aging Research, 10*, 221–223.

Erber, J.T., Botwinick, J., & Storandt, M. (1981). The impact of memory on age differences in digit symbol performance. *Journal of Gerontology, 36*, 586–590.

Eslinger, P.J., & Benton, A.L. (1983). Visuoperceptual performances in aging and dementia: Clinical and theoretical implications. *Journal of Clinical Neuropsychology, 5*, 213–220.

Farver, P.F., & Farver, T.B. (1982). Performance of normal older adults on tests designed to measure parietal lobe functions. *American Journal of Occupational Therapy, 36*, 444–449.

Feher, E., Swihart, A.A., & Largen, J.W. (1987). WAIS subtest scores: A typical pattern in Alzheimer's disease? *Clinical Neuropsychologist, 1*, 96.

Feier, C.D., & Gertsman, L.J. (1980). Sentence comprehension abilities throughout the life span. *Journal of Gerontology, 35*, 722–728.

Ferrier, I.N., Cross, A.J., Johnson, J.A., Roberts, G.W., Crow, T.J., Corsellis, J.A.N., Lee, Y.C., O'Shaughnessy, D., Adrian, T.E., McGregor, G.P., Baracese-Hamilton, A.J., & Bloom, S.R. (1983). Neuropeptides in Alzheimer type dementia. *Journal of the Neurological Sciences, 62*, 159–170.

Ferris, S.H., Crook, T., Clark, E., McCarthy, M., & Rae, D. (1981). Facial recognition memory deficits in normal aging and senile dementia. *Journal of Gerontology, 35*, 707–714.

Finch, C.E. (1980). The relationships of aging changes in the basal ganglia to manifestations of Huntington's chorea. *Annals of Neurology, 7*, 406–411.

Flowers, K.A., Pearce, I., & Pearce, J.M.S. (1984). Recognition memory in Parkinson's disease. *Journal of Neurology, Neurosurgery, and Psychiatry, 47*, 1174–1181.
Folstein, M.F., & McHugh, P.R. (1978). Dementia syndrome of depression. In R. Katzman, R.D. Terry, & K.L. Bick (Eds.), *Alzheimer's disease: Senile dementia and related disorders* (pp. 87–96). New York: Raven Press.
Foster, N.L., Chase, T.N., Fedio, P., Patronas, N.J., Brooks, R.A., & Di Chiro, G. (1983). Alzheimer's disease: Focal cortical changes shown by positron emission tomography. *Neurology, 33*, 961–965.
Fozard, J.L., Wolf, E., Bell, B., McFarland, R.A., & Podolsky, S. (1977). Visual perception and communication. In J.E. Birren & K.W. Schaie (Eds.), *Handbook of the psychology of aging* (pp. 497–534). New York: Van Nostrand Reinhold.
Francis, P.T., Palmer, A.M., Sims, N.R., Bowen, D.M., Davison, A.N., Esiri, M.M., Neary, D., Snowden, J.S., & Wilcock, G.K. (1985). Neurochemical studies of early-onset Alzheimer's disease: Possible influence on treatment. *New England Journal of Medicine, 313*, 7–11.
Freedman, M., Knoefel, J., Naeser, M., & Levine, H. (1984). Computerized axial tomography in aging. In M. Albert (Ed.), *Clinical neurology of aging* (pp. 139–148). New York: Oxford University Press.
Fuld, P.A. (1982). Behavioral signs of cholinergic deficiency in Alzheimer's dementia. In S. Corkin, K.L. Davis, J.H. Growden, E. Usdin, & R.J. Wurtman (Eds.), *Alzheimer's disease: A report of progress* (pp. 193–196). New York: Raven Press.
Fuld, P.A. (1984). Test profile of cholinergic dysfunction and of Alzheimer-type dementia. *Journal of Clinical Neuropsychology, 6*, 380–392.
Gajdusek, D.C. (1986). Chronic dementia caused by small unconventional viruses apparently containing no nucleic acid. In A.B. Scheibel & A.F. Wechsler (Eds.), *The biological substrates of Alzheimer's disease* (pp. 33–54). Orlando, FL: Academic Press.
Garron, D.C., Klawans, H.L., & Narin, F. (1972). Intellectual functioning of persons with idiopathic Parkinsonism. *Journal of Nervous and Mental Disease, 154*, 445–452.
George, A.E., de Leon, M.J., Gentes, C.I., Miller, J., London, E., Budzilovich, G.N., Ferris, S., & Chase, N. (1986). Leukoencephalopathy in normal and pathologic aging: 1. CT of brain lucencies. *American Journal of Neuroradiology, 7*, 561–566.
George, A.E., de Leon, M.J., Kalnin, A., Rosner, L., Goodgold, A., & Chase, N. (1986). Leukoencephalopathy in normal and pathologic aging: 2. MRI of brain lucencies. *American Journal of Neuroradiology, 7*, 567–570.
Gilroy, J., & Meyer, J.S. (1979). *Medical neurology* (3rd ed.) New York: Macmillan.
Glenner, G.G. (1983). Alzheimer's disease: Multiple cerebral amyloidosis. In R. Katzman (Ed.), *Banbury Report 15: Biological aspects of Alzheimer's disease* (pp. 137–143). Cold Spring Harbor, NY: Cold Spring Harbor Laboratory.
Glorig, A. (1977). Auditory processing and age. In H. Shove & M. Ernst (Eds.), *Sensory processes and aging* (pp. 39–60). Denton, TX: University Center for Community Services.
Goldgaber, D., Lerman, M.I., McBride, O.W., Saffiotti, U., & Gajdusek, D.C. (1987). Characterization and chromosomal localization of a cDNA encoding brain amyloid of Alzheimer's disease. *Science, 235*, 877–880.
Goodglass, H. (1980). Naming disorders in aphasia and aging. In L.K. Obler & M.L. Albert (Eds.), *Language and communication in the elderly* (pp. 37–45). Lexington, MA: Lexington Books.
Goodin, D.S., Squires, K.C., & Starr, A. (1978). Long-latency event related components of the auditory evoked potential in dementia. *Brain, 191*, 635–648.

Goudsmit, J., Morrow, C.H., Asher, D.M., Yanagihara, R.T., Masters, C.L., Gibbs, C.J., & Gajdusek, D.C. (1980). Evidence for and against the transmissability of Alzheimer's disease. *Neurology, 30*, 945–950.

Granick, S., Kleban, M.H., & Weiss, A.D. (1976). Relationships between hearing loss and cognition in normally hearing aged persons. *Journal of Gerontology, 31*, 434–440.

Graveland, G.A., Williams, R.S., & DiFiglia, M. (1985). Evidence for degenerative and regenerative changes in neostriatal spiny neurons in Huntington's disease. *Science, 227*, 770–773.

Greenamyre, J.T., Penny, J.B., Young, A.B., D'Amato, C.J., Hicks, S.P., & Shoulson, I. (1985). Alterations in L-Glutamate binding in Alzheimer's and Huntington's diseases. *Science, 227*, 1496–1499.

Gurland, B.J., & Toner, J.A. (1982). Depression in the elderly: A review of recently published studies. *Annual Review of Gerontology and Geriatrics, 3*, 228–265.

Gustafson, L., & Hagberg, B. (1978). Recovery in hydrocephalic dementia after shunt operation. *Journal of Neurology, Neurosurgery, and Psychiatry, 41*, 940–947.

Gustafson, L., & Nilsson, L. (1982). Differential diagnosis of presenile dementia on clinical grounds. *Acta Psychiatricia Scandinavica, 65*, 195–209.

Haaland, K.Y., Linn, R.T., Hunt, W.C., & Goodwin, J.S. (1983). A normative study of Russell's variant of the Wechsler Memory Scale in a healthy elderly population. *Journal of Consulting and Clinical Psychology, 51*, 878–881.

Hachinski, V.C., Iliff, L.D., Zilhka, E., Du Boulay, G.H., McAllister, V.L., Marshall, J., Ross-Russell, R.W., & Symon, L. (1975). Cerebral blood flow in dementia. *Archives of Neurology, 32*, 632–637.

Hakim, A.M., & Mathieson, G. (1979). Dementia in Parkinson disease: A neuropathologic study. *Neurology, 29*, 1209–1214.

Hansch, E.C., Syndulko, K., Pirozzolo, F.J., Cohen, S.N., Tourtellotte, W.W., & Potvin, A.R. (1980). Electrophysiological measurement in aging and dementia. In G.J. Maletta & F.J. Pirozzolo (Eds.), *The aging nervous system* (pp. 187–210). New York: Praeger.

Harkins, S.W., & Chapman, R.C. (1976). Detection and decision factors in pain perception in young and elderly man. *Pain, 2*, 253–264.

Harkins, S.W., & Chapman, R.C. (1977). The perception of induced dental pain in young and elderly women. *Journal of Gerontology, 32*, 428–435.

Harrington, D.O. (1976). *The visual fields: A textbook and atlas of clinical perimetry* (p. 102). St. Louis: Mosby.

Hart, R.P., Kwentus, J.A., Taylor, J.R., & Harkins, S.W. (1987). Rate of forgetting in dementia and depression. *Journal of Consulting and Clinical Psychology, 55*, 101–105.

Hartmann, A., & Alberti, E. (1977). Differentiation of communicating hydrocephalus and presenile dementia by continuous recording of cerebrospinal fluid pressure. *Journal of Neurology, Neurosurgery, and Psychiatry, 40*, 630–640.

Hasher, L., & Zacks, R.T. (1979). Automatic and effortful processes in memory. *Journal of Experimental Psychology: General, 108*, 356–388.

Hayes, D., & Jerger, J. (1984). Neurology of aging: The auditory system. In M.L. Albert (Ed.), *Clinical neurology of aging* (pp. 362–378). New York: Oxford University Press.

Heilig, C.W., Knopman, D.S., Mastri, A.R., & Frey, W. (1985). Dementia without Alzheimer pathology. *Neurology, 35*, 762–765.

Herman, G.E., Warren, L.R., & Wagener, J.W. (1977). Auditory lateralization: Age differences in sensitivity to dichotic time and amplitude cues. *Journal of Gerontology, 32*, 187–191.

Heston, L.L. (1980). Dementia associated with Parkinson's disease: A genetic study. *Journal of Neurology, Neurosurgery, and Psychiatry, 43,* 846–848.

Heston, L.L. (1983). Dementia of the Alzheimer's type: A perspective from family studies. In R. Katzman (Ed.), *Banbury Report 15: Biological aspects of Alzheimer's disease* (pp. 183–191). Cold Spring Harbor, NY: Cold Spring Harbor Laboratory.

Heston, L.L., Mastri, A.R., Anderson, E., & White, J. (1981). Dementia of the Alzheimer's type: Clinical genetics, natural history, and associated conditions. *Archives of General Psychiatry, 38,* 1085–1090.

Hochanadel, G., & Kaplan, E. (1984). Neuropsychology of normal aging. In M. Albert (Ed.), *Clinical neurology of aging* (pp. 231–244). New York: Oxford University Press.

Hollander, E., Mohs, R.C., & Davis, K.L. (1986). Antemortem markers of Alzheimer's disease. *Neurobiology of Aging, 7,* 367–387.

Horn, J.L. (1982). The theory of fluid and crystallized intelligence in relation to concepts of cognitive psychology of aging in adulthood. In F.I.M. Craik & S. Trehub (Eds.), *Advances in the study of communication and affect: Vol. 8. Aging and cognitive processes* (pp. 237–278). New York: Plenum Press.

Horn, J.L., & Cattell, R.B. (1967). Age differences in fluid and crystallized intelligence. *Acta Psychologica, 26,* 107–129.

Horn, J.L., Donaldson, G., & Engstrom, R. (1981). Apprehension, memory, and fluid intelligence decline through the "vital years" of adulthood. *Research on Aging, 3,* 33–84.

Hovestadt, A., de Jong, G.J., & Meerwaldt, J.D. (1987). Spatial disorientation as an early symptom of Parkinson's disease. *Neurology, 37,* 485–487.

Howard, D.V., Lasaga, M.I., & McAndrews, M.P. (1980). Semantic activation during memory encoding across the adult life span. *Journal of Gerontology, 35,* 884–890.

Huber, S.J., Shuttleworth, E.C., & Paulson, G.W. (1986). Dementia in Parkinson's disease. *Archives of Neurology, 43,* 967–990.

Hughes, C.P., Siegel, B.A., Coxe, W.S., Gado, M.H., Grubb, R.L., Coleman, R.E., & Berg, L. (1978). Adult idiopathic communicating hydrocephalus with and without shunting. *Journal of Neurology, Neurosurgery, and Psychiatry, 41,* 961–971.

Hutman, L.P., & Sekuler, R. (1980). Spatial vision and aging: II. Criterion effects. *Journal of Gerontology, 35,* 700–706.

Hynd, G.W., Pirozzolo, F.J., & Maletta, G.J. (1982). Progressive supranuclear palsy. *International Journal of Neuroscience, 16,* 87–98.

Jackson, J.A., Jankovic, J., & Ford, J. (1983). Progressive supranuclear palsy: Clinical features and response to treatment in 16 patients. *Annals of Neurology, 13,* 273–278.

Jacobs, L., Kinkel, W.R., Painter, F., Murawski, J., & Heffner, R.R. (1978). Computerized tomography in dementia with special reference to changes in size of normal ventricles during aging and normal pressure hydrocephalus. In R. Katzman, R.D. Terry, & K.L. Bick (Eds.), *Alzheimer's disease: Senile dementia and related disorders* (pp. 241–260). New York: Raven Press.

Jani, S.N. (1966). The age factor in stereopsis screening. *American Journal of Optometry, 43,* 653–655.

Jellinger, K., Riederer, P., & Tomonasa, M. (1980). Progressive supranuclear palsy: Clinico-pathological and biochemical studies. *Journal of Neural Transmission (Suppl.), 16,* 111–128.

Jerger, J., & Hayes, D. (1977). Diagnostic speech audiometry. *Archives of Otolaryngology, 103*, 216-222.

Josiassen, R.C., Curry, L.M., & Mancall, E.L. (1983). Development of neuropsychological deficits in Huntington's disease. *Archives of Neurology, 40*, 791-796.

Josiassen, R.C., Curry, L., Roemer, R.A., DeBease, C., & Mancall, E.L. (1982). Patterns of intellectual deficit in Huntington's disease. *Journal of Clinical Neuropsychology, 4*, 173-183.

Joynt, R.J., & McNeill, T.H. (1984). Neuropeptides in aging and dementia. *Peptides, 5*, 269-274.

Kaszniak, A.W., Garron, D.C., Fox, J.H., Bergen, D., & Huckman, M. (1979). Cerebral atrophy, EEG slowing, age, education, and cognitive functioning in suspected dementia. *Neurology, 29*, 1273-1279.

Katz, R.I., & Harner, R.N. (1984). Electroencephalography in aging. In M. Albert (Ed.), *Clinical neurology of aging* (pp. 114-138). New York: Oxford University Press.

Katzman, R. (1977). Normal pressure hydrocephalus. In C.E. Wells (Ed.), *Dementia* (2nd ed.) (pp. 69-92). Philadelphia: Davis.

Katzman, R. (1978). Normal pressure hydrocephalus. In R. Katzman, R.D. Terry, & K.L. Bick (Eds.), *Alzheimer's disease: Senile dementia and related disorders* (pp. 115-124). New York: Raven Press.

Katzman, R. (1986). Alzheimer's disease. *New England Journal of Medicine, 15*, 964-973.

Kaye, W.H., Sitaram, N., Weingartner, H., Egbert, M.G., Smallberg, S., & Gillin, J.C. (1982). Modest facilitation of memory in dementia with combined lecithin and anticholinesterase treatment. *Biological Psychiatry, 17*, 275-280.

Kemper, T.L. (1983). Organization of the neuropathology of the amygdala in Alzheimer's disease. In R. Katzman (Ed.), *Banbury Report 15: Biological aspects of Alzheimer's disease* (pp. 31-35). Cold Spring Harbor, NY: Cold Spring Harbor Laboratory.

Kemper, T. (1984). Neuroanatomical and neuropathological changes in normal aging and dementia. In M. Albert (Ed.), *Clinical neurology of aging* (pp. 9-52). New York: Oxford University Press.

Kendall, B.S. (1962). Memory-for-Designs performance in the seventh and eighth decades of life. *Perceptual and Motor Skills, 14*, 399-405.

Kenshalo, D.R. (1977). Age changes in touch, vibration, temperature, kinesthesis, and pain sensitivity. In J.E. Birren & K.W. Schaie (Eds.), *Handbook of the psychology of aging* (pp. 562-579). New York: Van Nostrand Reinhold.

Khachaturian, Z.S. (1985). Diagnosis of Alzheimer's disease. *Archives of Neurology, 42*, 1097-1105.

Kiloh, L.G. (1961). Pseudo-dementia. *Acta Psychiatrica Scandinavica, 37*, 336-351.

Kimura, D., Barnett, H.J.M., & Burkhart, G. (1981). The psychological test pattern in progressive supranuclear palsy. *Neuropsychologia, 19*, 301-306.

Kirshner, H.S. (1986). *Behavioral neurology: A practical approach* (pp. 161-163). New York: Churchill Livingstone.

Kirshner, H.S., Webb, W.G., Kelly, M.P., & Wells, C.E. (1984). Language disturbance: An initial symptom of cortical degeneration and dementia. *Archives of Neurology, 41*, 491-496.

Kline, D.W. (1984). Processing sense information. In J. Botwinick (Ed.), *Aging and behavior: A comprehensive integration of research findings* (3rd ed., pp. 207-228). New York: Springer.

Kopelman, M.D. (1985). Rates of forgetting in Alzheimer-type dementia and Korsakoff's syndrome. *Neuropsychologia, 23,* 623–638.
Kuhl, D.E., Metter, J., Riege, W.H., & Phelps, M.E. (1982). Effects of human aging on patterns of local cerebral glucose utilization determined by the [^{18}F]fluordeoxyglucose method. *Journal of Cerebral Blood Flow and Metabolism, 2,* 163–171.
Kushner, M., Younkin, D., Weinberger, J., Hurtig, H., Goldberg, H., & Reivich, M. (1984). Cerebral hemodynamics in the diagnosis of normal pressure hydrocephalus. *Neurology, 34,* 96–99.
LaBarge, E., Edwards, D., & Knesevich, J.W. (1986). Performance of normal elderly on the Boston Naming Test. *Brain and Language, 27,* 380–384.
Larrabee, G.J., Largen, J.W., & Levin, H.S. (1985). Sensitivity of age-decline resistant ("Hold") WAIS subtests to Alzheimer's disease. *Journal of Clinical and Experimental Neuropsychology, 7,* 497–504.
Larsson, L. (1982). Aging in mammalian skeletal muscle. In J.A. Mortimer, F.J. Pirozzolo, & G.J. Maletta (Eds.), *The aging motor system* (pp. 60–97). New York: Praeger.
Larsson, L., Grimby, G., & Karlsson, J. (1979). Muscle strength and speed of movement in relation to age and muscle morphology. *Journal of Applied Physiology, 46,* 451–456.
Lavy, S., Melamed, E., Cooper, G., Bentin, S., & Rinot, Y. (1979). Regional cerebral blood flow in patients with Parkinson's disease. *Archives in Neurology, 36,* 344–348.
Lees, A.J., & Smith, E. (1983). Cognitive deficits in the early stages of Parkinson's disease. *Brain, 106,* 257–270.
Leverenz, J., & Sumi, S.M. (1986). Parkinson's disease in patients with Alzheimer's disease. *Archives of Neurology, 43,* 662–664.
Lezak, M.D. (1983). *Neuropsychological assessment* (2nd ed.). New York: Oxford Press.
Liao, Y-C.J., Lebo, R.V., Clawson, G.A., & Smuckler, E.A. (1986). Human prion protein cDNA: Molecular cloning, chromosomal mapping, and biological implications. *Science, 233,* 364–367.
Lieberman, A., Dziatolowski, M., Kupersmith, M., Serby, M., Goodgold, A., Korein, J., & Goldstein, M. (1979). Dementia in Parkinson disease. *Annals of Neurology, 6,* 355–359.
Lyle, O.E., & Gottesman, I.I. (1977). Premorbid psychometric indicators of the gene for Huntington's disease. *Journal of Consulting and Clinical Psychology, 45,* 1011–1022.
Macht, M.L., & Buschke, H. (1983). Age differences in cognitive effort in recall. *Journal of Gerontology, 38,* 695–700.
Malatesta, C.Z., & Kalnok, M. (1984). Emotional experience in younger and older adults. *Journal of Gerontology, 39,* 301–308.
Mann, D.M.A., Yates, P.O., & Marcyniuk, B. (1984). A comparison of changes in the locus caeruleus in Alzheimer's disease. *Journal of Neurology, Neurosurgery, and Psychiatry, 47,* 201–203.
Martin, A., & Fedio, P. (1983). Word production and comprehension in Alzheimer's disease: The breakdown of semantic knowledge. *Brain and Language, 19,* 124–141.
Martin, J.B., & Gusella, J.F. (1986). Huntington's disease: Pathogenesis and management. *New England Journal of Medicine, 315,* 1267–1276.
Martin, W.E., Loewenson, R.B., Resch, J.A., & Baker, A.D. (1973). Parkinson's disease: Clinical analysis of 100 patients. *Neurology, 23,* 783–790.
Marttila, R.J., & Rinne, U.K. (1976). Dementia in Parkinsons disease. *Acta Neurologica Scandinavica, 54,* 431–441.
Matison, R., Mayeux, R., Rosen, J., & Fahn, S. (1982). "Tip-of-the-tongue" phenomenon in Parkinson disease. *Neurology, 32,* 567–570.

Mayeux, R., & Stern, Y. (1983). Intellectual dysfunction and dementia in Parkinson disease. In R. Mayeux & W.G. Rosen (Eds.), *The dementias* (pp. 211–227). New York: Raven Press.

Mayeux, R., Stern, Y., Rosen, J., & Leventhal, J. (1981). Depression, intellectual impairment, and Parkinson disease. *Neurology, 31,* 645–650.

McAllister, T.W. (1983). Overview: Pseudodementia. *American Journal of Psychiatry, 140,* 528–533.

McCarty, S.M., Siegler, I.C., & Logue, P.E. (1982). Cross-sectional and longitudinal patterns of three Wechsler Memory Scale subtests. *Journal of Gerontology, 37,* 169–175.

McCormack, P.D. (1981). Temporal coding by young and elderly adults. *Developmental Psychology, 17,* 509–515.

McCrae, R.R., Costa, P.T., & Arenberg, D. (1980). Constancy of adult personality structure in males: Longitudinal, cross-sectional, and times-of-measurement analyses. *Journal of Gerontology, 35,* 877–883.

McDuff, T., & Sumi, S.M. (1985). Subcortical degeneration in Alzheimer's disease. *Neurology, 35,* 123–126.

McKhann, G., Drachman, D., Folstein, M., Katzman, R., Price, D., & Stadlan, E.M. (1984). Clinical diagnosis of Alzheimer's disease: Report of the NINCDS-ADRDA Work Group under the auspices of the Department of Health and Human Services Task Force on Alzheimer's disease. *Neurology, 34,* 939–944.

McKinney, M., Davies, P., & Coyle, J.T. (1982). Somatostatin is not colocalized in cholinergic neurons innervating the rat cerebral cortex-hippocampal formation. *Brain Research, 243,* 169–172.

Meyer, J.S., & Shaw, T.G. (1984). Cerebral blood flow in aging. In M. Albert (Ed.), *Clinical neurology of aging* (pp. 178–196). New York: Oxford University Press.

Michalewski, H.J., Thompson, L.W., Smith, D.B.D., Patterson, J.V., Bowman, T.E., Litzelman, D., & Brent, G. (1980). Age differences in the Contingent Negative Variation (CNV): Reduced frontal activity in the elderly. *Journal of Gerontology, 35,* 542–549.

Miller, E. (1971). On the nature of the memory disorder in presenile dementia. *Neuropsychologia, 9,* 75–81.

Morris, R.G. (1986). Short-term forgetting in senile dementia of the Alzheimer's type. *Cognitive Neuropsychology, 3,* 77–97.

Morrison, J.H., Rogers, J., Scherr, S., Benoit, R., & Bloom, F.E. (1985). Somatostatin immunoreactivity in neuritic plaques of Alzheimer's patients. *Nature, 314,* 90–92.

Mortimer, J.A., Pirozzolo, F.J., Hansch, E.C., & Webster, D.D. (1982). Relationship of motor symptoms to intellectual deficits in Parkinson disease. *Neurology, 31,* 645–650.

Mortimer, J.A., Pirozzolo, F.J., & Maletta, G.J. (1982). Overview of the aging motor system. In J.A. Mortimer, F.J. Pirozzolo, & G.J. Maletta (Eds.), *The aging motor system* (pp. 1–6). New York: Praeger.

Mortimer, J.A., Schuman, L.M., & French, L.R. (1981). Epidemiology of dementing illness. In J.A. Mortimer & L.M. Schuman (Eds.), *The epidemiology of dementia* (pp. 3–23). New York: Oxford University Press.

Mortimer, J.A., & Webster, D.D. (1982). Comparison of extrapyramidal motor function in normal aging and Parkinson's disease. In J.A. Mortimer, F.J. Pirozzolo, & G.J. Maletta (Eds.), *The aging motor system* (pp. 217–241). New York: Praeger.

Moscovitch, M. (1982). A neuropsychological approach to perception and memory in normal and pathological aging. In F.I.M. Craik & S. Trehub (Eds.), *Advances in the study of communication and affect: Vol. 8. Aging and cognitive processes* (pp. 55–78). New York: Plenum Press.

Muramoto, O. (1984). Selective reminding in normal and demented aged people: Auditory verbal versus visual spatial task. *Cortex, 20,* 461–478.

Murphy, C. (1983). Age-related effects on the threshold, psychophysical function, and pleasantness of menthol. *Journal of Gerontology, 38,* 217–222.

Naritomi, H., Meyer, J.S., Sakai, F., Yamaguchi, F., & Shaw, T. (1979). Effects of advancing age on regional cerebral blood flow: Studies in normal subjects and subjects with risk factors for atherothrombotic stroke. *Archives of Neurology, 36,* 410–416.

Nebes, R.D., Boller, F., & Holland, A. (1986). Use of semantic context by patients with Alzheimer's disease. *Psychology and Aging, 1,* 261–269.

Nebes, R.D., Martin, D.C., & Horn, L.C. (1984). Sparing of semantic memory in Alzheimer's disease. *Journal of Abnormal Psychology, 93,* 321–330.

Neugarten, B.L. (1977). Personality and aging. In J.E. Birren & K.W. Schaie (Eds.), *Handbook of the psychology of aging* (pp. 626–649). New York: VanNostrand Reinhold.

Nissen, M.J., Corkin, S., Buonanno, F.S., Growdon, J.H., Wray, S.H., & Bauer, J. (1985). Spatial vision in Alzheimer's disease: General findings and a case report. *Archives of Neurology, 42,* 667–671.

Ober, B.A., Dronkers, N.F., Koss, E., Delis, D.C., & Friedland, R.P. (1986). Retrieval from semantic memory in Alzheimer-type dementia. *Journal of Clinical and Experimental Neuropsychology, 8,* 75–92.

Obler, L.K. (1980). Narrative discourse style in the elderly. In L.K. Obler & M.L. Albert (Eds.), *Language and communication in the elderly* (pp. 75–90). Lexington, MA: Lexington Books.

Obler, L.K., & Albert, M.L. (1984). Language in aging. In M.L. Albert (Ed.), *Clinical neurology of aging* (pp. 245–253). New York: Oxford University Press.

Ordy, J.M., Brizzee, K.R., & Beavers, T.L. (1980). Sensory function and short-term memory in aging. In G.J. Maletta & F.J. Pirozzolo (Eds.), *The aging nervous system* (pp. 40–78). New York: Praeger.

Parkinson, S.R., Lindholm, J.M., & Inman, V.W. (1982). An analysis of age differences in immediate recall. *Journal of Gerontology, 37,* 425–431.

Parkinson, S.R., & Perey, A. (1980). Aging, digit span, and the stimulus suffix effect. *Journal of Gerontology, 35,* 736–742.

Patterson, J.V., Michalewski, H.J., Thompson, L.W., Bowman, T.E., & Litzelman, D.K. (1981). Age and sex differences in the human auditory brainstem response. *Journal of Gerontology, 36,* 455–562.

Pearson, R.C.A., Gatter, K.C., & Powell, T.P.S. (1983). Retrograde cell degeneration in the basal nucleus in monkey and man. *Brain Research, 261,* 321–326.

Pearson, R.C.A., Sofroniew, M.V., Cuello, A.C., Powell, T.P.S., Eckstein, F., Esiri, M.M., & Wilcock, G.K. (1983). Persistence of cholinergic neurons in a brain with senile dementia of the Alzheimer's type demonstrated by immunohistochemical staining for choline acetyltransferase. *Brain Research, 289,* 375–379.

Pedley, T.A., & Miller, J.A. (1983). Clinical neurophysiology of aging and dementia. In R. Mayeux & W.G. Rosen (Eds.), *The dementias* (pp. 31–49). New York: Raven Press.

Perl, D.P. (1983). Aluminum and Alzheimer's disease: Intraneuronal x-ray spectrometry studies. In R. Katzman (Ed.), *Banbury Report 15: Biological aspects of Alzheimer's disease* (pp. 425–431). Cold Spring Harbor, NY: Cold Spring Harbor Laboratory.

Perlmutter, M., & Mitchell, D.B. (1982). The appearance and disappearance of age differences in adult memory. In F.I.M. Craik & S. Trehub (Eds.), *Advances in the study of communication and affect: Vol. 8. Aging and cognitive processes* (pp. 127–144). New York: Plenum Press.

Perry, E.K., Blessed, G., Tomlinson, B.E., Perry, R.H., Crow, T.J., Cross, A.J., Dockray, G.J., Dimaline, R., & Arregui, A. (1981). Neurochemical activities in human temporal lobe related to aging and Alzheimer-type changes. *Neurobiology of Aging, 2,* 251–256.

Perry, E.K., Curtis, M., Dick, D.J., Candy, M., Atack, J.R., Bloxham, C.A., Blessed, G., Fairbairn, A., Tomlinson, B.E., & Perry, R.H. (1985). Cholinergic correlates of cognitive impairment in Parkinson's disease: Comparisons with Alzheimer's disease. *Journal of Neurology, Neurosurgery, and Psychiatry, 48,* 413–421.

Perry, E.K., & Perry, R.H. (1985a). A review of the neuropathological and neurochemical correlates of Alzheimer's disease. *Danish Medical Bulletin, 32* (Suppl. 1), 27–34.

Perry, E.K., & Perry, R.H. (1985b). New insights into the nature of senile (Alzheimer-type) plaques. *Trends in Neuroscience, 8,* 301–303.

Perry, E.K., Tomlinson, B.E., Blessed, G., Perry, R.H., Cross, A.J., & Crow, T.J. (1981). Neuropathological and biochemical observations on the noradrenergic system in Alzheimer's disease. *Journal of the Neurological Sciences, 51,* 279–287.

Pfefferbaum, A., Ford, J., Roth, W., & Kopell, B. (1980). Age-related changes in auditory event-related potentials. *Electroencephalography and Clinical Neurophysiology, 49,* 266–276.

Pincus, J.H., & Tucker, G.J. (1985). *Behavioral neurology* (3rd ed.) (p. 242). New York: Oxford University Press.

Pirozzolo, F.J. (1982). Neuropsychological assessment of dementia. *Neurology Clinics, 4,* 12–18.

Pirozzolo, F.J., & Hansch, E.C. (1981). Oculomotor reaction time in dementia reflects degree of cerebral dysfunction. *Science, 214,* 349–351.

Pirozzolo, F.J., Hansch, E.C., Mortimer, J.A., Webster, D.D., & Kuskowski, M.A. (1982). Dementia in Parkinson disease: A neuropsychological analysis. *Brain and Cognition, 1,* 72–83.

Polich, J., & Starr, A. (1984). Evoked potentials in aging. In M. Albert (Ed.), *Clinical neurology of aging* (pp. 149–177). New York: Oxford University Press.

Poon, L.W. (1985). Differences in human memory with aging: Nature, causes, and clinical implications. In J.E. Birren & K.W. Schaie (Eds.), *The handbook of the psychology of aging* (2nd ed., pp. 427–462). New York: VanNostrand Reinhold.

Potvin, A.R., Syndulko, K., Tourtellotte, W.W., Goldberg, Z., Potvin, J.H., & Hansch, E.C. (1981). Quantitative evaluation of normal age-related changes in neurologic function. In F.J. Pirozzolo & G.J. Maletta (Eds.), *Behavioral assessment and psychopharmacology* (pp. 13–57). New York: Praeger.

Prusiner, S.B. (1984a). Some speculations about prions, amyloid, and Alzheimer's disease. *New England Journal of Medicine, 310,* 661–663.

Prusiner, S.B. (1984b). Prions. *Scientific American, 251,* 50–59.

Puglisi, J.T. (1980). Semantic encoding in older adults as evidenced by release from proactive inhibition. *Journal of Gerontology, 35,* 743–745.

Rabinowitz, J.C., & Ackerman, B.P. (1982). General encoding of episodic events by elderly adults. In F.I.M. Craik & S. Trehub (Eds.), *Advances in the study of communication and affect: Vol. 8. Aging and cognitive processes* (pp. 145–154). New York: Plenum Press.

Rae-Grant, A., Blume, W., Lau, C., Hachinski, V.C., Fisman, M., & Mersky, H. (1987). The electroencephalogram in Alzheimer-type dementia. *Archives of Neurology, 44,* 50–54.

Rafal, R.D., & Grimm, R.J. (1981). Progressive supranuclear palsy: Functional analysis of the response to methysergide and antiparkinson agents. *Neurology, 31,* 1507–1518.

Rapoport, S.E., Duara, R., London, E.D., Margolin, R.A., Schwartz, M., Cutler, N.R., Partanen, M., & Shinowara, N.L. (1983). Glucose metabolism of the aging nervous system. In D. Samuel, S. Algeri, S. Gershon, V.E. Grimm, & G. Toffano (Eds.), *Aging: Vol. 22. Aging of the brain* (pp. 111-121). New York: Raven Press.
Riege, W.H., & Inman, V. (1981). Age differences in nonverbal memory tasks. *Journal of Gerontology, 36,* 51-58.
Robakis, N.K., Wisniewski, H.M., Jenkins, E.C., Devine-Gage, E.A., Houck, G.E., Yao, X-L., Ramakrishna, N., Wolfe, G., Silverman, W.P., & Brown, W.T. (1987). Chromosome 21q 21 sublocalization of gene encoding beta-amyloid peptide in cerebral vessels and neuritic (senile) plaques of people with Alzheimer disease and Down syndrome. *Lancet, i,* 384-385.
Roberts, G.W., Crow, T.J., & Polak, J.M. (1985). Location of neuronal tangles in somatostatin neurones in Alzheimer's disease. *Nature, 314,* 92-94.
Roberts, G.W., Lofthouse, R., Brown, R., Crow, T.J., Barry, R.A., & Prusiner, S.B. (1986). Prion-protein immunoreactivity in human transmissible dementias. *New England Journal of Medicine, 315,* 1231-1233.
Rocca, W.A., Amaducci, L.A., & Schoenberg, B.S. (1986). Epidemiology of clinically diagnosed Alzheimer's disease. *Annals of Neurology, 19,* 415-524.
Ron, M.A., Toone, B.K., Garralda, M.E., & Lishman, W.A. (1979). Diagnostic accuracy in presenile dementia. *British Journal of Psychiatry, 134,* 161-168.
Rosen, W.G. (1980). Verbal fluency in aging and dementia. *Journal of Clinical Neuropsychology, 2,* 135-146.
Rosen, W.G., Terry, R.D., Fuld, P.A., Katzman, R., & Peck, A. (1980). Pathological verification of Ischemic Score in differentiation of dementia. *Annals of Neurology, 7,* 486-488.
Rosser, M.N., Emson, P.C., Mountjoy, C.Q., Roth, M., & Iverson, L.L. (1980). Reduced amounts of immunoreactive somatostatin in the temporal cortex in senile dementia of Alzheimer type. *Neuroscience Letters, 20,* 373-377.
Salthouse, T.A. (1985). Speed of behavior and its implications for cognition. In J.E. Birren & K.W. Schaie (Eds.), *The handbook of psychology of aging* (2nd ed., pp. 400-426). New York: VanNostrand Reinhold.
Sanders, R.E., Murphy, M.D., Schmitt, F.A., & Walsh, K.K. (1980). Age differences in free recall rehearsal strategies. *Journal of Gerontology, 35,* 550-558.
Sattler, J.M. (1982). Age effects on Wechsler Adult Intelligence Scale-Revised tests. *Journal of Consulting and Clinical Psychology, 50,* 785-786.
Sax, D.S., O'Donnell, B., Butters, N., Menzer, L., Montgomery, K., & Kayne, H.L. (1983). Computed tomographic, neurologic, and neuropsychological correlates of Huntington's disease. *International Journal of Neuroscience, 18,* 21-36.
Schaie, K.W. (1980). Cognitive development in aging. In L.K. Obler & M.L. Albert (Eds.), *Language and communication in the elderly* (pp. 7-25). Lexington, MA: Lexington Books.
Schaie, K.W., & Labouvie-Vief, G. (1974). Generational versus ontogenetic components of change in adult cognitive behavior: A fourteen-year cross-sequential study. *Developmental Psychology, 10,* 305-320.
Schiffman, S.S., & Covey, E. (1984). Changes in taste and smell with age: Nutritional aspects. In J.M. Ordy, D. Harmon, & R. Alfin-Slate (Eds.), *Nutrition in gerontology* (pp. 43-64). New York: Raven Press.
Schlaepfer, W.W. (1983). Neurofilaments and the abnormal filaments of Alzheimer's disease. In R. Katzman (Ed.), *Banbury Report 15: Biological aspects of Alzheimer's disease* (pp. 107-113). Cold Spring Harbor, NY: Cold Spring Harbor Laboratory.

Schlotterer, G., Moscovitch, M., & Crapper-McLachlan, D. (1983). Visual processing deficits as assessed by spatial frequency contrast sensitivity and backward masking in normal aging and Alzheimer's disease. *Brain, 107,* 309-325.

Schneck, M.K., Reisberg, B., & Ferris, S.H. (1982). An overview of current concepts of Alzheimer's disease. *American Journal of Psychiatry, 139,* 165-172.

Schoenfeld, M., Meyers, R.H., Cupples, L.A., Berkman, B., Sax, D.S., & Clark, E. (1984). Increased rate of suicide among patients with Huntington's disease. *Journal of Neurology, Neurosurgery, and Psychiatry, 47,* 1283-1287.

Schonfield, D. (1969). Age and remembering. *Duke University Council on Aging and Human Development, Proceedings of Seminars.* Durham, NC: Duke University.

Schulz, R. (1982a). Emotionality and aging. In K.R. Blankstein & J. Polivy (Eds.), *Advances in the study of communication and affect: Vol. 7. Self-control and self-modification of emotional behavior* (pp. 71-100). New York: Plenum Press.

Schulz, R. (1982b). Emotionality and aging: A theoretical and empirical analysis. *Journal of Gerontology, 37,* 42-51.

Scott, S., Caird, F.I., & Williams, B. (1984). Evidence for an apparent sensory speech disorder in Parkinson's disease. *Journal of Neurology, Neurosurgery, and Psychiatry, 47,* 840-843.

Sekuler, R., & Hutman, L.P. (1980). Spatial vision and aging: I. Contrast sensitivity. *Journal of Gerontology, 35,* 692-695.

Selby, G. (1968). Cerebral atrophy in Parkinsonism. *Journal of the Neurological Sciences, 6,* 517-559.

Shelton, M.D., Parsons, O.A., & Leber, W.R. (1982). Verbal and visuospatial performance and aging: A neuropsychological approach. *Journal of Gerontology, 37,* 336-341.

Siegler, I.C., McCarty, S.M., & Logue, P.E. (1982). Wechsler Memory Scale scores, selective attrition, and distance from death. *Journal of Gerontology, 37,* 176-181.

Soininen, H., Puranen, M., & Riekkinen, P.J. (1982). Computed tomography findings in senile dementia and normal aging. *Journal of Neurology, Neurosurgery, and Psychiatry, 45,* 50-54.

Spokes, E.G.S. (1981). The neurochemistry of Huntington's chorea. *Trends in Neuroscience, 4,* 115-118.

Squire, L.R. (1974). Remote memory as affected by aging. *Neuropsychologia, 12,* 429-435.

Sroka, H., Elizan, T.S., Yahr, M.D., Burger, A., & Mendoza, M.R. (1981). Organic mental syndrome and confusional states in Parkinson's disease: Relationship to computerized tomographic signs of cerebral atrophy. *Archives of Neurology, 38,* 339-342.

St. George-Hyslop, P.H., Tanzi, R.E., Polinsky, R.J., Haines, J.L., Nee, L., Watkins, P.C., Myers, R.H., Feldman, R.G., Pollen, D., Drachman, D., Growdon, J., Bruni, A., Foncin, J.F., Salmon, D., Frommelt, P., Amaducci, L., Sorbi, S., Piacentini, S., Stewart, G.D., Hobbs, W.J., Conneally, P.M., & Gusella, J.F. (1987). The genetic defect causing familial Alzheimer's disease maps on chromosome 21. *Science, 235,* 885-890.

Steele, J.C. (1972). Progressive supranuclear palsy. *Brain, 95,* 693-704.

Steele, J.C., Richardson, J.C., & Olszewski, J. (1964). Progressive supranuclear palsy. *Archives of Neurology, 10,* 333-359.

Steingart, A., Hachinski, V.C., Lau, C., Fox, A.J., Diaz, F., Cape, R., Lee, D., Inzitari, D., & Mersky, H. (1987). Cognitive and neurologic findings in subjects with diffuse white matter lucencies on computed tomographic scan (Leuko-Araiosis). *Archives of Neurology, 44,* 32-35.

Steingart, A., Hachinski, V.C., Lau, C., Fox, A.J., Fox, H., Lee, D., Inzitari, D., & Mersky, H. (1987). Cognitive and neurologic findings in demented patients with diffuse white matter lucencies on computed tomographic scan (Leuko-Araiosis). *Archives of Neurology, 44,* 36–39.
Stern, Y. (1983). Behavior and the basal ganglia. In R. Mayeux & W.G. Rosen (Eds.), *The dementias* (pp. 195–209). New York: Raven Press.
Stern, Y., Mayeux, R., Rosen, J., & Ilson, J. (1983). Perceptual motor dysfunction in Parkinson's disease: A deficit in sequential and predictive voluntary movement. *Journal of Neurology, Neurosurgery, and Psychiatry, 46,* 145–151.
Storandt, M. (1976). Speed and coding effects in relation to age and ability level. *Developmental Psychology, 12,* 177–178.
Storandt, M. (1977). Age, ability level, and method of administering and scoring the WAIS. *Journal of Gerontology, 32,* 175–178.
Storandt, M., Grant, E.A., & Gordon, B.C. (1978). Remote memory as a function of age and sex. *Experimental Aging Research, 4,* 365–375.
Struble, R.G., Cork, L.C., Whitehouse, P.J., & Price, D.L. (1982). Cholinergic innervation in neuritic plaques. *Science, 216,* 413–415.
Sulkava, R., Haltia, M., Paetau, A., Wikstrom, J., & Palo, J. (1983). Accuracy of clinical diagnosis in primary degenerative dementia: Correlation with neuropathological findings. *Journal of Neurology, Neurosurgery, and Psychiatry, 46,* 9–13.
Summers, W.K., Majovski, L.V., Marsh, G.M., Tachiki, K., & Kling, A. (1986). Oral tetrahydroaminoacridine in long-term treatment of senile dementia, Alzheimer-type. *New England Journal of Medicine, 315,* 1241–1245.
Tachibana, H., Meyer, J.S., Okayasu, H., Shaw, T.G., Kandula, P., & Rodgers, R.L. (1984). Xenon contrast CT-CBF scanning of the brain differentiates normal age-related changes from multi-infarct dementia and senile dementia of the Alzheimer type. *Journal of Gerontology, 39,* 415–423.
Tamminga, C.A., Foster, N.L., Fedio, P., Bird, E.D., & Chase, T.N. (1987). Alzheimer's disease: Low cerebral somatostatin levels correlate with impaired cognitive function and cortical metabolism. *Neurology, 37,* 161–165.
Tanzi, R.E., Gusella, J.F., Watkins, P.C., Bruns, G.A.P., St. George-Hyslop, P., van Keuren, M.L., Patterson, D., Pagan, S., Kurnit, D.M., & Neve, R.L. (1987). Amyloid beta protein gene: cDNA, mRNA distribution, and genetic linkage near the Alzheimer locus. *Science, 235,* 880–884.
Terry, R.D. (1983). Cortical morphometry in Alzheimer's disease. In R. Katzman (Ed.), *Banbury Report 15: Biological aspects of Alzheimer's disease* (pp. 95–99). Cold Spring Harbor, NY: Cold Spring Harbor Laboratory.
Thomas, P.D., Hunt, W.C., Garry, P.J., Hood, R.B., Goodwin, J.M., & Goodwin, J.S. (1983). Hearing acuity in a healthy elderly population: Effect on emotional, cognitive, and social status. *Journal of Gerontology, 38,* 321–325.
Thomsen, A.M., Borgesen, S.E., Bruhn, P., & Gjerris, F. (1986). Prognosis of dementia in normal-pressure hydrocephalus after a shunt operation. *Annals of Neurology, 20,* 304–310.
Thornbury, J., & Mistretta, C.M. (1981). Tactile sensitivity as a function of age. *Journal of Gerontology, 36,* 34–39.
Till, R.E. (1985). Verbatim and inferential memory in young and elderly adults. *Journal of Gerontology, 40,* 316–323.
Tweedy, J.R., Langer, K.G., & McDowell, F.H. (1982). The effect of semantic relations on the memory deficit associated with Parkinson's disease. *Journal of Clinical Neuropsychology, 4,* 235–247.

Uhl, G.R., Hilt, D.C., Hedreen, J.C., Whitehouse, P.J., & Price, D.L. (1983). Pick's disease (lobar sclerosis): Depletion of neurons in the nucleus basalis of Meynert. *Neurology, 33,* 1470–1473.

Verrillo, R.T. (1980). Age related changes in sensitivity to vibration. *Journal of Gerontology, 35,* 185–193.

Warren, L.R., Butler, R.W., Katholi, C.R., & Halsey, J.H. (1985). Age differences in cerebral blood flow during rest and during mental activation measurements with and without monetary incentive. *Journal of Gerontology, 40,* 53–59.

Warrington, E.K., & Sanders, H.I. (1971). The fate of old memories. *Quarterly Journal of Experimental Psychology, 23,* 432–442.

Warrington, E.K., & Silberstein, M. (1970). A questionnaire technique for investigating very long term memory. *Quarterly Journal of Experimental Psychology, 22,* 508–512.

Waugh, N.C., & Norman, D.A. (1965). Primary memory. *Psychological Review, 72,* 89–104.

Wechsler, A.F., Verity, M.A., Rosenschein, S., Fried, I., & Scheibel, A.B. (1982). Pick's disease: A clinical, computed tomographic, and histological study with Golgi impregnation observations. *Archives of Neurology, 39,* 287–290.

Weingartner, H., Grafman, J., Boutelle, W., Kaye, W., & Martin, P.R. (1983). Forms of memory failure. *Science, 221,* 380–382.

Weingartner, H., Kaye W., Smallberg, S.A., Ebert, M.H., Gillin, J.C., & Sitaran, N. (1981). Memory failures in progressive idiopathic dementia. *Journal of Abnormal Psychology, 90,* 187–196.

Welford, A.T. (1977). Motor performance. In J.E. Birren & K.W. Schaie (Eds.), *Handbook of the psychology of aging* (pp. 450–496). New York: VanNostrand Reinhold.

Wells, C. (1979). Pseudodementia. *American Journal of Psychiatry, 136,* 895–900.

Wells, C. (1982). Chronic brain disease: An update on alcoholism, Parkinson's disease, and dementia. *Hospital and Community Psychiatry, 33,* 111–126.

Whitehouse, P.J., Hedreen, J.C., White, C.L., & Price, D.L. (1983). Basal forebrain neurons in dementia of Parkinson's disease. *Annals of Neurology, 13,* 243–248.

Whitehouse, P.J., Price, D.L., Struble, R.G., Clark, A.W., Coyle, J.T., & DeLong, M.R. (1982). Alzheimer's disease and senile dementia: Loss of neurons in the basal forebrain. *Science, 215,* 1237–1239.

Wilcock, G.K., & Esiri, M.M. (1982). Plaques, tangles, and dementia: A quantitative study. *Journal of Neurological Sciences, 56,* 343–356.

Wilson, R.S., Bacon, L.D., Kramer, R.L., Fox, J.H., & Kaszniak, A.W. (1983). Word frequency effect and recognition memory in dementia of the Alzheimer type. *Journal of Clinical Neuropsychology, 5,* 97–104.

Wilson, R.S., Kaszniak, A.W., Bacon, L.D., Fox, J.H., & Kelly, M.P. (1982). Facial recognition memory in dementia. *Cortex, 18,* 329–336.

Wilson, R.S., Kaszniak, A.W., & Fox, J.H. (1981). Remote memory in senile dementia. *Cortex, 17,* 41–48.

Wilson, R.S., Kaszniak, A.W., Klawans, H.L., & Garron, D.C. (1980). High speed memory scanning in Parkinsonism. *Cortex, 16,* 67–72.

Winograd, E., Smith, A.D., & Simon, E.W. (1982). Aging and the picture superiority effect in recall. *Journal of Gerontology, 37,* 70–75.

Wisniewski, H.M., & Merz, G.S. (1983). Neuritic and amyloid plaques in senile dementia of the Alzheimer type. In R. Katzman (Ed.), *Banbury Report 15: Biological aspects of Alzheimer's disease* (pp. 145–152). Cold Spring Harbor, NY: Cold Spring Harbor Laboratory.

Wolozin, B.L., & Davies, P. (1986). Characterization of the Alz-50 antigen. *Society for Neuroscience (Abstracts), 12,* 944.

Wolozin, B.L., Pruchnicki, A., Dickson, D.W., & Davies, P. (1986). A neuronal antigen in the brains of Alzheimer patients. *Science, 232,* 648–650.

Wong, D.F., Wagner, H.N., Dannals, R.F., Links, J.M., Frost, J.J., Ravert, H.T., Wilson, A.A., Rosenbaum, A.E., Gjedde, A., Douglass, K.H., Petronis, J.D., Folstein, M.F., Toung, J.K.T., Burns, D.H., & Kuhar, M.J. (1984). Effects of age on dopamine and serotonin receptors measured by positron tomography in the living human brain. *Science, 226,* 1393–1396.

Wood, J.H., Bartlet, D., James, A.E., & Udvarhelyi, G.B. (1974). Normal-pressure hydrocephalus: Diagnosis and patient selection for shunt surgery. *Neurology, 24,* 517–526.

Woollacott, M.H., Shumway-Cook, A., & Nasher, L. (1982). Postural reflexes and aging. In J.A. Mortimer, F.J. Pirozzolo, & G.J. Maletta (Eds.), *The aging motor system* (pp. 98–119). New York: Praeger.

Wright, R.E. (1981). Aging, divided attention, and processing capacity. *Journal of Gerontology, 36,* 605–614.

Wright, R.E. (1982). Adult age similarities in free recall output order and strategies. *Journal of Gerontology, 37,* 76–79.

Wurtman, R.J. (1985). Alzheimer's disease. *Scientific American, 252,* 62–74.

Zacks, R.T. (1982). Encoding strategies used by young and elderly adults in a keeping track task. *Journal of Gerontology, 37,* 203–211.

Zetusky, W.J., Jankovic, J., & Pirozzolo, F.J. (1985). The heterogeneity of Parkinson's disease: Clinical and prognostic implications. *Neurology, 35,* 522–526.

2 Neuropsychological and Computed Tomographic Identification in Dementia

ERIN D. BIGLER

The presence of cortical atrophy, as demonstrated by computed tomographic (CT) imaging, is associated with a variety of neuropathological conditions, including progressive degenerative diseases, cerebral trauma, secondary effects of cerebrovascular disease, and anoxia (see Figure 2.1). Although the presence of cortical atrophy in the patient presenting with symptoms of dementia is considered to be one of the diagnostic signs associated with Alzheimer's disease (AD) (Cutler et al., 1984; Scheibel & Wechsler, 1986), the mere presence of atrophy of CT imaging is not a *sine qua non* indicator of dementia or AD.

Cortical atrophy also is seen in "normal" aging in the senescent individual who may be completely asymptomatic for neurological and cognitive disorder (Creasy & Rapoport, 1985; Jacoby & Levy, 1980; Schwartz et al., 1985). Because of this etiological diversity, the presence of atrophy may suggest a neuropathological state, but such findings may lack diagnostic specificity. Thus, the significance of cortical atrophy comes only in its relationship with other neurological and behavioral findings. This is in contrast to other conditions in which CT scanning has demonstrated diagnostic specificity (i.e., characteristic appearance of density changes associated with cerebral neoplasm or edema).

It is possible that the lack of diagnostic specificity of atrophy on CT images is due to inappropriate means of assessing atrophy. Initial rating scales (see Bird, 1982, for review) were unsuccessful in demonstrating significant relationships between CT-documented atrophy and dementia. However, these rating scales used either visual inspection, simple linear measurements, or radiographic rating scales. Such negative findings certainly could be questioned because of technique oversimplification, but it was surprising that even with more specific measurement techniques (such as Evans ratio, summed sulcal width measurements, ventrical/brain ratios; see Figure 2.2), greater reliability was not achieved (Fox, Kaszniak, & Huckman, 1979; Ramani, Loewenson, & Gold, 1979; Roberts, Caird, Grossart, & Steven, 1976).

Researchers in this area (Albert, Naeser, Levine, & Garvey, 1984a, 1984b; Eslinger, Damasio, Graff-Radford, & Damasio, 1984; Turkheimer et al., 1984) continued to speculate that a relationship did exist, but the lack of significant findings or inconsistent findings was related to measurement error. Thus, with

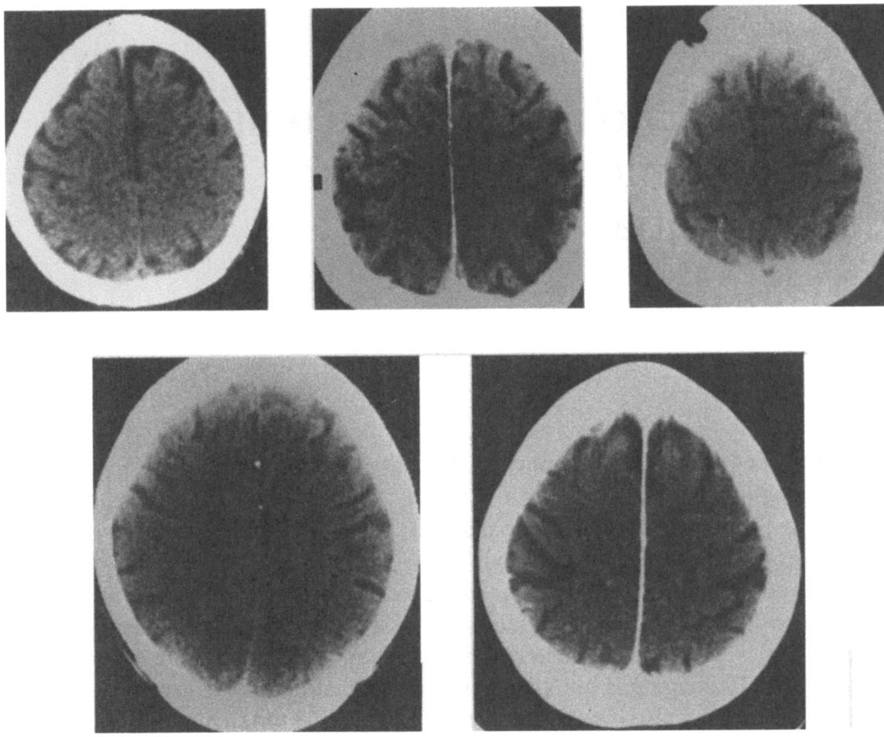

FIGURE 2.1. The five scans depict significant pericerebral atrophy, but are associated with different etiologies as follows: *top row*—(*left*) anoxia, (*center*) Alzheimer's disease, (*right*) cerebral trauma; *bottom row*—(*left*) demyelinating disease, (*right*) cerebral arteriosclerosis. Such diverse etiologies that all produce cortical atrophy clearly indicate the lack of diagnostic specificity that the finding of atrophy represents.

improvement in measuring techniques it was thought that greater reliability might be achieved in the assessment of the relationship between cortical atrophy, cortical functioning, and behavior. Since the relatively simple methods of assessment had proven to be unreliable, the next logical step was to pursue more precise volumetric measures. Such studies using actual volumetric estimates of brain or cerebral structure size have been quite promising and are described in the following section. The studies are based on patients with AD because of the relationship of this disease to the development of cortical atrophy (Cummings & Benson, 1983).

Quantifying Cerebral Measurements

The benchmark of psychobiological technique in examining brain-behavior relationships has been a precise measurement of lesion size and location in relationship to function (cf. Gazzaniga & Blakemore, 1975). Along these lines, it was

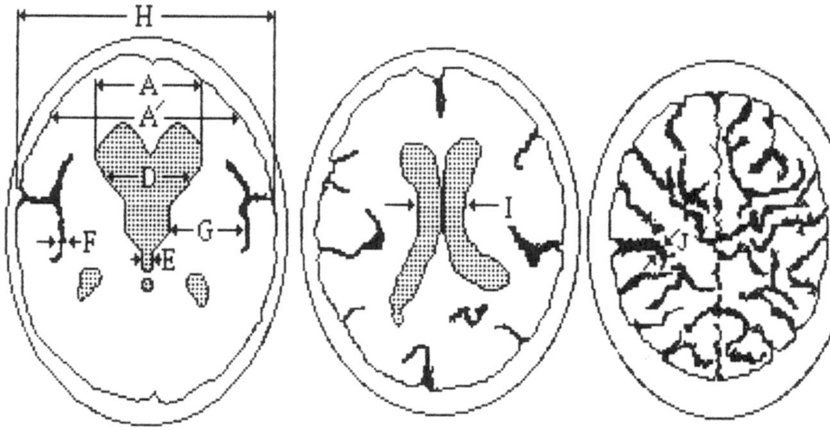

FIGURE 2.2. Diagrammatic outline of various procedures for assessing morphological measures from CT data. A, bifrontal span of the lateral ventricles; A′, brain width correction for measurement A; D, bicaudate diameter; E, width of the third ventricle; F, width of the left Sylvian fissure; G, distance between the third ventricle and the Sylvian fissure; H, width of the cortex at the widest lateral cut; I, minimal width of the ventricular bodies; J, width of an enlarged sulcus. Anterior Horn Index (Evans Ratio) = A/H. Bicaudate Index = D/H. Huckman Number = A + D. (Adapted from Bird [1982, p. 94] and DeLeon and George [1983, p. 108].)

assumed that by increasing the precision of measurement of neuropathological findings on the CT image, similar precision could be given to human brain-behavior relationships. Postmortem studies of atrophic brains have long demonstrated the relationship between gyral shrinkage, sulcal enlargement and ventricular dilation. By adapting partial volume estimation techniques (Turkheimer, Yeo, & Bigler, 1983) and direct volumetric measurement (Creasy, Schwartz, Frederickson, Haxby, & Rapoport, 1986), in vivo size and volume of cerebral structures can now be accomplished, as is described as follows.

Cerebral Atrophy

In the normal brain, the outer mantle of the cerebral cortex interfaces with the inner surface of the skull, being separated only by the width of the meninges and surrounding vasculature (i.e., arachnoid and subarachnoid space). Likewise, in the normal brain, the gyral pattern is such that the amount of space accounted for by the sulcal cleft is minimal. Thus, the actual volume accounted for by the meninges, sulcal space, and vasculature in the normal brain is quite a minimal amount, and thus an estimate of original brain volume can be obtained by taking the volume of the skull cavity by using inner circumference measures. By then taking the accumulative size of the sulcal width and subtracting this from the estimate of the original brain size, an estimation of the "shrinkage" can be obtained

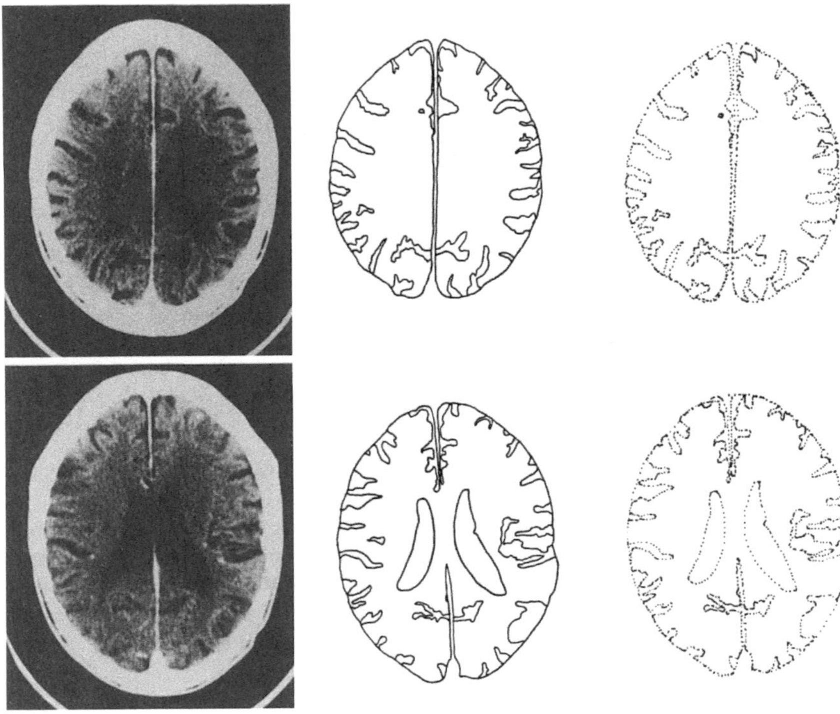

FIGURE 2.3. This illustration demonstrates the tracing technique utilized in this study. The CT scan (*on the left*) was first manually traced (*middle figure*) with special attention given to tracing the details of all sulci that were visible, as well as the ventricular system. The tracings were then digitized using a Summagraphics Bit Pad by moving a cursor manually around the perimeter of all relevant structures traced. The bit pad recorded X/Y plot coordinates of the cursor every 0.2 second. A computer-generated representation is present in the *far right figure* based on the X/Y plot coordinates. These data were then used to compute ventricular volume, brain volume, and cranial volume, as has been previously described.

(see Figure 2.3). This actually permits two measurement estimates: the estimate of the atrophied brain volume (direct estimate of brain size) and an estimate of the space or volume left by the atrophy (i.e., the space between the outer surface of the brain including the accumulated sulcal cleft area from the inner skull surface or a measure of the pericerebral space). Head size needs to be corrected for, so that greater atrophy is not related to larger head size alone. This is easily accomplished by utilizing ratio scores between brain size and skull volume.

Another problem that needs to be accounted for is positioning of the brain and partial volume effects. Since the CT sections are not continuous but separated by 5 to 10 mm, the volume has to be estimated between each slice. A starting point also needs to be defined, and in our studies we have used eight sequential CT slices (separated by 10 mm) starting at the base of the temporal lobes where the inferior horn of the lateral ventricular system can be first visualized and then proceeding dorsally. Although this ensures uniformity across patients, some cerebral tissue will be excluded from analysis, including the more ventral aspects of the temporal, and at times frontal areas, and the most dorsal aspect of the posterior frontal and parietal areas. Using this technique, the brain stem and most of the cerebellum also are omitted. While some areas are omitted, by using this standardized approach approximately two thirds of brain volume is accounted for and the critical areas of interest in degenerative disease are fully included (i.e., third and lateral ventricles, Sylvian fissure and frontal interhemispheric fissure).

Ventricular Enlargement

Ventricular volumetric measures are somewhat more straightforward. By using a volumetric estimation technique, the ventrical/brain interface surface can be traced and volume estimates established (see Figure 2.3). On current generation CT scanners, because of the distinct contrast between cerebral spinal fluid and cerebral tissue, the ventricular system typically is easily visualized, and tracing of the ventricular system and degree of cortical atrophy has been shown to have a high interrater reliability score (Turkheimer et al., 1984). One problem does exist, however, with this technique, and that deals with the border zone interface between ventricle and brain surface on the face of the ventricle. The CT picture elements (i.e., pixels) surrounding the ventricles are partially volumed—that is, they are neither all brain nor all ventricle, but part of both. Thus, using a simple tracing technique may slightly over- or underestimate actual volume size. Albert et al. (1984a, 1984b) have shown that this problem can be minimized by using an automated program based on CT density number configuration. The problem with this is that few laboratories store such data directly from the digitization of original CT information and typically only keep as a "hard" copy the x-ray film itself. Thus, the advantage of the tracing techniques, as described herein, is that it can be done directly from the CT film image, even though there may be some sacrifice with respect to accuracy.

Cortical Atrophy and Ventricular Enlargement Findings in Alzheimer's Disease

Utilizing the above techniques for estimating brain size and ventricular volume, the author studied such estimations in 42 patients with suspected Alzheimer's disease (Bigler, Hubler, Cullum, & Turkheimer, 1985). The mean values of the cranial, cerebral, and ventricular measurements are presented in Table 2.1. As can be seen by the total estimate of brain volume (858.6 cc), this is only a partial estimate (mean estimate for total brain is 1333 cc according to Blinkov and Glezer [1968]). One needs to take into account that, as discussed previously, the most dorsal aspect of the posterior frontal and anterior parietal areas are absent

TABLE 2.1. Mean cranial, brain, and ventricular volumes.

	Mean (cc)	*SD*
Cranial volume	910.97	87.41
Right cranial volume	455.56	47.45
Left cranial volume	455.42	47.51
Brain volume	858.60	83.98
Right brain volume	432.44	42.05
Left brain volume	426.16	44.26
Total ventricular volume	65.56	27.95
Right ventricular volume	32.03	12.90
Left ventricular volume	33.42	15.67
Lateral ventricular volume	61.27	27.25
III Ventricle volume	3.22	1.47
IV Ventricle volume	1.29	2.40

from analysis as well as the most ventral aspect of the temporal lobes and, in some cases, the most ventral aspect of the frontal area as well as most infratentorial regions. As indicated, though, this technique does account for approximately two thirds of the cerebral volume and includes the critical structures of importance to the documentation of cortical atrophy.

For the purpose of the study reported, the individual brain volumes were corrected for head size by taking ratio scores of brain volume to skull volume. Precise cutoff scores for what are "normal" and "abnormal" degrees of atrophy are not available for several reasons. The major factor here is that a "normal" degree of atrophy that occurs with age, as assessed by CT scan analysis, may be indistinct from atrophy associated with AD (Schwartz et al., 1985). Thus, rather than focusing on "cutoff" scores of normal versus abnormal, the analysis centered on examining the correlational relationships between the degree of cortical atrophy and cognitive functioning.

In this sample, the mean ventricular volume was 65.56 cc. Although there is considerable variability in what is considered normal ventricle size, Blinkov and Glezer (1968) have suggested 39 cc as an estimate of the upper limit of normal volume. Thus, the mean ventricular volume in this sample of suspect Alzheimer's patients is approximately 60% greater than the upper limit of normal. The relationship between these various brain volumetric analyses and neuropsychological performance is discussed in the following sections.

Neuropsychological Findings in Dementia

The presence of dementia implies that there has been some detectable decline in cognitive functioning from presumed premorbid levels (Albert, 1984; Friedland, Budinger, Brant-Zawadski, & Jagust, 1984; Wells, 1984). Along these lines, the standard intellectual assessment has utilized the Wechsler Adult Intelligence Scale (WAIS) (Wechsler, 1955) in the analysis of intellectual deterioration. There has been a plethora of WAIS studies (see Russell, 1979) that examine the relationship between organic brain disorders and intellectual functioning. The consensus from these studies has shown that verbal subtests on the WAIS tend to be related to more overlearned and therefore "crystallized" cognitive functions, and typically are less affected by generalized cerebral dysfunction (Cullum, Steinman, & Bigler, 1984). Performance subtests, while being not only more spatial and motor oriented, tend to tap new learning skills and, accordingly, more "fluid" cognitive processes. Hence, WAIS Verbal IQ (VIQ) scores in a demented individual tend to be more intact than Performance IQ (PIQ), and inversely, significantly lower PIQ (one standard deviation or more; see Fuld, 1984) in relationship to VIQ may be a more discriminating measure of intellectual deterioration (Bigler, 1984; Brinkman & Braun, 1984).

In addition to VIQ and PIQ comparisons, examinations of subtest performance can assist in determining the extent and degree of intellectual decline. Again, the verbal subtests tend to represent "hold" tests that may not be affected much by cerebral damage/dysfunction and thereby permit an estimate of premorbid ability levels (see Wechsler, 1958). For this purpose, the most useful verbal subtests are Information and Vocabulary. The performance-based subtests, with the exception of Picture Completion, tend to be "don't hold" measures and, in particular, the Block Design and Digit Symbol subtests are typically the subtests that are most impaired in patients with organic cerebral disorders, irrespective of whether the damage/dysfunction is diffuse, lateralized, or focal (Bigler, 1984; Russell, 1979).

In terms of measured memory functioning, the Wechsler Memory Scale (WMS) (Wechsler, 1945) has probably been the most researched and standardized test of memory functioning, although it has been criticized as being too dependent on verbal memory and language functions, and does not assess intermediate recall (Russell, 1981). Nonetheless, the WMS continues to be used and is the standard memory battery in the assessment of memory decline in the demented individual. Based on the results of the WMS, a Memory Quotient (MQ) can be derived that has an identical mean and standard deviation as the WAIS IQ scores. This permits direct comparison of the patient's MQ with IQ, and since they are highly intercorrelated, examination of MQ relative to IQ can render memory and intellectual comparisons. With respect to subtest analysis, the Logical Memory, Visual Memory, and Paired Associate subtests have been shown to be particularly impaired in dementing illnesses (Albert, 1984; Bigler, 1984; Storandt, Botwinick, Danziger, Berg, & Hughes, 1984).

From the psychometric assessment standpoint, the presence of dementia originally was thought to be a rather uniform decline in intellectual functioning (Wechsler, 1958). However, this unitary concept of decline has been abandoned for the concept of heterogeneity and diversity in declining function, at least in the early stages of AD. For example, Rosen, Mohs, and Davis (1984) have demonstrated four cognitive (memory, word recognition, language functions, and motor/constructional praxic functions) and two noncognitive dimensions (mood state and behavioral disorders) that differentiate patients with AD from non-AD patients. Such findings suggest that the appropriate neuropsychological assessment in patients with dementing illness needs to tap a variety of cognitive and behavioral measures.

Along these lines, Storandt et al. (1984) were able to correctly classify 98% of patients with senile dementia of the Alzheimer's type using only neuropsychological measures. Using the discriminant analysis technique, four neuropsychometric measures were identified by Storandt et al. as providing such a high differentiation. These four tests were: The Mental Control and Logical Memory subtests of the WMS; Trail Making, Part A (Reitan & Davison, 1974); and word fluency for the letters S and P. The discriminant function that was utilized demonstrated significant impairment on the Logical Memory, Trail Making A, and word fluency subtests in the AD patients, with intact level of performance on Mental Control for the normals (thus the Mental Control results functioned as a suppressor variable—that is, they positively correlated with normalcy and not with dementia). This work suggests that by examining neuropsychological function over a spectrum of tasks that tap new learning and memory (e.g., Logical Memory subtest), verbal fluency (which requires expressive and receptive language, and immediate recall as well as recall from long-term storage), and sequential cognition (the verbal sequencing of information on the WMS Mental Control subtest and visual motor sequencing on the Trail Making Test, Part A), cognitive deficits in dementia may not only be delimited, but highly discriminatory with respect to the disorder (see also Eslinger, Damasio, Benton, & Van Allen, 1985).

Neuropsychological–CT Scan Interrelationships

Creasy et al. (1986), Damasio et al. (1983), de Leon and George (1983), Eslinger et al. (1984), and Albert et al. (1984a, 1984b) have demonstrated increased ventricular dilation and cortical atrophy in patients with suspected Alzheimer's disease using volumetric CT scan analyses. By using volumetric size estimates alone, they were able to classify correctly most patients with Alzheimer's disease. These studies have focused mainly on the properties of the ventricular dilation seen in Alzheimer's patients, and concomitant neuropsychological findings were not thoroughly evaluated. To this end, the author has examined (see Bigler et al., 1985) the relationship between neuropsychological performance on the Wechsler Adult Intelligence Scale and the Wechsler Memory Scale and volumetric CT findings in the group of 42 patients previously described who met the criteria for probable AD.

As reported earlier, CT volume estimates of ventricular enlargement in this group of AD patients indicated a mean enlargement nearly twice the size of what is considered to be normal. Despite these very significant findings of ventricular enlargement, there were no significant correlations between ventricular enlargement and neuropsychological performance. Thus, ventricular dilation appears to be a highly discriminating neuroanatomical factor for the presence of AD (see Damasio et al., 1983), and in patients who meet the behavioral and neuropsychological criteria for AD, studies have shown that correct classification can be made in greater than 95% of such patients in contrast to normal controls,

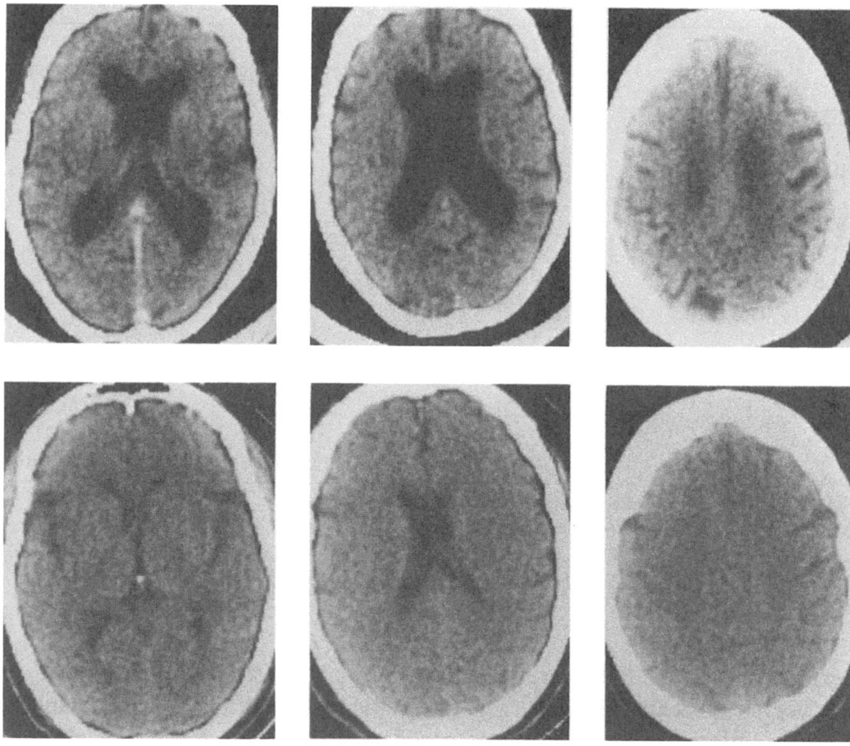

FIGURE 2.4. These CT films present representative films of the patient with the largest ventricular system (total volume) irrespective of atrophy (*top scans*) and the corresponding patient (*bottom scans*) with the smallest ventricular volume in the study of 42 patients with AD. The patient depicted in the top scans was a 74-year-old female. Her intellectual scores on the WAIS were: Verbal IQ Score (VIQ) = 74, Performance IQ Score (PIQ) = 67, Fullscale IQ Score (FSIQ) = 69. Her WMS Memory Quotient (MQ) was 72. She had a high school education and was a homemaker. The patient depicted in the bottom scans was a 53-year-old male. His WAIS results were: VIQ = 105, PIQ = 91, FSIQ = 99. His WMS MQ was 70. It is of interest to note in these scans that even though the top scans demonstrate marked ventricular dilation, cortical atrophy for her age is minimal. Oppositely, the individual in the bottom scans has very small ventricles, but prominent Sylvian fissures (a sign of frontotemporal atrophy). Despite these great differences in the degree of ventricular dilation, there is no difference in MQ. Accordingly, it is not surprising that there is little relationship between MQ and ventricular volume in AD.

based on ventricular size alone. However, there appears to be little relationship between ventricular dilation itself, and WAIS and WMS performance. The apparent confounding factor here is the marked variability that may occur not only in terms of ventricular size, but the type and degree of cognitive impairments present. This is demonstrated quite eloquently by the cases that are presented in Figure 2.4. In this illustration, two patients with nearly identical

TABLE 2.2. Correlation matrix between ATVOL and neuropsychological performance.

Neuropsychological measure	ATVOL	ATVOL-Right	ATVOL-Left
VIQ	−0.15	−0.17	−0.12
	(0.16)	(0.14)	(0.22)
PIQ	−0.47	−0.45	−0.41
	(0.001)	(0.002)	(0.005)
FSIQ	−0.38	−0.36	−0.34
	(0.008)	(0.01)	(0.02)
VIQD	0.06	0.08	0.03
	(0.36)	(0.29)	(0.41)
PIQD	0.43	0.41	0.36
	(0.03)	(0.004)	(0.01)
FSIQD	0.30	0.29	0.26
	(0.03)	(0.03)	(0.05)
MQ	−0.24	−0.25	−0.21
	(0.07)	(0.06)	(0.10)

Note. Significance levels are in parentheses.
ATVOL = Cranial Volume − Brain Volume/Cranial Volume; VIQ = Verbal IQ; PIQ = Performance IQ; FSIQ = Fullscale IQ; VIQD = Verbal IQ Deterioration; PIQD = Performance IQ Deterioration; FSIQD = Fullscale IQ Deterioration; MQ = Memory Quotient.

performance on the WMS are presented, but they show striking differences in the degree of ventricular enlargement. With such high degree of variability, there is little chance of systematic correlations between ventricular size and cognitive impairment.

The cortical atrophy measures, however, were found to correlate with a number of neuropsychological measures, and the results of this analysis are presented in Table 2.2. VIQ measures were not correlated with the degree of atrophy, but PIQ measures were, regardless of hemisphere. As previously indicated, the performance subtests and the conglomerate PIQ scores are considered to tap new learning and are thereby more sensitive to the presence of organic dysfunction. This finding was corroborated by these studies and suggested that there was a significant relationship between increasing cortical atrophy and impaired manipulo-spatial/visual-motor functioning as assessed by the WAIS Performance subtests.

To examine further the relationship between the degree of atrophy and neuropsychological performance, an atrophy index measure was used to divide the patients into two groups, one with a higher degree of atrophy and one with a lower degree. The results of this analysis are presented in Table 2.3. Inspection of these findings indicates that the group with greater atrophy did indeed exhibit greater impairment on most measures. These results have also been substantiated by Creasy et al. (1986). The subtests that were not significantly different likely were so because of "floor" effects in that both groups did very poorly on these particular measures (i.e., Digit Span, Logical Memory, and Visual Memory subtests). These particular subtests are the ones that tap new learning and short-term memory functioning and have likewise been demonstrated to consistently be impaired in patients with AD (see Storandt et al., 1984).

TABLE 2.3. Neuropsychological performance comparisons between high and low ATVOL groups.

Neuropsychological measure	High ATVOL		Low ATVOL		t test significance
	Mean	*SD*	Mean	*SD*	($p <$)
VIQ	90.5	11.8	100.4	17.2	0.04
PIQ	80.1	10.9	93.2	18.6	0.01
FSIQ	85.3	10.6	98.6	16.0	0.01
Information	6.9	2.1	9.5	3.8	0.01
Comprehension	7.1	2.5	9.7	4.1	0.02
Arithmetic	6.4	2.4	7.4	3.9	0.32
Similarities	6.5	3.5	8.7	4.1	0.07
Digit Span	6.9	3.2	7.0	2.8	0.88
Vocabulary	8.3	3.5	9.7	3.3	0.20
Picture Completion	4.1	2.2	7.2	3.5	0.01
Block Design	3.6	2.8	5.7	4.3	0.07
Picture Arrangement	3.9	2.2	5.7	3.0	0.04
Object Assembly	3.9	2.8	6.1	3.7	0.05
Digit Symbol	3.0	2.6	4.0	3.2	0.28
VIQD	23.6	13.5	18.2	12.1	0.26
PIQD	31.5	11.8	22.1	16.8	0.04
FSIQD	28.2	12.2	19.2	14.6	0.04
MQ	78.5	15.1	84.4	19.9	0.31
Logical Memory	4.2	3.1	5.6	3.4	0.18
Digits	8.6	2.6	8.9	1.3	0.62
Visual Memory	2.8	2.7	3.6	3.7	0.41
Associate Learning	6.2	3.6	9.3	4.9	0.03

Note. ATVOL = Cranial Volume − Brain Volume/Cranial Volume; VIQ = Verbal IQ; PIQ = Performance IQ; FSIQ = Fullscale IQ; VIQD = Verbal IQ Deterioration; PIQD = Performance IQ Deterioration; FSIQD = Fullscale IQ Deterioration; MQ = Memory Quotient.

It is of interest to note in this analysis between groups of higher and lower atrophy that there was not a significant difference between WMS MQ scores. Although memory deficits often are considered to be the hallmarks of AD, and the MQ values were indicative of overall memory disturbance, there was no significant difference between groups with higher and lower atrophy in terms of MQ results. The only significant WMS difference between these groups was on the Associate Learning subtest. It is of interest to compare these findings with Storandt's previously discussed findings in which the Logical Memory subtest of the WMS in comparison to the other subtests was found to be one of the neuropsychological measures in their discriminant analysis that delineated AD patients from normals. However, between AD groups with high and low atrophy, Logical Memory was not found to relate systematically to morphological brain change, but was rather uniformly affected independent of the degree of atrophy.

It also is interesting to note that there were not more significant findings relating to changes in brain morphology and neuropsychological performance in patients with AD. These results suggest there may be some relationship between

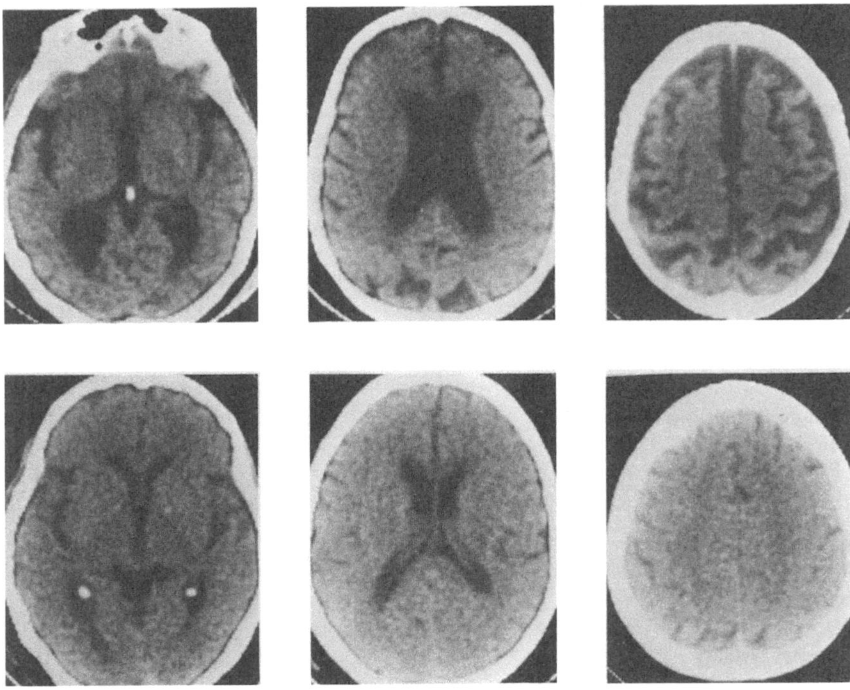

FIGURE 2.5. These CT films present representative films of the patient with the greatest degree of pericerebral atrophy (*top scan*) irrespective of ventricular volume and the corresponding patient (*bottom scan*) with the least degree of atrophy in the study of 42 patients with AD. The patient depicted in the top scan was a 78-year-old female. Her WAIS and WMS scores were: VIQ = 97, PIQ = 73, FSIQ = 85, MQ = 87. She was a retired school teacher and had a college education. The patient depicted in the bottom scans was a 74-year-old female. Her WAIS and WMS scores were: VIQ = 93, PIQ = 82, FSIQ = 88, MQ = 68. She had a high school education and was a homemaker. These results indicate that there was considerable range in the extent of pericerebral atrophy in this group of AD patients.

cognitive deficits and morphological brain change, but the relationship clearly is not a linear one (see Figure 2.5).

A major factor in this lack of linearity is the gap between the more molar measure that the CT image represents and the microscopic neuronal changes seen in AD. For example, in preliminary studies of five patients with AD, Hyman, Van Hoesen, Damasio, and Barnes (1984) found specific cellular pathology of the subiculum of the hippocampal formation and Layers II and IV of the entorhinal cortex. They suggest that this level of pathology may be responsible for the memory deficit in AD because degeneration at this level would disconnect the hippocampus from association cortices, the basal forebrain, thalamus, and hypothalamus (see also Hyman, Van Hoesen, Kromer, & Damasio, 1986;

McDuff & Sumi, 1985). Complete behavioral data are still lacking in such studies, and specific conclusions correlating these findings with morphological brain changes are still not available. At the cortical level, Sajdel-Sulkowska and Marotta (1984) have demonstrated decreased protein synthesis associated with RNA aberrations in AD. They suggest that this downward regulation of protein synthesis may specifically affect neurotransmitter enzymes, in particular choline (see Kitt et al., 1984), as well as the survival of neurons. Because of decreased acetylcholine in AD (Appel, 1981; Kitt et al., 1984; McGeer, McGeer, Suzuki, Dolman, & Nagai, 1984), speculation has been directed to the nucleus basalis of Meynert because of its role in acetylcholine production (Appel, 1981). However, in a recent study of Nakano and Hirano (1984) they failed to demonstrate consistent AD even with significant neuronal degeneration of the nucleus basalis of Meynert. Thus, at this time, neuronal pathology in AD may involve a variety of pathological states in addition to the traditional pathology of diffusely distributed neuritic plaques and neurofibrillary tangles that are diagnostic of AD. As such, it is not surprising that the more molar measures obtained from CT imaging would show only a few significant relationships.

Another factor accounting for lack of a greater relationship between WAIS and WMS performance and CT finding in AD is that these measures may not be accurately assessing the nature of dysfunction in AD (Massman, Bigler, Cullum, & Naugle, 1986). For example, Albert et al. (1984) and Eslinger et al. (1984) have shown more robust correlations between ventricular enlargement and memory disturbance in AD by using more complex short-term measures than the WMS. So there may be more of a relationship present depending on the complexity of the cognitive task.

Subgroup Analysis and Dementia: Neuropsychological, CT Scan, and Presenting Symptom Analysis

As eluded to earlier, there is considerable heterogeneity in the presenting symptomatology with AD and related forms of dementing illnesses. Like the speculation of a relationship between cerebral atrophy and cognitive impairment in AD, it also has been considered that a relationship may exist between present symptomatology and morphological brain change in AD and other degenerative diseases (Brouwers, Cox, Martin, Chase, & Fedio, 1984; Direnfeld et al., 1984; Fuld, 1984). For example, it has been speculated that more lateralized or focal atrophy may indeed have a direct bearing upon the presenting symptomatology. For example, Wechsler (1977) (see also Wechsler, Verity, Rosenschein, Fried, & Scheibel, 1982; Bigler, 1984, p. 141) argues by the use of case illustrations that prominent language disturbance in the early stages of a dementing illness suggests a greater lateralization of atrophy to the dominant hemisphere, and in some cases such findings may be more suggestive of Pick's disease than AD (see also Morris, Cole, Banker, & Wright, 1984; Munoz-Garcia & Ludwin, 1984). Gustafson, Hagberg, and Ingvar (1978) reported that demented patients in their study with nonfluent dysphasic deficits had focal cerebral blood flow abnormalities in the frontal lobe of the dominant hemisphere (see also Duara et al., 1984; Foster et al., 1984; Kitagawa, Meyer, Tachibana, Mortel, & Rogers, 1984; MacInnes et al., 1984). Mesulam (1982) also presents a case study of slowly progressive aphasia without concomitant generalized cognitive deterioration in dementia, implicating a lateralized atrophic process. Crystal, Horoupian, and Katzman (1982) have reported on a case of histologically verified Alzheimer's disease that presented initially with focal right parietal symptomatology (sensory-perceptual/visuospatial deficits) in the absence of significant language disturbance or other cognitive impairment. Based on these studies, it appears quite convincingly that on an individual basis focal atrophic processes may result in focal symptomatology.

To study this possibility further, Naugle, Cullum, Bigler, and Massman (1985) examined the relationship between initial symptomatology, cognitive impairment, and CT volumetric findings in dementia. One hundred thirty-eight patients were identified who had a dementing disorder, most likely AD. The patients were classified in terms of their presenting complaints as outlined in Table 2.4. All patients in this study received a detailed neuropsychological examination including the following tests: Wechsler Adult Intelligence Scale (WAIS), Wechsler Memory Scale (WMS), Reitan-Klove Sensory Perceptual Examination, Reitan-Indiana Aphasia Screening Test, Trail Making Parts A and B, Finger Oscillation Test, and Strength of Grip (see Reitan & Davison, 1974, for test description). By using these neuropsychometric measures, the data could be grouped into the following areas: motor, language, IQ, memory, and spatial-perceptual functioning. CT scan results were analyzed using volumetric measures as previously outlined.

To eliminate errors due to arbitrary or subjective classification of patients, the neuropsychological data were subjected to cluster analysis in addition to examination by presenting complaint. This statistical procedure permits the "clustering" of patients into similar groups based upon the statistical properties of related patient groupings in terms of test performance. A variety of cluster solutions are generated and a "best" cluster solution is then established (Spath, 1980). In this sample, a five-cluster solution was found to clearly differentiate the groups along a variety of lines without producing any redundancy in classification. The five-cluster solution (see Figure 2.6) could be best characterized in terms of verbal and visuospatial functioning. The following clusters were derived: Cluster 1 (N = 42, mean age = 70.8 years)—this group displayed generalized deficits on all measures and differed from the others with respect to severity of impairment;

TABLE 2.4. Presenting symptomatology of the 138 AD patients in the cluster analysis.

Memory dysfunction (memory loss, confusion, disorientation)	51.1%
Affective alterations (depression, anxiety, emotional lability)	12.4%
Psychotic symptomatology (delusions, hallucinations, bizarre behavior)	22.6%
Language dysfunction (dysphasic deficits)	3.8%
Motoric impairment (coordination problems, balance disturbance, gait problems, falling, weakness, tremor)	10.2%

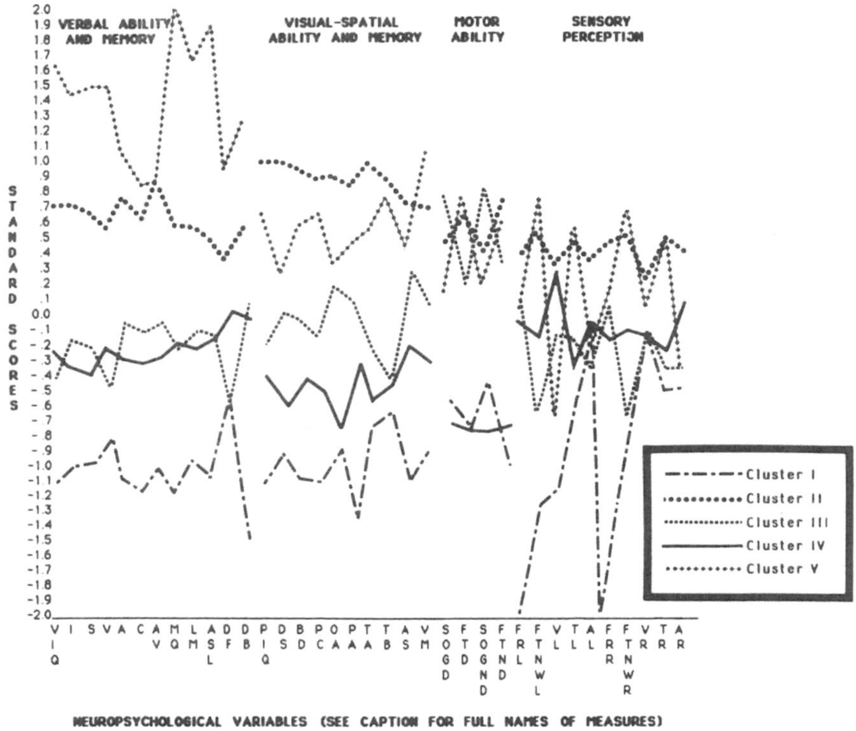

FIGURE 2.6. Neuropsychological profiles of the five clusters. All values are given in z-score form. Variables abbreviated along the abscissa are: VIQ, Verbal IQ; I, Information; S, Similarities; V, Vocabulary; A, Arithmetic; C, Comprehension; AV, Aphasia Screening Test, Verbal Score; MQ, Memory Quotient; LM, Logical Memory; ASL, Associate Learning; DF, Digits Forward; DB, Digits Backwards; PIQ, Performance IQ; DS, Digit Span; BD, Block Design; PC, Picture Completion; OA, Object Assembly; PA, Picture Arrangement; TA, Trail Making Test, Form A; TB, Trail Making Test, Form B; AS, Aphasia Screening Test, Spatial Score; VM, Visual Memory; SOGD, Strength of Grip, Dominant Hand; FTD, Finger Oscillation Test, Dominant Hand; SOGND, Strength of Grip, Nondominant Hand; FTND, Finger Oscillation Test, Nondominant Hand; FRL, Finger Recognition on the Left Hand; FTNWL, Finger Tip Number Writing on the Left Hand; VL, Visual Extinctions in the Left Visual Field; TL, Tactile Extinctions on the Left Body Side; AL, Auditory Extinctions of the Left Ear; FRR, Finger Recognition on the Right Hand; FTNWR, Finger Tip Number Writing on the Right Hand; VR, Visual Extinctions in the Right Visual Field; TR, Tactile Extinctions on the Right Hand; and AR, Auditory Extinctions of the Right Ear. Raw score means for all of the variables are given in Table 2.1.

Cluster 2 ($N = 39$, mean age = 63.4 years)—this group was found to be intact on visuospatial tasks, but in comparison had lowered functioning on verbal language measures; Cluster 3 ($N = 21$, mean age = 66.3 years) and Cluster 4 ($N = 42$, mean age = 74.7) were considered to be intermediate subgroups that were virtually indistinguishable in terms of verbal and memory functioning, but that did exhibit significant differences on visuospatial functioning, with the latter group having more prominent deficits (it should also be noted that these two groups made more verbal language-related errors than Group 2); Cluster 5 (N = 11, mean age = 69.4)—this group had relatively intact verbal language and memory abilities, superior to all of the other clusters, but had distinctly lowered functioning on visuospatial tasks in comparison.

Based on these groupings, if lateralized atrophy affects symptomatology in a systematic fashion, it would be predicted that CT results would show that Group 1 would have generalized atrophy, Group 2 lateralized left hemisphere atrophy, and Group 5 lateralized right hemisphere involvement. Similarly, based on presenting symptomatology as outlined in Table 2.4, the relationship between such symptoms and CT findings was examined. The results of volumetric analysis, however, showed no such relationship. There was a significant relationship between greater atrophy and age. Ventricular size measurements were uniformly insignificant in relation to cognitive deficits or symptomatology. Accordingly, there were no significant morphological features that corresponded with presenting symptomatology or cluster group by using this methodological approach.

Across the five subgroups, subjects did differ significantly with regard to age. The patients in Clusters 2 and 3 were younger. Both had visuospatial scores consistently higher than verbal memory scores, suggesting a relative lowering of verbal memory abilities in comparison. Combining these two groups yields a mean age of 64.4. Combining Groups 4 and 5, which had the opposite combination (visuospatial scores lower than verbal memory), resulted in a mean age of 73.6. This finding is consistent with the observation of Seltzer and Sherwin (1983) that suggested a greater prevalence of language dysfunction with presenile onset. However, even with combining these groups there was no significant difference with respect to morphological features, and no lateralization effects were noted. Age was related to greater ventricular dilation, but not cortical atrophy. These results were consistent with previous studies (see Schwartz et al., 1985) that demonstrate increased ventricular size with age. Along these lines, it is of interest to note that McDuff and Sumi (1985) have found greater degrees of subcortical degeneration in presenile than senile onset AD patients. Naugle, Cullum, Bigler, and Massman (1986), as well as others (see Albert & Stafford, 1986; Filley, Kelly, & Heaton, 1986; Loring & Largen, 1985), have also found some tentative support for the early onset course of AD to be associated with greater cognitive impairment.

The clusters also differed with respect to sex differences. Despite the greater number of females in the total sample, males outnumbered females in Groups 2 and 3 (intact visuospatial groups relative to verbal functioning by a factor of 2:1 (40 males to 20 females), whereas when combining the two groups (4 and 5) with intact verbal memory abilities relative to visuospatial, there was an equally disproportionate number, but in the opposite direction, 37 females to 16 males. Several avenues of research have suggested that females may show less of a deficit with lateralized injury than do males (see review by Corballis,

1983; Springer & Deutsch, 1981) and may show greater facility with language-based functions, whereas males may have greater facility with spatial abilities (Yeo, Turkheimer, & Bigler, 1984; however, see Bornstein & Matarazzo, 1984). These results suggest that there may be some relationship associated with presenting symptomatology, sex, and neuropsychological impairment in AD, but this did not systematically relate to any greater or lateralized atrophy, in this study.

Although the groups were studied as to their performance on a number of motor tasks, none of the motor findings differentiated among the groups and there was no consistent relationship seen between cortical atrophy, ventricular enlargement, and motor disturbances. This is consistent with recent findings that have suggested little relationship between motor deficits and presentation or progression of Alzheimer's disease (Koller, Wilson, Glatt, & Fox, 1984).

In a separate study, Raz et al. (in press) sought to better differentiate lateralized brain atrophy in AD patients by obtaining ratio scores of the degree of atrophy of the hemisphere displaying the greatest atrophy versus the hemisphere with the least amount of atrophy, irrespective of presenting symptom as was done in the Naugle et al. (1985) study. Also, this approach afforded a more direct index of lateralized atrophy than was utilized in the previous studies. There was some modest support that in some AD patients there may be a relationship between lateralized degenerative patterns and corresponding cognitive asymmetries of dysfunction (i.e., greater left hemisphere atrophy was associated with greater VIQ decline in comparison to PIQ). However, the relationship was far from linear, and considerable intersubject variability was present.

In conclusion, although case studies have clearly demonstrated that focal symptomatology may relate to focal atrophy in dementia, the current studies, using a group analysis, suggest that this is not uniformly the case, and that broad conclusions cannot be made from these case studies. Along these lines, Kirschner, Webb, Kelly, and Wells (1984) reviewed six cases of patients with clear dementia without focal or lateralized CT findings, but who had language disturbance as the more prominent initial symptom. Thus, even though they had what appeared to be focal presenting symptomatology (i.e., dysphasia), this was not associated with lateralized findings on CT scan analysis. However, a very important finding was discovered on a 1-year follow-up with one of the patients, and that was that subsequent left perisylvian atrophy did develop. It may be that the nature of the progressive deterioration with dementing illness is such that there is a critical time period for the expression of symptoms, but that the onset of such symptoms may not correspond to observable CT changes. Obviously, for cortical degeneration to occur sufficient to be noted on CT scanning, it will take weeks to months to develop, and within this time frame, it may be that it does not correspond well with presenting symptoms. Microstructural degenerative changes obviously would occur before more gross atrophic changes could be visualized. Thus, there may be little relationship between initial symptomatology, CT analysis, and subsequent cognitive symptomatology due to the imprecise relationship between atrophy and neuropsychological status.

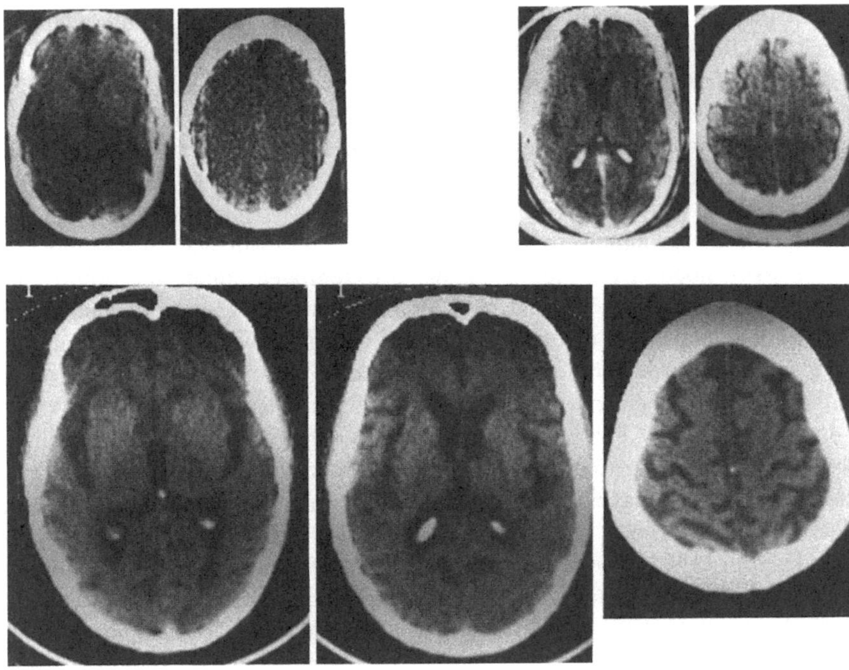

FIGURE 2.7. These scans depict the course of cerebral atrophy in Alzheimer's disease. This patient was first diagnosed in 1977 (*top left scan*) as having AD. CT scan findings showed some prominence of the Sylvian fissures bilaterally and slight prominence of the anterior aspect of the frontal interhemispheric fissure. Otherwise, the scan was within normal limits for this 55-year-old college-educated engineer. In that year, his WAIS and WMS results indicated the following: VIQ = 93, PIQ = 87, FSIQ = 90, MQ = 63. Eighteen months later, there were some changes noted on CT examination (*top right scan*), namely in the presence of sulcal enlargement. His WAIS and WMS at that time indicated the following scores: VIQ = 85, PIQ = 72, FSIQ = 79, MQ = 57. He was seen again in 1981 (no CT performed that year), and the following WAIS and WMS results were obtained: VIQ = 59, PIQ = 62, FSIQ = 57, MQ = 48 (he could perform no aspect of the WMS). Prior to this writing he was seen again (1984), and there was a complete absence of any higher mental functions and the patient was likewise with a generalized paresis. CT scanning (*bottom pictures*) depicts advanced cortical atrophy and widespread sulcal enlargement and very prominent bilateral Sylvian fissures. It is of interest to note that there is relatively little change in the size of the ventricular system from 1978 to 1984.

Prediction of Deterioration

Many of the dementing illnesses are progressive in nature, with both progressive deterioration in mental as well as physical status. Initial studies using CT scan ratings to predict progression have been disappointing (Kaszniak et al. 1978), whereas neuropsychological studies have been quite promising. To date, the most comprehensive study has been that by Berg et al. (1984), who found that two neuropsychological measures, the Digit Symbol subtest of the WAIS and an aphasia battery, correctly predicted the stage of dementia 1 year later in 95% of their patients studied. CT scan and electrophysiological (EEG and evoked potential) were not predictive. Based on their findings, the greater the neuropsychological impairment on these measures, the greater the severity of dementia and rapidity in progression within a year. The case study detailed in Figure 2.7 demonstrates these various points.

Using the more detailed procedures for volumetric analysis, Bigler et al. (1985) have examined deterioration indices in AD and found modest correlations, but only with the degree of cortical atrophy and then with just PIQ measures. Taken together, it appears that cognitive measures alone, particularly those based on complex short-term memory, manipulospatial abilities, and certain verbal language functions are better predictors of deterioration in AD than are a variety of CT measures (see also Botwinick, Storandt, & Berg, 1986).

Relationship of CT with Magnetic Resonance Imaging and Positron Emission Tomography Scanning Techniques

Magnetic resonance imaging (MRI) studies of the brain of the AD victim may provide a more precise definition of cerebral structures than can be obtained by CT (see Figure 2.8). MRI scanning techniques permit a better delineation of white versus gray matter, eliminate bone artifact problems that plague some CT views, and can be readily performed in the coronal and sagittal planes. Despite these advances with MRI over traditional CT in the identification of gross pathology and degree of cortical atrophy/ventricular enlargement, both procedures offer a reliable index of cortical atrophy (see McGeer et al., 1986).

MRI studies are considerably more sensitive to tissue density differences than are traditional CT measures and have provided an improved in vivo method in the identification of small infarcts that may lead to multi-infarct dementia (Hershey, Modic, Greenough, & Jaffe, 1987). MRI studies will provide better diagnostic guidelines in AD research because they will permit the elimination of AD patients with multi-infarct dementia and related white matter degenerative changes—the so-called condition of leukoaraiosis (Steingart, Hachinski, Lau, Fox, Diaz, et al., 1987; Steingart, Hachinski, Lau, Fox, Fox, et al., 1987). It may be that some of the past inconsistent CT findings in AD patients may be because of undetected lucency changes from etiologies other than AD.

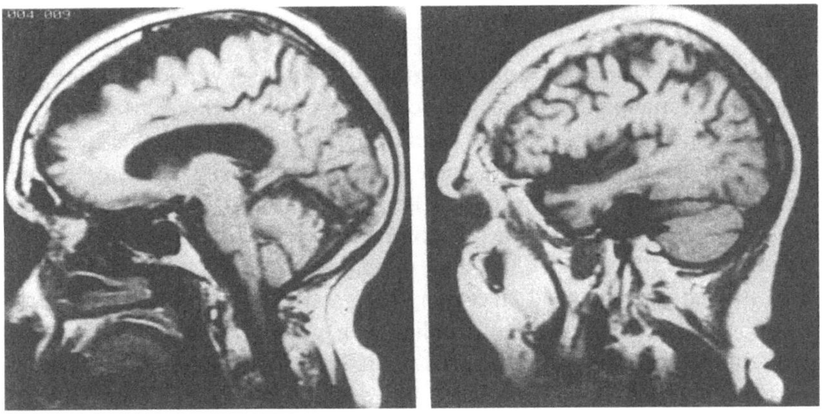

FIGURE 2.8. Sagittal MRI views of a 76-year-old female with senile dementia. Note how clearly the sulcal patterns can be identified. There is marked atrophy of the frontal and temporal regions. This patient was originally seen at age 71 at which time her intellectual studies were intact (VIQ = 123, PIQ = 119, FSIQ = 122), but memory was impaired (MQ = 93). Two years later there had been intellectual deterioration (VIQ = 123, PIQ = 114, FSIQ = 113) with particular decline in memory (MQ = 87). Five years later, at the time the MRI was taken, further intellectual deterioration had occurred (VIQ = 76, PIQ = 87, FSIQ = 80) with marked impairment in memory (MQ = 66).

Because positron emission tomography (PET) findings provide an index of underlying metabolic activity, it may be the more sensitive measure. For example, McGeer et al. (1986) recently demonstrated that PET scanning of a patient with AD, which was later confirmed at autopsy, correlated best with the underlying microscopic findings of neuronal loss and glial proliferation. It may be that future PET neuroimaging studies may provide a more robust relationship between cognitive deficit and brain imaging since it will permit more specific correlations of degenerative changes in AD and concomittant cognitive changes.

However, PET scanning techniques are not widely available because of the problems attending the creation of the radioactive isotopes necessary to perform the test. Because of the cost factors in the use of MRI (MRI studies cost more), CT scanning will likely remain the routine neuroradiological procedure in the evaluation of the dementia patient, for at least the immediate future.

Summary

This chapter reviews the current status of various objective CT measures in relationship to cognitive functioning in AD. Although ventricular dilation is a consistent finding in AD, it correlates poorly with cognitive status, with the degree of cortical atrophy being a better index. Presenting symptomatology, likewise, did not correlate with CT findings. Age does systematically relate to some factors of presenting symptomatology and degree of cortical atrophy and ventricular enlargement in AD. Lastly, estimations of deterioration and predicting the degree of deterioration is best accomplished by neuropsychological measures rather than by CT analysis.

References

Albert, M. (1984). Assessment of cognitive function in the elderly. *Psychomatics, 25*, 310–317.

Albert, M., & Stafford, J.L. (1986). CT scan and neuropsychological relationships in aging and dementia. In G. Goldstein & R.E. Tarter (Eds.), *Advances in clinical neuropsychology*. New York: Plenum Press.

Albert, M., Naeser, M.A., Levine, H.L., & Garvey, A.J. (1984a). Ventricular size in patients with presenile dementia of the Alzheimer's type. *Archives of Neurology, 41*, 1258–1263.

Albert, M., Naeser, M.A., Levine, H.L., & Garvey, A.J. (1984b). CT density numbers in patients with senile dementia of the Alzheimer's type. *Archives of Neurology, 41*, 1264–1269.

Appel, S.H. (1981). A unifying hypothesis for the cause of amyotrophic lateral sclerosis, Parkinsonism and Alzheimer's disease. *Annals of Neurology, 10*, 499–505.

Berg, L., Danziger, W.L., Storandt, M., Cohen, L.A., Gado, M., Hughes, C.P., Knesevich, J.W., & Botwinick, J. (1984). Predictive features in mild senile dementia of the Alzheimer type. *Neurology, 34*, 563–569.

Bigler, E.D. (1984). *Diagnostic clinical neuropsychology*. Austin, TX: University of Texas Press.

Bigler, E.D., Hubler, D.W., Cullum, C.M., & Turkheimer, E. (1985). Intellectual and memory impairment: CT volume correlations. *Journal of Nervous and Mental Disease, 173*, 347–355.

Bird, J.M. (1982). Computerized tomography, atrophy and dementia: A review. *Progress in Neurobiology, 19*, 91–115.

Blinkov, S.M., & Glezer, I.I. (1968). *The human brain in figures and tables*. New York: Basic Books.

Bornstein, R.A., & Matarazzo, J.D. (1984). Relationship of sex and the effects of unilateral lesions on the Wechsler Intelligence Scales. *Journal of Nervous and Mental Disease, 172*, 707–710.

Botwinick, J., Storandt, M., & Berg, L. (1986). A longitudinal behavioral study of senile dementia of the Alzheimer type. *Archives of Neurology, 43*, 1124–1127.

Brinkman, S.D., & Braun, P. (1984). Classification of dementia patients by a WAIS profile related to central cholinergic deficiencies. *Journal of Clinical Neuropsychology, 6*, 393–400.

Brouwers, P., Cox, C., Martin, A., Chase, T., & Fedio, P. (1984). Differential perceptual-spatial impairment in Huntington's and Alzheimer's dementias. *Archives of Neurology, 41*, 1073–1076.

Corballis, M.D. (1983). *Human laterality*. New York: Academic Press.

Creasy, H., & Rapoport, S.I. (1985). The aging human brain. *Annals of Neurology, 17*, 2–10.

Creasy, H., Schwartz, M., Frederickson, H., Haxby, J.V., & Rapoport, S.I. (1986). Quantitative computed tomography in dementia of the Alzheimer type. *Neurology, 36*, 1563–1568.

Crystal, H.A., Horoupian, D.S., & Katzman, R. (1982). Biopsy-proved Alzheimer disease presenting as a right parietal lobe syndrome. *Annals of Neurology, 12*, 186–188.

Cullum, C.M., Steinman, D.R., & Bigler, E.D. (1984). Relationship between "fluid" and "crystallized" cognitive function using Category and WAIS test scores. *Clinical Neuropsychology, 6*, 172–174.

Cummings, J.L., & Benson, D.F. (1983). *Dementia: A clinical approach*. Boston: Butterworths.

Cutler, N.R., Duara, R., Creasy, H., Grady, C.L., Haxby, J.V., Schapiro, M.B., & Rapoport, S.I. (1984). Brain imaging: Aging and dementia. *Annals of Internal Medicine, 101*, 355–369.

Damasio, H., Eslinger, P., Damasio, A.R., Rizzo, M., Huang, H.K., & Demeter, S. (1983). Quantitative computer tomographic analysis in the diagnosis of dementia. *Archives of Neurology, 40*, 715–719.

de Leon, M.J., & George, A.E. (1983). Computed tomography in aging and senile dementia of the Alzheimer's type. In R. Mayeux & W.G. Rosen (Eds.), *The dementias* (pp. 103–122). New York: Raven Press.

Direnfeld, L.K., Albert, M.L., Volice, L., Langlais, P.J., Marquis, J., & Kaplan, E. (1984). Parkinson's disease: The possible relationship of laterality to dementia and neurochemical findings. *Archives of Neurology, 41*, 935–941.

Duara, R., Grady, C., Haxby, J., Ingvar, D., Sokoloff, L., Margolin, R.A., Manning, R.G., Cutler, N.R., & Rapoport, S.I. (1984). Human brain glucose utilization and cognitive function in relation to age. *Annals of Neurology, 16*, 702–713.

Eslinger, P.J., Damasio, A.R., Benton, A.L., & Van Allen, M. (1985). Neuropsychologic detection of abnormal mental decline in older persons. *Journal of the American Medical Association, 253*, 670–674.

Eslinger, P.J., Damasio, H., Graff-Radford, N., & Damasio, A.R. (1984). Examining the relationship between computed tomography and neuropsychological measures in normal and demented elderly. *Journal of Neurology, Neurosurgery, and Psychiatry, 47*, 1319–1325.

Filley, C.M., Kelly, J., & Heaton, R.K. (1986). Neuropsychologic features of early- and late-onset Alzheimer's disease. *Archives of Neurology, 43*, 574–576.

Foster, N.L., Chase, T.N., Mansi, L., Brooks, R., Fedio, P., Patronas, H.J., & DiChiro, G. (1984). Cortical abnormalities in Alzheimer's disease. *Annals of Neurology, 16*, 649–654.

Fox, J.H., Kaszniak, A.W., & Huckman, M. (1979). Computerized tomographic screening not very helpful in dementia—nor in craniopharyngioma. *New England Journal of Medicine, 300*, 437.

Fox, J.H., Topel, J.L., & Huckman, M.S. (1975). Use of computed tomography in senile dementia. *Journal of Neurology, Neurosurgery, and Psychiatry, 38*, 948–953.

Friedland, R.P., Budinger, T.F., Brant-Zawadzki, M., & Jagust, W.J. (1984). The diagnosis of Alzheimer-type dementia: A preliminary comparison of positron emission tomography and proton magnetic resonance. *Journal of the American Medical Association, 252*, 2750–2752.

Fuld, P.A. (1984). Test profile of cholinergic dysfunction and of Alzheimer-type dementia. *Journal of Clinical Neuropsychology, 6*, 380–392.

Gazzaniga, M.S., & Blakemore, C. (1975). *Handbook of psychobiology.* New York: Academic Press.

Gustafson, L., Hagberg, B., & Ingvar, D. (1978). Speech disturbances in presenile dementia related to local cerebral blood flow abnormalities in the dominant hemisphere. *Brain and Language, 5,* 103–118.

Hershey, L.A., Modic, M.T., Greenough, G., & Jaffe, D.F. (1987). Magnetic resonance imaging in vascular dementia. *Neurology, 37,* 29–36.

Hyman, B.T., Van Hoesen, G.W., Damasio, A.R., & Barnes, C.L. (1984). Alzheimer's disease: Cell-specific pathology isolates the hippocampal formation. *Science, 225,* 1168–1170.

Hyman, B.T., Van Hoesen, G.W., Kromer, L.J., & Damasio, A.R. (1986). Perforant pathway changes and memory impairment of Alzheimer's disease. *Annals of Neurology, 20,* 472–481.

Jacoby, R., & Levy, R. (1980). CT scanning and the investigation of dementia: A review. *Journal of the Royal Society of Medicine, 73,* 366–369.

Kaszniak, A.W., Fox, J., Gandell, D.L., Garron, D.C., Huckman, M.S., & Ramsey, R.G. (1978). Predictors of mortality in presenile and senile dementia. *Annals of Neurology, 3,* 246–252.

Kirshner, H.S., Webb, W.G., Kelly, M.P., & Wells, C.E. (1984). Language disturbance: An initial symptom of cortical degenerations and dementia. *Archives of Neurology, 41,* 491–496.

Kitagawa, Y., Meyer, J.S., Tachibana, H., Mortel, K.F., & Rogers, R.L. (1984). CT-CBF correlations of cognitive deficits in multi-infarct dementia. *Stroke, 15,* 1000–1009.

Kitt, C.A., Price, D.L., Struble, R.G., Cork, L.C., Wainer, B.H., Becher, M.W., & Mobley, W.C. (1984). Evidence for cholinergic neurites in senile plaques. *Science, 226,* 1443–1445.

Koller, W.C., Wilson, R.S., Glatt, S.L., & Fox, J.H. (1984). Motor signs are infrequent in dementia of the Alzheimer type. *Annals of Neurology, 16,* 514–516.

Loring, D.W., & Largen, J.W. (1985). Neuropsychological patterns of presenile and senile dementia of the Alzheimer's type. *Neuropsychologia, 23,* 351–357.

MacInnes, W.D., Golden, C.J., Gillen, R.W., Sawicki, R.F., Quaife, M., Uhl, H.S.M., & Greenhouse, A.J. (1984). Aging, regional cerebral blood flow, and neuropsychological functioning. *Journal of the American Geriatric Society, 32,* 712–718.

Massman, P.J., Bigler, E.D., Cullum, C.M., & Naugle, R.I. (1986). The relationship between cortical atrophy and ventricular volume in Alzheimer's disease and closed head injury. *International Journal of Neuroscience, 30,* 87–99.

McDuff, T., & Sumi, S.M. (1985). Subcortical degeneration in Alzheimer's disease. *Neurology, 35,* 123–126.

McGeer, P.L., Kamo, H., Harrop, R., McGeer, E.G., Martin, W.R.W., Pate, B.D., & Li, D.K.B. (1986). Comparison of PET, MRI, and CT with pathology in a proven case of Alzheimer's disease. *Neurology, 36,* 1569–1574.

McGeer, P.L., McGeer, E.G., Suzuki, J., Dolman, C.E., & Nagai, T. (1984). Aging, Alzheimer's disease and the cholinergic system of the basal forebrain. *Neurology, 34,* 741–745.

Mesulam, M.M. (1982). Slowly progressive aphasia without generalized dementia. *Annals of Neurology, 11,* 592–598.

Morris, J.C., Cole, M., Banker, B.Q., & Wright, D. (1984). Hereditary dysphasic dementia and the Pick-Alzheimer spectrum. *Annals of Neurology, 16,* 455–466.

Munoz-Garcia, D., & Ludwin, S.K. (1984). Classic and generalized variants of Pick's disease: A clinicopathological, ultrastructural, and immunocytochemical comparative study. *Annals of Neurology, 16*, 467–480.
Nakano, I., & Hirano, A. (1984). Parkinson's disease: Neuron loss in the nucleus basalis without concomitant Alzheimer's disease. *Annals of Neurology, 15*, 415–418.
Naugle, R.I., Cullum, C.M., Bigler, E.D., & Massman, P. (1985). Neuropsychological and CT volume characteristics of empirically derived dementia subgroups. *Journal of Nervous and Mental Disease, 173*, 596–604.
Naugle, R.I., Cullum, C.M., Bigler, E.D., & Massman, P. (1986). Neuropsychological characteristics of atrophic brain changes in senile and presenile dementia. *Archives of Clinical Neuropsychology, 1*, 219–230.
Ramani, S.V., Loewenson, R.B., & Gold, L. (1979). Computerized tomographic scanning and the diagnosis of dementia. *New England Journal of Medicine, 300*, 1336–1337.
Raz, N., Raz, S., Yeo, R.A., Turkheimer, E., Bigler, E.D., & Cullum, C.M. (In press). Relationship between cognitive and morphological asymmetry in dementia of the Alzheimer type: At CT scan study. *International Journal of Neuroscience.*
Reitan, R.M., & Davison, L.A. (1974). *Clinical neuropsychology: Current status and applications*. Washington, DC: Winston.
Roberts, M.A., Caird, F.L., Grossart, K.W., & Steven, J.L. (1976). Computerized tomography and the diagnosis of cerebral atrophy. *Journal of Neurology, Neurosurgery, and Psychiatry, 39*, 909–915.
Rosen, W.G., Mohs, R.C., & Davis, K.L. (1984). A new rating scale for Alzheimer's disease. *American Journal of Psychiatry, 141*, 1356–1364.
Russell, E.W. (1979). Three patterns of brain damage on the WAIS. *Journal of Clinical Psychology, 35*, 611–620.
Russell, E.W. (1981). The pathology and clinical examination of memory. In S.B. Filskov, & T.J. Boll (Eds.), *Handbook of clinical neuropsychology* (pp. 287–319). New York: Wiley.
Sajdel-Sulkowska, E.M., & Marotta, C.A. (1984). Alzheimer's disease brain: Alterations in RNA levels and in a ribonuclease-inhibitor complex. *Science, 225*, 947–949.
Scheibel, A.B., & Wechsler, A.F. (1986). *The biological substrates of Alzheimer's disease.* New York: Academic Press.
Schwartz, M., Creasy, H., Grady, C.L., deLeo, J.M., Frederickson, H.A., Cutler, N.R., & Rapoport, S.I. (1985). Computed tomographic analysis of brain morphometrics in 30 healthy men, aged 21 to 81 years. *Annals of Neurology, 17*, 146–157.
Seltzer, B., & Sherwin, I. (1983). A comparison of clinical features in early- and late-onset primary degenerative dementia. *Archives of Neurology, 40*, 143–146.
Spath, H. (1980). *Cluster analysis algorithms*. Chichester, England: Ellis Harwood.
Springer, S.P., & Deutsch, G. (1981). *Left brain, right brain*. San Francisco: Freeman.
Steingart, A., Hachinski, V.C., Lau, C., Fox, A.J., Diaz, F., Cape, R., Lee, D., Inzitari, D., & Merskey, H. (1987). Cognitive and neurologic findings in subjects with diffuse white matter lucencies on computed tomographic scan (Leuko-Araiosis). *Archives of Neurology, 44*, 32–35.
Steingart, A., Hachinski, V.C., Lau, C., Fox, A.J., Fox, H., Lee, D., Inzitari, D., & Merskey, H. (1987). Cognitive and neurologic findings in demented patients with diffuse white matter lucencies on computed tomographic scan (Leuko-Araiosis). *Archives of Neurology, 44*, 36–39.
Storandt, M., Botwinick, J., Danziger, W.L., Berg, L., & Hughes, C.P. (1984). Psycho-

metric differentiation of mild senile dementia of the Alzheimer's type. *Archives of Neurology, 41*, 497–499.

Turkheimer, E., Cullum, C.M., Hubler, D.W., Paver, S.W., Yeo, R.A., & Bigler, E.D. (1984). Quantifying cortical atrophy. *Journal of Neurology, Neurosurgery, and Psychiatry, 47*, 1314–1318.

Turkheimer, E., Yeo, R., & Bigler, E.D. (1983). Digital planimetry in APLSF. *Behavioral Research Methods and Instrumentation, 15*, 471–473.

Wechsler, A.F. (1977). Presenile dementia presenting as aphasia. *Journal of Neurology, Neurosurgery, and Psychiatry, 40*, 303–305.

Wechsler, A.F., Verity, M.A., Rosenschein, S., Fried, I., & Scheibel, A.B. (1982). Pick's disease: A clinical, computed tomographic and histologic study with golgi impregnation observations. *Archives of Neurology, 39*, 287–290.

Wechsler, D. (1945). A standardized memory scale for clinical use. *Journal of Psychology, 19*, 87–93.

Wechsler, D. (1955). *Wechsler Adult Intelligence Scale: Manual*. New York: Psychological Corp.

Wechsler, D. (1958). *The measurement and appraisal of adult intelligence*. Baltimore: Williams & Wilkins.

Wells, C.E. (1984). Diagnosis of dementia: A reassessment. *Psychosomatics, 25*, 183–190.

Yeo, R.A., Turkheimer, E., & Bigler, E.D. (1984). The influence of sex and age on unilateral cerebral lesion sequelae. *International Journal of Neuroscience, 24*, 299–301.

3
Dementia of the Alzheimer Type: Challenges of Definition and Clinical Diagnosis

JEFFREY L. CUMMINGS

Dementia of the Alzheimer type (DAT) has become the focus of increasing interest and study in recent years. This intensified attention reflects the increased prevalence of dementia in a society with a rapidly expanding geriatric population and the fact that DAT is among the most common causes of intellectual deterioration in the aged. As clinicians have devoted more study to DAT and to other etiologies of acquired intellectual decline, many conceptual and definitional problems have emerged and currently remain unresolved. Among the most pressing of these issues are the following: Are the clinical manifestations of DAT sufficiently uniform to allow accurate clinical identification? What clinical features should be present before a diagnosis of DAT is warranted? How accurate are current clinical criteria in predicting a pathological diagnosis of DAT? What correlations exist between the pathological alterations of DAT and the clinical manifestations? Is DAT a single disease or should it be regarded as a clinical syndrome with a few or many etiologies? Answers to these questions are crucial to an understanding of DAT and dementia. Accurate prevalence figures cannot be obtained until criteria for the clinical diagnosis of DAT are agreed upon. The prognosis of individual patients with dementia cannot be determined unless the etiology of their dementia can be correctly established. Research regarding the treatment, progression, laboratory correlates, and neuropsychological manifestations of DAT are meaningless if homogenous groups of DAT patients cannot be identified in life. Conclusions based on clinically diagnosed DAT patients must be regarded skeptically if the correlation between clinical and pathological diagnosis is poor.

This chapter examines the difficulties of clinical definition and diagnosis of DAT. A brief history of ideas concerning the clinical identification of DAT is presented, a profile of clinical findings typical of DAT is advanced, problems raised by atypical presentations of DAT are discussed, correlations between the cardinal features of DAT and the neuropathological changes of the disorder are reviewed, and the usefulness of a standard DAT clinical profile in differential diagnosis of similar dementia syndromes is discussed. Finally, implications of DAT-related observations for understanding brain-behavior relationships and the neurological basis of thought are briefly considered.

History of Clinical Diagnosis of DAT

In 1907, Alois Alzheimer reported the disease that came to bear his name (Alzheimer, 1907). He described a woman who presented at the age of 51 with paranoia and progressive memory impairment. She made paraphasic errors when asked to name objects, had difficulty comprehending spoken and written language, and could not write correctly. She was impaired in the appropriate utilization of objects, but her motor and reflex functions remained undisturbed. She died 4 years after onset of symptoms. At autopsy, Alzheimer found abundant neurofibrillary tangles, and "miliary foci" (senile or neuritic plaques) as well as extensive cell loss in the cerebral cortex of the hemispheres. Alzheimer concluded his brief report with the following optimistic prediction (in translation): "Over a period of time we will come to the point where we can isolate single clinical cases from the larger classifications and thus more clearly define each clinical entity" (p. 43). Alzheimer's goal was thus to identify clinical features that would correlate with and correctly predict pathological findings, and he regarded the disorder that he described as an important example of the ability to make such correlations.

Alzheimer's report raised two important questions that are still debated. First, what is the relationship between DAT, senile dementia, and normal aging? Second, can DAT be identified on the basis of clinical findings or does accurate diagnosis depend on pathological examination?

Before Alzheimer's report, senile dementia was considered a normal and expected part of the aging process. In his 1895 textbook *The Pathology of the Mind*, Henry Maudsley classified the nonsyphilitic "chronic dementias" as follows: 1) dementia as a residual of mental illness; 2) dementia due to habitual alcoholic excess; 3) dementia produced by frequent epileptic seizures; 4) dementia secondary to physical damage such as trauma, tumors, or stroke; and 5) senile dementia (Maudsley, 1895/1979). The latter was explicitly considered a natural part of the aging process. In Maudsley's eloquent words: "But old age is virtually the slow natural disease of which a man dies at last when he has no other disease . . . and if that answer will not serve, there is the unanswerable argument that it [old age and dementia] is secondary to the feverish disease of life" (pp. 347–348). Alzheimer's description of a disorder characterized pathologically by excessive neurofibrillary tangles and senile plaques added another element to this nosology, but the relationships between senile dementia and DAT remained undefined, and they were regarded as separate entities with the latter beginning before age 65 and the former after age 65.

In the 1922 edition of his widely used textbook, Kraepelin noted that anatomic findings suggested that DAT might be a severe form of senile dementia, but its occasional onset in the presenium indicated that DAT was at least a precocious form of senility and possibly an independent condition (quoted by Malamud & Lowenberg, 1929). McMenemey, in 1940, championed the idea that DAT and senile dementia were age-related variants of the same disorder, and he also suggested that the underlying disturbance might be a product of various combinations of endogenous-genetic and exogenous-toxic-infective abnormalities. McMenemey also observed that the pathology of DAT–neurofibrillary tangles and neuritic plaques–occurred in clinically diverse circumstances and, therefore, the diagnosis of DAT should be based on pathological rather than clinical findings (McMenemey, 1940). This emphasis on pathological diagnosis was widely accepted and continued until the recent resurgence of interest in the clinical identification of DAT (Newton, 1948; Raskin & Ehrenberg, 1956). As information has accumulated, there has been a general, although not unanimous, consensus that DAT is correlated with specific pathological characteristics and that DAT and senile dementia are related, if not identical, disorders.

At the same time that general agreement has been achieved regarding the pathological features of DAT and the identity of DAT and senile dementia, the clinical attributes of DAT have received progressively less attention and their diagnostic relevance has been challenged. Most early reports of DAT included thorough clinical descriptions, and clinicians agreed that DAT presented with an identifiable clinical syndrome. When summarizing the cases described in the first 20 years following Alzheimer's report, Gruenthal emphasized the homogenous nature of the clinical findings. He noted that (in translation): "If we were to describe as a typical case an artificial average in which the chief features of every single case would be represented, we would hardly get anything that would differ materially from the description of any one case" (quoted by Malamud & Lowenberg, 1929, p. 805). The concurrence regarding the clinical features of DAT was sustained through the 1930s and early 1940s (English, 1942; Jervis, 1937; Rothschild, 1934) but gave way to the emphasis on pathological diagnosis after the mid-1940s.

The surrender of clinical to pathological criteria for the diagnosis of DAT became incorporated into many textbooks and dementia classifications. For example, the 2nd edition of the *Diagnostic and Statistical Manual of Mental Disorders* (American Psychiatric Association, 1968) enumerated the clinical features of senile dementia and DAT as "self-centeredness, difficulty in assimilating new experiences, and childish emotionality" (p. 24). It is little wonder that such descriptions failed to aid in differentiating DAT from other causes of dementia and reinforced the belief that identification of the etiologies of dementia depended on histological investigation.

Recently, neuropsychological and neurobehavioral studies have refocused on DAT and have resurrected the possibility of establishing clinical criteria for the recognition of DAT in the living victim.

DAT Diagnostic Criteria

Currently, the most widely accepted criteria for the diagnosis of DAT are those proposed in the 3rd edition of the *Diagnostic and Statistical Manual of Mental Disorders (DSM-III)* (American Psychiatric Association, 1980) for Primary Degenerative Dementia (PDD) (Table 3.1). To warrant the diagnosis of PDD, the

TABLE 3.1. DSM-III criteria for the diagnosis of dementia and of primary degenerative dementia.

I. Dementia
  A. Loss of intellectual abilities of sufficient severity to interfere with social or occupational functioning
  B. Memory impairment
  C. At least one of the following:
    1. Impairment of abstract thinking, as manifested by concrete interpretation of proverbs, inability to find similarities and differences between related words, difficulty in defining words and concepts, and other similar tasks
    2. Impaired judgment
    3. Other disturbances of higher cortical functions such as:
      a. Aphasia
      b. Apraxia
      c. Agnosia
      d. Constructional difficulty
    4. Personality change
  D. Consciousness not clouded
  E. One of the following:
    1. Evidence of an etiologically related disturbance
    2. Organic factors reasonably suspected and other conditions excluded

II. Primary degenerative dementia
  A. Meet above criteria for dementia (I)
  B. Insidious onset with uniformly progressive deteriorating course
  C. Exclusion of all other specific causes of dementia by history, physical examination, and laboratory tests

Note: Adapted from *Diagnostic and Statistical Manual of Mental Disorders*, 3rd ed., 1980, Washington, DC: American Psychiatric Association.

patient must meet the criteria for dementia and the dementia must be gradually progressive. Unfortunately, neither the *DSM-III* features of dementia nor those of PDD are sufficiently restrictive to confidently support the intended diagnoses. For example, Wernicke-Korsakoff patients are occupationally disabled, have memory impairments, and exhibit personality changes, thus meeting criteria for dementia. Most clinicians, however, regard the Wernicke-Korsakoff syndrome as an amnestic syndrome, not a dementia, and Wernicke-Korsakoff patients share with other amnestic patients the existence of lesions in the medial limbic circuits, not the more widespread changes characteristic of most dementias. Pick's disease, on the other hand, is generally regarded as a dementia syndrome, but does not exhibit memory impairment until the later phases of the disease course and would not meet *DSM-III* criteria for dementia until the disease is in an advanced stage (Cummings & Benson, 1983). In an effort to avoid some of these definitional pitfalls, Cummings and Benson and colleagues (Cummings & Benson, 1983; Cummings, Benson, & LoVerme, 1980) have proposed that dementia be defined as a syndrome of acquired intellectual impairment with disturbances in at least three of the following spheres of mental activities: language, memory, visuospatial skills, personality, and cognition (e.g., abstraction, calculation). This definition excludes amnestic syndromes (such as the Wernicke-Korsakoff syndrome) by demanding that at least three areas of neuropsychological activity be compromised and include dementias such as Pick's disease by allowing different combinations of intellectual impairment to be encompassed within the dementia syndrome.

Problems also arise with the *DSM-III* criteria for PDD. For the diagnosis of PDD, *DSM-III* requires that the patient meet the criteria for dementia and that the disorder be insidiously progressive (Table 3.1). Many non-DAT dementias, however, are encompassed in such a definition. Examples of non-DAT dementia syndromes that would meet criteria for PDD include alcohol-related dementias when the alcoholism is denied or inapparent, the dementia syndrome of depression if the cognitive disturbances are manifest and the affective alterations are modest, and vascular dementias if the individual infarctions have been subtle (Cummings & Benson, 1983; Hachinski et al., 1975; Ron, 1973). Pick's disease patients would also meet all criteria for PPD once the disease is sufficiently advanced to produce memory impairment (Cummings, 1982). Autopsy studies have shown that at least 18% of patients diagnosed as PDD are suffering from non-DAT dementing disorders (Sulkava, Haltia, Paetau, Wikstrom, & Palo, 1983), and long-term follow-up investigations demonstrate that 30% to 60% of patients diagnosed as suffering from degenerative dementia are eventually shown to have alternate diagnoses (e.g., depression) that accounted for the intellectual impairment (Nott & Fleminger, 1975; Ron, Toone, Garralda, & Lishman, 1979). Thus, PPD cannot be equated with DAT and more restrictive criteria allowing better correlation between clinical and pathological diagnoses of DAT are needed.

Based on recorded clinical observations of autopsy-proven DAT patients reported in the literature, Cummings and Benson (1986) suggested that DAT produces a specific clinical profile characterized by abnormal intellectual function and motor integrity throughout most of the clinical course (Table 3.2). Mental state changes include fluent aphasia, impairment of recent and remote memory, constructional disturbances, abnormal abstraction and calculation skills, and an indifferent personality. Motor abilities including speech, gait, posture, coordination, and psychomotor speed remain normal until the terminal phases of the disease. Operationalizing these criteria such that classical DAT features received a score of 2 and non-DAT manifestations received a score of 0 or 1 (depending on how much they deviated from the standard characteristics), Cummings and Benson (1986) retrospectively reviewed 50 dementia patients and identified 14 DAT patients with 100% accuracy and 36 non-DAT patients with 94% accuracy. The DAT versus non-DAT scores differed with a .005 level of significance, suggesting that it was possible to distinguish DAT from non-DAT dementias on the basis of clinical characteristics. Preliminary validation of the DAT and non-DAT diagnoses suggested by the inventory had been accomplished by neurobehavioral and neuropsychological assessments, laboratory studies (serological test for syphilis, serum calcium

TABLE 3.2. Inventory of DAT clinical features.

Function	Non-DAT (0)	Intermediate clinical features (1)	DAT (2)
1. Memory	Normal or forgetfulness that improves with clues	Recalls 1–2/3 words; aided only partially by prompting	Disoriented; unable to learn 3 words in 3 minutes; recall not aided by prompting
2. Language	Normal	Anomia; mild comprehension defects may be present	Fluent aphasia, anomia, decreased comprehension, paraphasia
3. Visuospatial	Normal or clumsy; minimal distortions	Flattening, omissions, distortions	Disorganized, unrecognizable
4. Cognition	Normal or impairment in solving complex problems	Fails to abstract proverbs and has difficulty with mathematical problems	Concrete interpretation of simple proverbs and idioms; acalculia
5. Personality	Apathetic or depressed	Appropriately concerned	Unaware or indifferent
6. Speech	Mute, severely dysarthric	Slurred, amelodic, hypophonic	Normal
7. Psychomotor	Slow, long latency to response	Hesitant replies	Normal, prompt answers
8. Posture	Distorted; flexed or extended	Stooped	Erect, normal
9. Gait	Abnormal; hemiparetic, ataxic, apraxic, or hyperkinetic	Shuffling	Normal
10. Movements	Tremor, akinesia, rigidity, chorea	Imprecise; uncoordinated	Normal

Note. Modified from Cummings and Benson, 1986, *Journal of the American Geriatrics Society, 34*, 12–19.

and phosphorus levels, liver and thyroid function studies, erythrocyte sedimentation rate, and vitamin B_{12} and folate levels), electroencephalography, and computed tomography as well as a limited number of positron emission tomography studies and autopsy investigations. Each of the features used to distinguish the DAT from the non-DAT dementias is discussed and their specific manifestations in DAT are described.

Memory Impairment

There is near-universal agreement that memory is affected early in the clinical course of DAT and remains one of the most severely impaired intellectual functions. Memory impairment is a cardinal component of all existing sets of diagnostic criteria for DAT (American Psychiatric Association, 1980; Eisdorfer & Cohen, 1980; McKhann et al., 1984; Shuttleworth, 1982). Psychometric testing of DAT patients reveals deficits in all aspects of memory functioning and demonstrates that the Logical Memory subtest of the Wechsler Memory Scale is among the most sensitive indices for distinguishing DAT patients from normal elderly individuals (Berg et al., 1984; Storandt, Botwinick, Danziger, Berg, & Hughes, 1984). Experimental investigations suggest that the major abnormality in DAT is a failure to adequately encode the stimulus material for later retrieval (Davis & Mumford, 1984; Miller, 1971, 1972). The memory impairment of DAT is such a consistent and ubiquitous feature that the diagnosis of DAT must be regarded skeptically in any individual without significant memory deficits.

Language Abnormalities

Most sets of diagnostic criteria for DAT regard aphasia as an optional component of the syndrome, but several recent studies suggest that language abnormalities are present in most if not all DAT patients (Albert, 1981; Appell, Kertesz, & Fisman, 1982; Bayles, 1982; Bayles & Tomoeda, 1983; Cummings, Benson, Hill, & Read, 1985; Skelton-Robinson & Jones, 1984). The language disturbance does not affect all functions uniformly but produces a distinctive pattern of linguistic compromise characterized by fluent verbal output, poor auditory comprehension, poor naming with paraphasia, writing impairment, and poor reading comprehension. Repetition and reading aloud are relatively spared throughout most of the disease course (Appell et al., 1982; Martin & Fedio, 1983; Schwartz, Marin, & Saffran, 1979). Poor word list generation (number of animals named in 1 minute or number of words beginning with a designated letter produced in 1 minute) and intrusion of words from one portion of the mental state examination into a later portion of the testing are also noted in DAT patients (Fuld, Katzman, Davies, et al., 1982; Martin & Fedio, 1983; Rosen, 1980). Cummings and coworkers (1985), using modified portions of the Boston Diagnostic Aphasia Examination (Goodglass & Kaplan, 1976) and the Western Aphasia Battery (Kertesz, 1979), found that DAT patients had their maximum abnormalities on the subscales measuring information content of spontaneous speech, auditory comprehension of complex commands, confrontation naming, narrative writing and writing to dictation, nursery rhyme completion, and word list generation (Table 3.3). Repetition of words, oral reading, and counting were minimally impaired. The resulting pattern of verbal output resembled transcortical sensory aphasia but contained less paraphasia and less echolalia, exhibited less of the completion phenomenon, and manifested more impairment of automatic speech production than classical transcortical sensory aphasia associated with focal posterior left

TABLE 3.3. Language abnormalities of DAT subjects.

Language characteristic	Mean scale score (standard error)
Most abnormal parameters	
Spontaneous speech	
Information content	3.83 (0.29)
Auditory comprehension	
Complex commands	3.09 (0.43)
Naming (confrontation)	3.03 (0.34)
Writing	
Dictation	3.20 (0.42)
Narrative	4.63 (0.39)
Automatic speech	
Nursery rhyme completion	3.17 (0.42)
Least abnormal parameters	
Repetition	
Words	0.80 (0.32)
Numbers	0.97 (0.36)
Phrases	1.87 (0.40)
Speech intelligibility	1.17 (0.27)
Oral reading	
Words	1.47 (0.45)
Sentences	1.97 (0.47)

Note. All scores derived from rating scales with 0=normal and 6=maximum abnormality. Only those parameters with scores greater than 3 and less than 2 are listed (Cummings et al., 1985).

hemisphere lesions (Benson, 1979). Thus, DAT usually produces a unique syndrome of language impairment that resembles, but can be distinguished from, other aphasic syndromes.

There have been relatively few longitudinal studies of the linguistic changes in DAT as they progress over the course of the disorder. The language abnormalities described previously are most characteristic of the middle phases of the illness (Table 3.4). In the initial stage of the disease, DAT patients tend to initiate less conversation, exhibit fluent empty speech, are mildly anomic, and have difficulty generating lists of words. As the disease progresses, they become less easily engaged in conversation, are anomic, manifest paraphasic errors that have increasingly less relation to the target word, exhibit shorter phrase length, have impaired comprehension of auditory and written material, and make aphasic errors in their writing. Repetition and reading aloud are relatively preserved in this stage of the disease. In the final phase, the remaining verbal output is largely incoherent and is marked by echolalia, prominent palilalia, and logoclonia. Articulatory precision may be compromised, and terminally, the patient may be mute. A mechanical agraphia replaces the aphasic agraphia (Cummings & Benson, 1983). The linguistic alterations undergo a predictable course of increasing deterioration, and the language changes correlate well with the progressive intellectual decline.

TABLE 3.4. Progressive changes in linguistic abilities in DAT.

Stage I	
	Empty, fluent speech
	Poor word list generation
	Mild anomia
	Lack of spontaneously initiated conversation
Stage II	
	Anomia
	Paraphasia with increasingly little relation to target word
	Impaired auditory comprehension
	Impaired comprehension of written language
	Aphasic agraphia
	Relative preservation of repetition and reading aloud
	Poor engagement in conversation
Stage III	
	Incoherent verbal output
	Echolalia, palilalia, logoclonia
	Diminished articulatory agility
	Terminal mutism
	Mechanical agraphia

Note. Modified and reprinted with permission of the publisher from Cummings and Benson, 1983, *Dementia: A clinical approach*, Boston: Butterworths.

Some have objected to the use of the word *aphasia* to describe the language changes of DAT. In this presentation, *aphasia* is used as a generic term to describe language changes produced by brain damage (Benson, 1979). Moreover, as described in the following section, the pathological changes of DAT are most abundant in the temporo-parieto-occipital junction region, coinciding with the site of lesions producing fluent aphasia in the more traditional aphasic syndromes associated with focal brain damage. The combination of memory, visuospatial, and cognitive deterioration with language impairment, however, produces meta-aphasic abnormalities that go beyond the changes seen with focal lesions. These meta-aphasic alterations contribute to the DAT patient's impairment of conversational initiation and engagement, progressive incoherence of verbal output, and increasing difficulty finding words within specific target categories.

Visuospatial Disturbances

Visuospatial abnormalities, along with memory and language disturbances, occur early in the course of DAT. Getting lost in familiar neighborhoods, driving the wrong direction in unidirectional lanes, and difficulty solving spatial problems (e.g., elementary mechanical tasks) are common presenting complaints, and formal testing confirms the visuospatial impairment. Patients have difficulty copying model figures and producing spontaneous drawings (Brouwers, Cox, Martin, Chase, & Fedio, 1976). Performance items of the

Wechsler Adult Intelligence Scale discriminate DAT patients from normal controls, and DAT subjects also perform significantly worse on these subtests than patients with multi-infarct dementia (Perez et al., 1975; Storandt et al., 1984). Visuospatial disturbances worsen as the disease advances (Berg et al., 1984).

Cognitive Deficits

Cognitive deficits including disturbances of abstraction and calculation are also common in DAT. Initially, patients have difficulty grasping the nuances of meanings and relationships, are impaired in the ability to abstract proverbs, and cannot solve complex mathematical problems. As the disease advances, these abnormalities become more profound and the patients cannot abstract simple idioms or solve elementary arithmetic problems (Cummings & Benson, 1983; Perez et al., 1975).

Personality, Affect, and Psychosis

Alterations of personality and behavior are more difficult to quantitate and have received less systematic study. Indifference and lack of concern are the most common personality changes noted in DAT and a majority of DAT patients manifest such alterations. Of the 377 patients studied by Larsson, Sjogren, and Jacobson (1963), 69% had "simple dementia," 18% were paranoid, 10% had affective disturbances, and 3% had a combination of paranoid and affective features. Similarly, of the 71 patients studied by Sulkava (1982), 13% were paranoid and 7% were depressed. Using a more structured approach with depression rating scales, Knesevich, Martin, Berg, and Danzinger (1983) found no measurable depression among DAT patients at the time of entry into the study or 1 year later. Other studies have found higher incidence rates of depression in DAT, but criteria for identifying DAT patients appear to have been less discriminating (Breen, Larson, Reifler, Vitaliano, & Lawrence, 1984; Kral, 1983; Reifler, Larson, & Hanley, 1982). Cummings, Miller, Hill, and Neshkes (1987) found that 20% of their DAT patients exhibited symptoms of depression but had not had a major depressive episode; 50% of the patients manifested delusions at some point in the course of their illness. Cummings (1985) investigated the delusions of DAT and found them to be loosely held, poorly structured persecutory ideas involving feelings of being endangered or having one's belongings stolen.

Motor System Changes

Abnormalities of motor function are rare in DAT (Koller, Wilson, Glatt, & Fox, 1984; Pomara, Reisberg, Albers, Ferris, & Gershon, 1981). Posture, gait, and coordination remain normal throughout most of the course of the disease, although rigidity may occur late in the disorder (Molsa, Martilla, & Rinne, 1984). Chorea, tremor, and dystonia do not occur in DAT, but myoclonus is not uncommon and may be noted in a substantial number of patients with advanced disease (Faden & Townsend, 1976; Gimenez-Roldan, Peraita, Lopez Agreda,

Abad, & Esteban, 1971; Jacob, 1970; Mayeux, Hunter, & Fahn, 1981; Wilkins, Hallett, Berardelli, Walshe, & Alvarez, 1984). Like other motor system functions, speech is not affected in DAT and articulation remains normal through most of the course (Cummings et al., 1985). Primitive reflexes such as grasp and suck also emerge in the final stages of the disease. Ophthalmoplegia and nystagmus are not apparent in DAT patients, but measurement of smooth pursuit and saccadic latencies reveal subtle abnormalities (Hershey, et al., 1983; Hutton, Nagel, & Loewenson, 1984).

Atypical DAT

So little systematic study has been devoted to the clinical features of DAT that the full variety of presentations has not been determined. Although patients in the middle and late phases of DAT have the stereotyped pattern of deficits discussed above, in the initial stages they may manifest disproportionate involvement of almost any neuropsychological faculty. Patients may exhibit predominant memory deficits, aphasia, or visuospatial abnormalities (Chase et al., 1984; Crystal, Horoupian, Katzman, & Jotkowitz, 1982; Folstein & Breitner, 1981; Foster et al., 1983). The emphasis on the standard profile of deficits described here may compromise the ability to diagnose these atypical presentations. However, most patients manifesting isolated mental status defects will be found to be suffering from non-DAT disorders and insistence on multifaculty involvement for the diagnosis helps avoid the overdiagnosis of DAT. If DAT accounts for the specific neuropsychological impairments, other abnormalities will emerge as the disorder progresses, and the correct diagnosis will become apparent during a longitudinal observation period.

Pathophysiological Correlates of DAT Clinical Manifestations

DAT has often been regarded as a diffuse or global disease, but recent studies of the geography of the histopathological changes demonstrate a distinctive pattern of distribution. Brun and Gustafson (1978) investigated the regional distribution of senile plaques, neurofibrillary tangles, granulovacuolar degeneration, neuronal loss, and cortical gliosis and found these degenerative changes to be most abundant in the medial temporal and the temporo-parieto-occipital junction region (Figure 3.1). Primary motor, somatosensory, and visual cortex were relatively spared and frontal convexity was moderately affected. A similar distribution of loss of cholinergic system enzymes was found by Davies (1978). Compared with controls, the brains of DAT patients showed greater than 80% reduction of choline acetylase activity in hippocampus, mid-temporal gyrus, parietal cortex, and cortex of frontal convexity. No significant reductions were found in basal ganglia, brain stem, precentral gyrus, postcentral gyrus, occipital lobe cortex, or cerebellum.

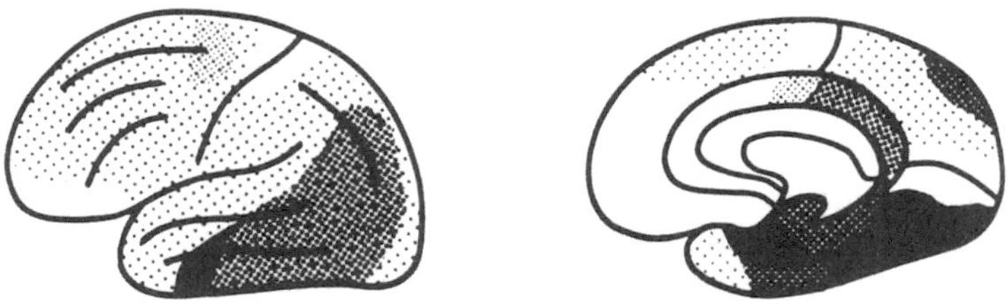

FIGURE 3.1. Relative distributions of pathological changes in patients with DAT. Darker areas are more severely involved. (Reproduced with permission of the publisher from Brun and Gustafson, 1978, *Archiv fur Psychiatie und Nervenkrankheiten, 226*, 79–93.)

Positron emission tomography (PET) provides a means for assessing cerebral metabolism in vivo. After intravenous injection of the positron-emitting radiolabeled substance, scanning and computerized reconstruction results in a map of cerebral metabolic activity. Using 18-F-fluorodeoxyglucose to investigate glucose metabolism in DAT, Benson et al. (1983) and Foster et al. (1984) found a pattern of metabolism reflecting the distribution of pathological changes discussed previously. The temporo-parieto-occipital junction and frontal lobe showed the least metabolic activity, whereas the primary motor and sensory areas showed no metabolic decrement (Figure 3.2). Most of the metabolic alterations were symmetric in the two hemispheres, but in some patients there was

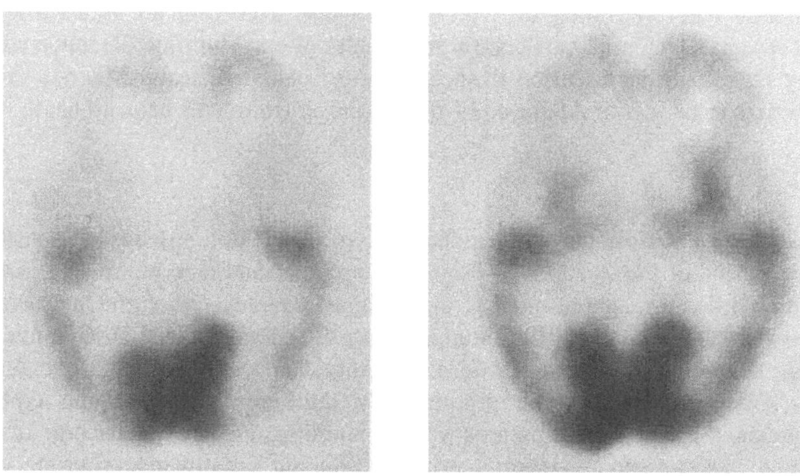

FIGURE 3.2. PET of patient with DAT showing regional alterations in glucose metabolism (horizontal section, normal metabolism appears dark, hypometabolic areas are less dense). (Reproduced with permission of the publisher from Cummings and Benson, 1983, *Dementia: A clinical approach*, Boston: Butterworths.)

greater left or right hemispheric involvement, and these asymmetries were reflected in greater verbal or performance deficits, respectively (Chase et al., 1984; Foster et al., 1983). The pattern of metabolism noted in DAT differs from that of multi-infarct dementia, Jakob-Cruetzfeldt disease, obstructive hydrocephalus, Huntington's disease, and angular gyrus syndrome (Benson et al., 1983; Cummings & Benson, 1983).

Cerebral blood flow studies support and conform to the regional pattern noted in pathological and PET studies. Cerebral blood flow is maximally reduced in the parietal regions and the frontal convexity (Gustafson, Hagberg, & Ingvar, 1978; Perez, Matthew, Stumpf, & Meyer, 1977). The flow pattern is distinguishable from that of multi-infarct dementia (Perez et al., 1977).

Thus, neuropathological investigations reveal a consistent pattern of anatomical and functional alterations with maximal involvement in the temporo-parietal junction region and the convexity of the frontal lobe. This pattern correlates well with the cardinal DAT features discussed previously, including transcortical sensory aphasia, acalculia, major visuospatial deficits, indifferent personality, and normal motor and sensory function. DAT produces a specific pattern of neuropathological alterations, and this pattern is reflected in a distinctive profile of clinical characteristics.

Differential Diagnosis of DAT

One product of an improved clinical definition of DAT is an enhanced ability to distinguish DAT from disorders that have similar clinical presentations. The two dementia syndromes most difficult to distinguish from DAT are Pick's disease and vascular dementia, particularly the angular gyrus syndrome. Recent studies have suggested that attention to specific neurobehavioral features allows these disorders to be identified and to be distinguished from DAT prior to death.

Pick's Disease

Pick's disease shares many clinical features with DAT. Both diseases begin in the same period of life, manifest a prominent aphasia, and lack motor or sensory abnormalities throughout most of their clinical courses. Other characteristics, however, can be used to differentiate the two disorders (Table 3.5) (Cummings, 1982; Cummings & Benson, 1983). Personality changes are particularly distinctive. DAT patients become progressively indifferent, whereas the typical behavior of Pick's disease patients is more extravagant. Patients become disinhibited, lack tact and judgment, may be facetious and socially inappropriate, and show a general coarsening of demeanor (Lishman, 1978). Components of the Kluver-Bucy syndrome also appear early in the course of Pick's disease and occur only late, if at all, in DAT. The Kluver-Bucy syndrome was first described in monkeys subjected to bilateral amputation of the anterior temporal lobes and is a behavioral complex consisting of placidity, hyperorality, bulimia, hyper-

TABLE 3.5. Features that distinguish DAT and Pick's disease.

Feature	DAT	Pick's disease
Behavior	Indifferent	Disinhibited
Klüver-Bucy syndrome	Late	Early
Language	Transcortical sensory aphasia; palilalia	Stereotyped verbal output; echolalia; mutism
Memory	Impaired early	Impaired late
Visuospatial skills	Impaired early	Impaired late
Calculation abilities	Impaired early	Impaired late
EEG	Normal or generalized slowing	Normal or fronto-temporal slowing
CAT scan	Normal or generalized atrophy	Fronto-temporal atrophy
Histopathology	Neurofibrillary tangles, senile plaques, granulo-vacuolar degeneration	Pick cells, Pick bodies, subcortical gliosis
Geography of pathological changes	Medial temporal and temporo-parieto-occipital junctions show most intense changes	Anterior temporal and inferior frontal regions have most intense changes

metamorphosis (forced attention to environmental stimuli), hypersexuality, and sensory agnosia (Kluver & Bucy, 1939). The syndrome has since been observed in humans with bilateral temporal lobe damage produced by a wide variety of conditions, and elements of the syndrome may be particularly prominent in Pick's disease (Cummings & Duchen, 1981; Lilly, Cummings, Benson, & Frankel, 1983).

Language disturbances occur in both DAT and Pick's disease. As noted previously, transcortical sensory aphasia is prominent throughout most of the course of DAT. Similar language changes may also occur in Pick's disease, but other linguistic alterations help to distinguish the two conditions. The anomia of Pick's disease is often of the semantic type with inability to recall the correct name and a concomitant inability to recognize the target word when supplied by the examiner. Pick's disease patients also have a greater tendency toward verbal stereotypes and an inclination to repeat the same story again and again. The latter phenomenon was labeled "gramophone syndrome" by Mayer-Gross (Mayer-Gross, Critchley, Greenfield, & Meyer, 1937–1938). In the later phases of the disease, Pick's disease patients are more likely than DAT patients to exhibit echolalia or to become completely mute (Cummings, 1982; Cummings & Benson, 1983). A few patients have retained the ability to read and write after auditory comprehension and intelligible spontaneous speech were lost (Holland, McBurney, Moossy, & Reinmuth, 1985).

Neuropsychological observations that distinguish DAT and Pick's disease involve memory, visuospatial abilities, and arithmetic skills. All of these functions are compromised early in the course of DAT, but in many cases are preserved until the middle or late stages of Pick's disease (Cummings & Benson, 1983; Robertson, le Roux, & Brown, 1958; Stengel, 1943; Wechsler, Verity, Rosenchein, Fried, & Scheibel, 1982). Thus, in contrast to DAT, Pick's disease patients may continue to remember examiners, keep appointments, find their way in familiar neighborhoods, and perform at least elementary computations at a time that behavioral and language changes are advanced.

Laboratory procedures can also help differentiate DAT and Pick's disease. The EEG may be normal in both diseases, but in some cases the tracing reveals bilateral frontal and/or temporal slowing in Pick's disease patients (Cummings & Duchen, 1981; Groen & Endtz, 1982; Munoz-Garcia & Ludwin, 1984). Likewise, computed axial tomographic (CAT) scanning in DAT is normal or reveals generalized atrophy; in Pick's disease the CAT scan frequently reveals restricted frontotemporal atrophy with relative sparing of other cortical regions (Cummings & Duchen, 1981; Groen & Endtz, 1982; McGeachie, Fleming, Sharer, & Hyman, 1979; Wechsler et al., 1982).

Pathological studies of Pick's disease demonstrate that the cell loss, gliosis, Pick bodies, and Pick cells characteristic of the disease preferentially involve the anterior temporal and orbitofrontal regions of the cerebral cortex (Brun & Gustafson, 1978). This distribution is reflected in the profound personality alterations, Kluver-Bucy symptoms, and relative sparing of visuospatial skills noted in Pick's disease. Thus, in general DAT reflects posterior hemispheric dysfunction, whereas Pick's disease correlates with anterior hemispheric alterations.

Angular Gyrus Syndrome

Multi-infarct dementia can usually be distinguished from DAT on the basis of clinical and historical characteristics such as abrupt onset, stepwise deterioration, history of previous strokes or transient ischemic attacks, depression, and focal neurological signs on examination (Hachinski et al., 1975). When a single stroke involves the posterior left hemisphere in the region of the angular gyrus, however, the resulting syndrome may closely resemble DAT (Benson, Cummings, & Tsai, 1982). The two conditions share the following characteristics: aphasia, alexia and agraphia, acalculia, right-left disorientation, finger agnosia, constructional disturbances, impaired learning of verbal material, poor abstraction skills, ideomotor apraxia, and relative paucity of motor and sensory abnormalities. Despite these similarities, other clinical features allow the two disorders to be distinguished (Table 3.6). Historically, DAT has an insidious onset, whereas the angular gyrus syndrome typically begins abruptly. Memory and topographic orientation are impaired in DAT; in angular gyrus syndrome spatial orientation and the nonverbal aspects of memory are preserved. DAT patients are unaware of their linguistic deficit, are difficult to engage in conversation, and make paraphasic errors that bear little relation to the target word. Patients with angular gyrus syndrome are often acutely aware of their deficits, do their best to converse despite their aphasia, and make within-category paraphasic

TABLE 3.6. Clinical features that distinguish DAT and the angular gyrus syndrome.

Feature	DAT	Angular gyrus syndrome
History	Insidiously progressive	Abrupt onset; vascular risk factors present
Memory	Impaired	Nonverbal memory spared
Topographic orientation	Impaired	Intact
Language		
Aware of deficit	No	Yes
Engaged	No	Yes
Paraphasia	Little relation to target word	Within-category naming errors
Reading aloud	Preserved	Impaired
Neurological examination	Normal	± Subtle right-sided abnormalities
EEG	Normal or diffuse slowing	± Left-sided slowing
CAT scan	Normal or diffuse atrophy	Normal or left-sided abnormality
PET scan	Bilateral frontal and parietal hypometabolism	Left posterior hypometabolism

Note. From Benson, Cummings, and Tsai, 1982, *Archives of Neurology, 39*, 616–620. Reprinted with permission of the American Medical Association.

substitutions. Paradoxically, DAT patients may be able to read aloud with more facility than patients with alexia with agraphia as part of their angular gyrus syndrome. In contrast to DAT, angular gyrus lesions may be associated with subtle right-sided motor or sensory defects, left-sided slowing on the EEG, or a left-sided lesion on CAT or PET images.

DAT and the Neurological Basis of Thought

Current understanding of the neurological basis of neuropsychological abilities is based largely on studies of patients with isolated focal lesions of the brain. Aphasia, amnesia, alexia, agnosia, acalculia, and apraxia are among the deficits produced by focal damage to the CNS and whose investigation has contributed to knowledge of language, memory, praxis, and arithmetic skills. Until recently, the study of dementia syndromes has been ignored as a possible model for investigation of human mental activity. Dementia was regarded as a global syndrome of progressive intellectual decline that, although tragic, was simply a matter of advancing brain failure.

Investigation of dementia syndromes such as DAT, however, has begun to influence concepts of psychological faculties and how they interact to produce the richness and complexity of human thought. The principal lesson emerging from the study of DAT is that the combination of several deficits (aphasia plus amnesia, etc.) results in a total impairment greater than the sum of the individual losses. With focal lesions, memory defects have little impact on verbal output and aphasia does not disturb memory abilities. In DAT, on the other hand, multiple defects interact to produce additive abnormalities: The memory deficit contributes to the impoverished linguistic output and the aphasia exaggerates the memory abnormalities. Language and memory abnormalities are further magnified by visuospatial and calculation deficits and together those disturbances make integrative abilities such as insight, strategy formulation, and anticipatory planning impossible. Thus, in dementia, individual abilities are compromised and the supraordinant cognitive organization that extends beyond the sum of the parts is also lost. This latter supraordinant function should not be regarded as a reformulation of a special "factor g" that represents an independent neuropsychological entity compromised in dementia. Rather, the loss of the supraordinant abilities is a product of the loss of the more basic skills and their interactions.

These considerations give rise to a tentative three-tiered model of human intellectual activity. *Fundamental functions* are basic activities such as arousal, attention, timing, and motivation mediated largely by subcortical structures (Albert, 1978). Dysfunction of these subcortical anatomic areas (basal ganglia, thalamus, and rostral brain stem nuclei) result in the clinical syndrome of "subcortical dementia" with memory impairment, cognitive dilapidation, psychomotor retardation, and prominent affective disturbances (Cummings & Benson, 1984). *Instrumental functions* are specific neuropsychological abilities such as language, memory, and calculation that are mediated by the cerebral cortex (Albert, 1978). These instrumental functions can be individually impaired by focal cortical lesions producing aphasia, amnesia, alexia, and acalculia. The instrumental abilities are coordinated through, and activities from numerous cortical areas are connected by, intra- and interhemispheric white matter tracts; these tracts may be interrupted by hemispheric lesions producing disconnection syndromes (Geschwind, 1965). Thus, instrumental disabilities may be produced by focal cortical lesions or by focal white matter lesions. Finally, there are *supraordinant functions* that result from the intactions of these more elementary abilities and are dependent on the integrity of both fundamental and instrumental functions. In DAT, fundamental functions dependent on subcortical structures are largely intact, but both instrumental abilities and their additive supraordinate functions are progressively impaired. Further investigation of DAT and other dementia syndromes will contribute to and extend an evolving conceptualization of the neurological basis of human intellectual function.

Acknowledgments. This manuscript was prepared by Joan Lopez and Norene Hiekel. Many of the studies described in this chapter were carried out in cooperation with D. Frank Benson, M.D., Augustus Rose Professor of Neurology, UCLA School of Medicine. This project was supported by the Veteran's Administration.

REFERENCES

Albert, M.L. (1978). Subcortical dementia. In R. Katzman, R.D. Terry, & K.L. Bick (Eds.), *Alzheimer's disease: Senile dementia and related disorders*. New York: Raven Press, pp. 173–180.

Albert, M.L. (1981). Changes in language with aging. *Seminars in Neurology, 1*, 43–46.

Alzheimer, A. (1907; translation, 1977). A unique illness involving the cerebral cortex. Translated by C.H. Hochberg & F.H. Hochberg. In D.A. Rottenberg & F.H. Hochberg (Eds.), *Neurological classics in modern translation*. New York: Hafner Press, pp. 41–43.

American Psychiatric Association. (1968). *Diagnostic and statistical manual of mental disorders* (2nd ed.). Washington, DC: Author.

American Psychiatric Association (1980). *Diagnostic and statistical manual of mental disorders* (3rd ed.). Washington, DC: Author.

Appell, J., Kertesz, A., & Fisman, M. (1982). A study of language functioning in Alzheimer patients. *Brain and Language, 17*, 73–91.

Bayles, K.A. (1982). Language function in senile dementia. *Brain and Language, 16*, 265–280.

Bayles, K.A., & Tomoeda, C.K. (1983). Confrontation naming impairment in dementia. *Brain and Language, 19*, 98–114.

Benson, D.F. (1979). *Aphasia, alexia, and agraphia*. New York: Churchill Livingstone.

Benson, D.F., Cummings, J.L., & Tsai, S. (1982). Angular gyrus syndrome simulating Alzheimer's disease. *Archives of Neurology, 39*, 616–620.

Benson, D.F., Kuhl, D.E., Hawkins, R.A., Phelps, M.E., Cummings, J.L., & Tsai, S.Y. (1983). The fluorodeoxyglucose 18F scan in Alzheimer's disease and multi-infarct dementia. *Archives of Neurology, 40*, 711–714.

Berg, L., Danziger, W., Storandt, M., Coben, L.A., Gado, M., Hughes, C.P., Knesevich, J.W., & Botwinick, J. (1984). Predictive features in mild senile dementia of the Alzheimer type. *Neurology, 34*, 563–569.

Breen, A.R., Larson, E.B., Reifler, B.V., Vitaliano, P.P., & Lawrence, G.L. (1984). Cognitive performance and functional competence in coexisting dementia and depression. *Journal of the American Geriatrics Society, 32*, 132–137.

Brouwers, P., Cox, C., Martin, A., Chase, T., & Fedio, P. (1984). Differential perceptual-spatial impairment in Huntington's and Alzheimer's dementias. *Archives of Neurology, 41*, 1073–1076.

Brun, A., & Gustafson, L. (1978). Limbic lobe involvement in presenile dementia. *Archiv fur Psychiatie und Nervenkrankheiten, 226*, 79–93.

Chase, T.N., Fedio, P., Foster, N.L., Brooks, R., Di Chiro, G., & Mansi, L. (1984). Wechsler adult intelligence scale performance. *Archives of Neurology, 41*, 1244–1247.

Crystal, H.A., Horoupian, D.S., Katzman, R., & Jotkowitz, S. (1982). Biopsy-proved Alzheimer disease presenting as a right parietal lobe syndrome. *Annals of Neurology, 12*, 186–188.

Cummings, J.L. (1982). Cortical dementias. In D.F. Benson & D. Blumer (Eds.), *Psychiatric aspects of neurologic disease* (Vol. 2). New York: Grune & Stratton, pp. 93–120.

Cummings, J.L. (1985). Organic delusions. *British Journal of Psychiatry, 146*, 184–197.

Cummings, J.L., & Benson, D.F. (1983). *Dementia: A clinical approach*. Boston: Butterworths.

Cummings, J.L., & Benson, D.F. (1984). Subcortical dementia. *Archives of Neurology, 41*, 874–879.
Cummings, J.L., & Benson, D.F. (1986). Dementia of the Alzheimer type: An inventory of diagnostic clinical features. *Journal of the American Geriatrics Society, 34*, 12–19.
Cummings, J.L., Benson, D.F., Hill, M.A., & Read, S. (1985). Aphasia in dementia of the Alzheimer type. *Neurology, 35*, 394–397.
Cummings, J.L., Benson, D.F., & LoVerme, S., Jr. (1980). Reversible dementia. *Journal of the American Medical Association, 243*, 2434–2439.
Cummings, J.L., & Duchen, L.W. (1981). Kluver-Bucy syndrome in Pick disease: Clinical and pathologic correlations. *Neurology, 31*, 1415–1422.
Cummings, J.L., Miller, B., Hill, M.A., & Neshkes, R. (1987). Neuropsychiatric aspects of multi-infarct dementia and dementia of the Alzheimer type. *Archives of Neurology, 44*, 389–393.
Davies, P. (1978). Studies on the neuro-chemistry of central cholinergic systems in Alzheimer's disease. In R. Katzman, R.D. Terry, & K.L. Bick (Eds.), *Alzheimer's disease: Senile dementia and related disorders*. New York: Raven Press.
Davis, P.E., & Mumford, S.J. (1984). Cued recall and the nature of the memory disorder in dementia. *British Journal of Psychiatry, 144*, 383–386.
Eisdorfer, C., & Cohen, D. (1980). Diagnostic criteria for primary neuronal degeneration of the Alzheimer's type. *Journal of Family Practice, 11*, 553–557.
English, W.H. (1942). Alzheimer's disease. *Psychiatric Quarterly, 16*, 91–106.
Faden, A.I., & Townsend, J.J. (1976). Myoclonus in Alzheimer disease. *Archives of Neurology, 33*, 278–280.
Folstein, M.F., & Breitner, J.C.S. (1981). Language disorder predicts familial Alzheimer's disease. *Johns Hopkins Medical Journal, 149*, 145–147.
Foster, N.L., Chase, T.N., Fedio, P., Patronas, N.J., Brooks, R.A., & Di Chiro, G. (1983). Alzheimer's disease: Focal cortical changes shown by positron emission tomography. *Neurology, 33*, 961–965.
Foster, N.L., Chase, T.N., Mansi, L., Brooks, R., Fedio, P., Patronas, N.J., & Di Chiro, G. (1984). Cortical abnormalities in Alzheimer's disease. *Annals of Neurology, 11*, 155–159.
Fuld, P.A., Katzman, R., Davies, P., & Terry, R.D. (1982). Intrusions as a sign of Alzheimer dementia: chemical and pathological verification. *Annals of Neurology, 11*, 155–159.
Geschwind, N. (1965). Disconnexion syndromes in animals and man. *Brain, 88*, 237–294, 585–644.
Gimenez-Roldan, S., Peraita, P., Lopez Agreda, J.M., Abad, J.M., & Esteban, A. (1971). Myoclonus and photic-induced seizures in Alzheimer's disease. *European Neurology, 5*, 215–224.
Goodglass, H., & Kaplan, E. (1976). *The assessment of aphasia and related disorders*. Philadelphia: Lea & Febiger.
Groen, J.J., & Endtz, L.J. (1982). Hereditary Pick's disease. *Brain, 105*, 443–459.
Gustafson, L., Hagberg, B., & Ingvar, D.H. (1978). Speech disturbances in presenile dementia related to local cerebral blood flow abnormalities in the dominant hemisphere. *Brain and Language, 5*, 103–118.
Hachinski, V.C., Iliff, L.D., Zilhka, E., Du Boulay, G.H., McAllister, V.L., Marshall, J., Russell, R.W.R., & Symon, L. (1975). Cerebral blood flow in dementia. *Archives of Neurology, 32*, 632–637.

Hachinski, V.C., Lassen, N.A., & Marshall, J. (1974). Multi-infarct dementia. A cause of mental deterioration in the elderly. *Lancet, 2*, 207–210.

Hershey, L.A., Whicker, L., Jr., Abel, L.A., Dell Osso, L.F., Traccis, S., & Grossniklaus, D. (1983). Saccadic latency measurements in dementia. *Archives of Neurology, 40*, 592–593.

Holland, A., McBurney, P.H., Moossy, J., & Reinmuth, O.M. (1985). The dissolution of language in Pick's disease with neurofibrillary tangles: A case study. *Brain and Language, 24*, 36–58.

Hutton, J.T., Nagel, J.A., & Loewenson, R.B. (1984). Eye tracking dysfunction in Alzheimer-type dementia. *Neurology, 34*, 99–102.

Jacob, H. (1970). Muscular twitchings in Alzheimer's disease. In G.E.W. Wolstenholme & M. O'Connor (Eds.), *Alzheimer's disease and related conditions*. London: J. and A. Churchill.

Jervis, G.A. (1937). Alzheimer's disease. *Psychiatric Quarterly, 11*, 5–18.

Kertesz, A. (1979). *Aphasia and associated disorders: Taxonomy, localization, and recovery*. New York: Grune & Stratton.

Kluver, H., & Bucy, P.C. (1939). Preliminary analysis of functions of the temporal lobes in monkeys. *Archives of Neurology and Psychiatry, 42*, 979–1000.

Knesevich, J.W., Martin, R.L., Berg, L., & Danziger, W. (1983). Preliminary report on affective symptoms in the early stages of senile dementia of the Alzheimer type. *American Journal of Psychiatry, 140*, 233–235.

Koller, W.C., Wilson, R.S., Glatt, S.L., & Fox, J.H. (1984). Motor signs are infrequent in dementia of the Alzheimer type. *Annals of Neurology, 16*, 514–516.

Kral, V.A. (1983). The relationships between senile dementia (Alzheimer type) and depression. *Canadian Journal of Psychiatry, 28*, 304–306.

Larsson, T., Sjogren, T., & Jacobson, G. (1963). Senile dementia: A clinical, sociomedical and genetic study. *Acta Psychiatrica Scandinavia* (Suppl. 167), 1–259.

Lilly, R., Cummings, J.L., Benson, D.F., & Frankel, M. (1983). The human Kluver-Bucy syndrome. *Neurology, 33*, 1141–1145.

Lishman, W.A. (1978). *Organic psychiatry*. London: Blackwell Scientific Publications.

Malamud, W., & Lowenberg, K. (1929). Alzheimer's disease. *Archives of Neurology and Psychiatry, 21*, 805–827.

Martin, A., & Fedio, P. (1983). Word production and comprehension in Alzheimer's disease: The breakdown of semantic knowledge. *Brain and Language, 19*, 124–141.

Maudsley, H. (1979). *The pathology of the mind* (based on 1895 ed.). London: Julian Freidmann.

Mayer-Gross, W., Critchley, M., Greenfield, J.G., & Meyer, A. (1937–1938). Discussion on the presenile dementias: Symptomatology, pathology, and differential diagnosis. *Proceedings of the Royal Society of Medicine, 31*, 1443–1454.

Mayeux, R., Hunter, S., & Fahn, S. (1981). More on myoclonus in Alzheimer disease. *Annals of Neurology, 9*, 200.

McGeachie, R.E., Fleming, J.O., Sharer, L.R., & Hyman, R.A. (1979). Diagnosis of Pick's disease by computer tomography. *Journal of Computer Assisted Tomography, 3*, 113–114.

McKhann, G., Drachman, D., Folstein, M., Katzman, R., Price, D., & Stadlan, E.M. (1984). Clinical diagnosis of Alzheimer's disease: Report of the NINCDS-ADRDA work group under the auspices of Department of Health and Human Services Task Force on Alzheimer's disease. *Neurology, 34*, 939–944.

McMenemey, W.H. (1940). Alzheimer's disease. *Journal of Neurology and Psychiatry, 3*, 211-240.
Miller, E. (1971). On the nature of the memory disorder in presenile dementia. *Neuropsychologia, 9*, 75-81.
Miller, E. (1972). Efficiency of coding and short-term memory defect in presenile dementia. *Neuropsychologia, 1*, 133-136.
Molsa, P.K., Martilla, R.J., & Rinne, U.K. (1984). Extrapyramidal signs in Alzheimer's disease. *Neurology, 34*, 1114-1116.
Munoz-Garcia, D., & Ludwin, S.K. (1984). Classic and generalized variants of Pick's disease: A clinicopathological, ultrastructural and immunocytochemical comparative study. *Annals of Neurology, 16*, 467-480.
Newton, R.D. (1948). The identity of Alzheimer's disease and senile dementia and their relationship to senility. *Journal of Mental Science, 94*, 225-249.
Nott, P.N., & Fleminger, J.J. (1975). Presenile dementia: The difficulties of early diagnosis. *Acta Psychiatrica Scandinavia, 51*, 210-217.
Perez, F.I., Matthew, N.T., Stump, D.A., & Meyer, J.S. (1977). Regional cerebral blood flow statistical patterns and psychological performance in multi-infarct dementia and Alzheimer's disease. *Canadian Journal of Neurological Science, 4*, 53-62.
Perez, F.I., Rivera, V.M., Meyer, J.S., Gay, J.R.A., Taylor, R.L., & Matthew, N.T. (1975). Analysis of intellectual and cognitive performance in patients with multi-infarct dementia, vertebrobasilar insufficiency with dementia, and Alzheimer's disease. *Journal of Neurology, Neurosurgery, and Psychiatry, 38*, 533-540.
Pomara, N., Reisberg, B., Albers, S., Ferris, S., & Gershon, S. (1981). Extrapyramidal symptoms in patients with primary degenerative dementia. *Journal of Clinical Psychopharmacology, 1*, 398-400.
Raskin, N., & Ehrenberg, R. (1956). Senescence, senility, and Alzheimer's disease. *American Journal of Psychiatry, 113*, 133-137.
Reifler, B.V., Larson, E., & Hanley, R. (1982). Coexistence of cognitive impairment and depression in geriatric outpatients. *American Journal of Psychiatry, 139*, 623-626.
Robertson, E.E., le Roux, A., & Brown, J.H. (1958). The clinical differentiation of Pick's disease. *Journal of Mental Science, 104*, 1000-1024.
Ron, M.A. (1973). Brain damage in chronic alcoholism: A neuropathological, neuroradiological and psychological review. *Psychological Medicine, 7*, 103-112.
Ron, M.A., Toone, B.K., Garralda, M.E., & Lishman, W.A. (1979). Diagnostic accuracy in presenile dementia. *British Journal of Psychiatry, 134*, 161-168.
Rosen, W.G. (1980). Verbal fluency in aging and dementia. *Journal of Clinical Neuropsychology, 2*, 135-146.
Rothschild, D. (1934). Alzheimer's disease. *American Journal of Psychiatry, 91*, 485-518.
Schwartz, M.F., Marin, O.S.M., & Saffran, E.M. (1979). Dissociations of language function in dementia: A case study. *Brain and Language, 7*, 277-306.
Shuttleworth, E.C. (1982). Memory function and the clinical differentiation of dementing disorders. *Journal of the American Geriatrics Society, 30*, 363-366.
Skelton-Robinson, M., & Jones, S. (1984). Nominal dysphasia and the severity of senile dementia. *British Journal of Psychiatry, 145*, 168-171.
Stengel, E. (1943). A study on the symptomatology and differential diagnosis of Alzheimer's disease and Pick's disease. *Journal of Mental Science, 89*, 1-20.
Storandt, M., Botwinick, J., Danziger, W.L., Berg, L., & Hughes, C.P. (1984). Psychometric differentiation of mild senile dementia of the Alzheimer type. *Archives of Neurology, 41*, 497-499.

Sulkava, R. (1982). Alzheimer's disease and senile dementia of the Alzheimer type. *Acta Neurologica Scandinavia, 65*, 636–650.

Sulkava, R., Haltia, M., Paetau, A., Wikstrom, J., & Palo, J. (1983). Accuracy of clinical diagnosis in primary degenerative dementia: Correlation with neuropathological findings. *Journal of Neurology, Neurosurgery, and Psychiatry, 46*, 9–13.

Wechsler, A.F., Verity, A., Rosenchein, S., Fried, I., & Scheibel, A.B. (1982). Pick's disease: A clinical computed tomographic and histologic study with Golgi impregnation observations. *Archives of Neurology, 39*, 287–290.

Wilkins, D.E., Hallett, M., Berardelli, A., Walshe, T., & Alvarez, N. (1984). Physiologic analysis of the myoclonus of Alzheimer's disease. *Neurology, 34*, 898–903.

4
Discourse Performance in Subjects with Dementia of the Alzheimer Type

HANNA K. ULATOWSKA, LEE ALLARD, ADRIENNE DONNELL, JEAN BRISTOW, SARA M. HAYNES, ADELAIDE FLOWER, and ALVIN J. NORTH

In recent years, there has been an increase in the number of investigations concerned with the language abilities of demented patients. These studies have suggested that the linguistic deficits in demented subjects may be specific rather than global. It appears that certain levels of language are disrupted, while others may be relatively spared. The majority of research has focused on lexical retrieval, although other aspects of linguistic functioning have been examined as well.

Difficulty with lexical retrieval has been reported on several types of tasks. Schwartz, Marin, and Saffran (1979), in a case study of a dementia patient, found severe impairments on picture-naming tasks and in object naming, although the patient was able to signal recognition of many items that she could not name. Naming errors were not random, but rather typically involved selection of a semantic distractor. Bayles (1982) also reported that patients with senile dementia showed deficits in a picture-naming task. Subjects produced both semantically related responses and completely unrelated responses. Bayles and Tomoeda (1983) investigated the naming impairment in dementia in more detail and found similar results: most of the subjects' naming errors were semantically related to the target; unrelated errors increased with severity of the dementia. Bayles and Tomoeda (1983) argued against a perceptual basis for the naming problem in dementia. Martin and Fedio (1983) examined both confrontation naming and verbal fluency in subjects with presumed Alzheimer's disease. In the naming task, errors typically consisted of semantically related items, similar to the results of Bayles and Tomoeda (1983). In the verbal fluency task, subjects produced fewer items and proportionately more superordinate items, compared to normals. Congruent with this body of research, Huff, Corkin, and Growdon (1986) reported that errors in object naming in presumed Alzheimer subjects usually consisted of semantically related responses.

Phonology and syntax appear to be relatively spared in dementia, at least in the mild to moderate stages. Preservation of these levels of language has been demonstrated by several researchers on several types of tasks. The patient studied by Schwartz et al. (1979) showed minimal impairments in phonology and syntax, despite marked impairments in naming and semantic knowledge. Bayles (1982) tested patients with senile dementia on a sentence correction task, in which both phonological and syntactic errors were introduced. Although patients showed some deficits relative to normals, their performance on these tasks was much better than their performance on tests of semantic competence. Similar results were reported by Bayles and Boone (1982). Appell, Kertesz, and Fisman (1982) administered the Western Aphasia Battery to presumed Alzheimer patients and reported that syntax was relatively intact. Hier, Hagenlocker, and Shindler (1985) administered a picture description task to patients with senile dementia and similarly reported that syntax was relatively preserved, although some reduction of grammatical complexity was evident.

The research reviewed above has focused on so-called "lower" levels of language, (i.e., phonology, syntax, and semantics), and has revealed marked deficits in the semantic system in the face of relatively preserved phonology and syntax. These findings are important from both a clinical perspective, insofar as they help to isolate and characterize the nature of linguistic deficits in dementia, and from a theoretical perspective, in that they help to clarify the relationship among various levels of language. However, it is also important to examine "higher" levels of language in dementia. How well do patients use language to communicate? The presence of mild semantic deficits does not in itself ensure communicative deficits, if, for example, patients are aware of and can compensate for these deficits. Nor does the presence of intact syntax imply that communication will be effective. It is, therefore, important to examine the ability of dementia patients to use language communicatively.

The results of several investigations of connected language suggest that the language of demented subjects is low in informativity (i.e., the amount of information conveyed relative to the overall amount of language produced). A picture description task used by Hier et al. (1985) revealed that demented patients, relative to normals, produced fewer relevant observations, more perseverations, and more incomplete sentences. Nicholas, Obler, Albert, and Helm-Estabrooks (1985), also using a picture description task, found that patients with presumed Alzheimer's disease produced more empty phrases and repetitions. Bayles, Tomoeda, Kaszniak, Stern, and Eagans (1985), using a verbal description task, reported that demented subjects, relative to normals, produced fewer relevant units of information and more perseverations. Appell et al. (1982) administered the Western Aphasia Battery to presumed Alzheimer patients. These authors reported that their subjects had high fluency and low information scores. They argued that their results are in accord with clinical descriptions of the speech of Alzheimer patients, in which their language is described as circuitous and verbose, while being empty and lacking meaningful content.

Another aspect of connected language that may be disrupted in dementia is use of reference. Hier et al. (1985) reported that as severity of dementia increased, their subjects produced a higher proportion of pronouns and empty words (like "thing"). However, in their overall sample, dementia patients did not produce significantly higher proportions of these items compared to normals. Nicholas et al. (1985) reported that presumed Alzheimer patients, compared to normals, produced a higher proportion of pronouns without antecedents, deictic terms (like "this" or "that"), and empty words. LeDoux, Blum, and Hirst (1983) found that dementia patients were impaired in comprehension of pronominal coreference.

The studies reviewed above have significantly increased our understanding of the language of demented subjects, but there are still gaps in our knowledge. In particular, there has been relatively little systematic research on the discourse performance of demented patients. Some of the studies mentioned above (particularly those dealing with reference or information content) did use tasks that elicited extended text (e.g., picture description or story retelling), but performance on a single task like these may not provide a very comprehensive picture of discourse abilities in dementia. Patients need to be examined on a range of discourse-eliciting tasks that vary in difficulty, degree of naturalness, and types of demands placed on subjects. The present study represents an initial attempt to analyze performance of demented subjects in connected discourse. Because of the exploratory nature of this study and the relative complexity of extended discourse, a large number of linguistic variables were selected for investigation. Also, analysis of multiple variables within the same subject sample may allow for a more precise specification of the nature of language deficits. This is especially important with demented subjects, who appear to show selective and not global deficits.

Several levels of analysis were selected. Lexical-semantic aspects of language were examined using standardized language tests. For other linguistic levels, patients' performance on several experimental language tasks was used. Syntax was studied using conventional measures of syntactic complexity; information content was examined using the number of relevant information units in each text; and reference was examined by determining the number and types of reference devices used and the number of reference errors committed. These aspects of language have been previously explored in the demented population, so the results of the current study allow for replication under different task demands. Additionally, subjects' use of narrative superstructure was examined in a number of tasks. The functional adequacy of patients' language was assessed by having listeners rate each text in terms of its communicative effectiveness and by questioning spouses (or other relatives) on various aspects of the patients' communicative behavior.

As indicated above, several experimental tasks were used in the study, to allow for replication of previous research findings in different types of tasks and to allow for direct comparison of subjects' performance in different types of communicative activity. On the basis of normal language performance, it might be expected that demented subjects would also show variability in their language performance on different tasks. Presumably, some types of tasks would be more subject to disruption than others. Therefore, in the present study, we selected tasks that we anticipated would vary in difficulty and in the types of demands placed on speakers. Also, the tasks chosen varied in their degree of naturalness, since it is reasonable to expect that demented patients may be differentially (and adversely) affected by artificial contexts for language use. All experimental tasks were intended to elicit connected discourse, appropriate for a study of communicative ability as well as linguistic performance.

The primary purpose of the present study, then, was to examine the ability of mildly and moderately impaired dementia patients to produce narrative and procedural discourse, and to isolate the linguistic levels at which deficits were evident. Additionally, we were interested in comparing the language performance of dementia patients to that of aphasics, who have been tested on similar tasks in other studies (Ulatowska, Doyel, Freedman-Stern, Macaluso-Haynes, & North, 1983; Ulatowska, Freedman-Stern, Doyel, Macaluso-Haynes, & North, 1983). Previous researchers have pointed out some similarities between the linguistic functions of demented and aphasic subjects. According to Appell et al. (1982) and Hier et al. (1985), the speech of persons with early senile dementia resembles anomic aphasia, whereas the speech of late-dementia subjects more closely resembles Wernicke's aphasia. Nicholas et al. (1985) also reported that their demented subjects, who ranged in severity from early-midstage to midstage, were not significantly different on any measure from patients with anomic aphasia.

Subjects

Ten subjects were selected for the investigation, six males and four females between the ages of 55 and 86 years (although only one subject was older than 75). Subjects were diagnosed by their neurologists as having dementia of the Alzheimer's type (DAT), based on neurological, cognitive, and behavioral testing and exclusion of alternative diagnoses. Five subjects were classified as mildly impaired and five as moderately impaired, based on clinical observation and the results of cognitive testing. Nine subjects lived in home environments with a family member; one lived in an independent-living retirement facility.

A control group of 10 subjects was matched to the experimental population in age, sex, and education. Table 4.1 shows the descriptive data for the two groups.

TABLE 4.1. Description of populations.

Measure (in years)	DAT subjects ($N = 10$)		Normal subjects ($N = 10$)	
	Mean	Range	Mean	Range
Age	68.8	55–86	68.4	56–84
Education	14.7	9–22	14.5	8–22

Materials and Methods

Cognitive and Language Tests

The test battery administered to the subjects consisted of cognitive tests and standardized language tests (see Table 4.2), as well as several experimental language tasks designed to elicit narrative and procedural discourse. The narrative tasks included: (a) a self-generated account of a memorable experience, (b) a "Cat Story" elicited by a series of pictures (Ulatowska, North, & Macaluso-Haynes, 1981), (c) a retelling of a "Wallet Story" (Bayles, 1982) immediately following the examiner's reading of the story, (d) a summary and moral for the Cat Story, and (e) a written version of the Cat Story. Procedural discourse was elicited by asking subjects to describe the routine procedures for making a sandwich, addressing and mailing a letter, and changing a light bulb.

The tests were administered in two 1½-hour sessions by the research team, which included a speech pathologist and psychologist. All testing was performed in the subject's home. Control subjects were given all tests with the exception of the Boston Diagnostic Aphasia Examination. All experimental narrative and procedural discourse tasks were tape-recorded and transcribed for analysis. The two test sessions were completed within 2 weeks of one another.

Interviews

In order to obtain preliminary information regarding language and everyday competencies or deficiencies of the DAT patients, an interview and a written questionnaire were given to each patient's spouse or other family member. The interview was administered by a member of the research team; it took 30 to 45 minutes. The spouse or other family member was interviewed without the patient being present. The interview dealt with cognitive function in such areas as orientation to place and time, recent memory, new learning, judgment, and problem solving. It also dealt with the subject's use of speech and language in

TABLE 4.2. Cognitive and standardized language tests.

I. Standardized tests to evaluate language functioning:
   A. Selected subtests of the Boston Diagnostic Aphasia Examination
   B. The Boston Naming Test
   C. The Verbal Fluency Test (number of words beginning with "s" that could be produced in 60 seconds)

II. Tests to evaluate cognitive functioning:
   A. The Mini-Mental Status Exam
   B. Sets A and B of the Raven Coloured Progressive Matrices Test
   C. The Block Design Subtest of the WAIS
   D. Symbol-Digit (modified from the WAIS by using symbol cues and digits as responses)
   E. Symbol-Digit Recall
   F. The Buschke Selective Reminding Test (Buschke, 1973)

everyday communication, including the patient's ability to comprehend others and the clarity of his or her language. Finally, strategies utilized by family members in giving directions or explanations to the subject were elicited. The interview probed for specific instances of competencies and deficiencies and was tape-recorded. The method of data reduction was to listen to the tape and write down the most salient characteristics of patients' behavior, either verbatim or in paraphrase.

Questionnaire

The questionnaire administered to family informants consisted of 48 items pertaining to the use of speech and language, 22 items pertaining to competencies in everyday life, and 10 items pertaining to social and personal behavior. The respondent was asked to judge the proportion of days that the behavior in question had been observed within the previous 2 weeks.

Methods for Data Analysis

The tape-recorded data from the experimental language tasks were transcribed verbatim with verification for accuracy by a second listener. The basic unit for segmenting the data was the T-unit, defined as one independent clause plus the dependent modifiers of that clause (Hunt, 1965). Comparisons between groups were statistically analyzed using Mann-Whitney U-Tests. A nonparametric technique was chosen because of the small sample size and large within-group variance on some parameters. For purposes of analysis, the three procedures were always treated in combination, that is, a composite score was derived. Generally, the three narrative tasks were analyzed separately, due to the differing demands imposed by each. The Cat Story involved a description of a series of pictures; this task therefore placed minimal demands on recent memory or retrieval of information from long-term memory. Furthermore, the pictures provided some degree of structure for the task. The Wallet Story, a retelling, placed heavier demands on recent memory but minimal demands on retrieval of old information. The structure of this text was completely provided. In the Memorable Experience, demands were placed on retrieval of information from long-term memory and minimal structure was provided. On sentence level and reference measures, the three narrative tasks (Cat Story, Wallet Story, and Memorable Experience) were combined for ease of presentation, since there were not marked differences among the tasks on these parameters. For certain sentential and reference measures having a low frequency of occurrence, results are reported only for all tasks combined (i.e., the three procedures and three narratives), to allow for more reliable statistical analysis. Results for the Written Cat Story are not presented in detail, since there were no significant group differences on this task for any parameter. Linguistic analyses were not performed on the Cat Story summary or moral, due to the very small amount of language produced for these tasks. The discourses were analyzed in terms of sentential grammar, content characteristics, discourse grammar, and reference.

Sentential Analysis

Variables dealing with sentential level characteristics included:

1. Length of T-units and clauses as measured by number of words
2. Complexity of language as measured by amount of embedding, expressed in number of clauses per T-unit
3. Disruption of language as measured by:
   a. Number of grammatically incorrect sentences
   b. Number of incomplete sentences (i.e., utterances in which the subject did not complete a thought)

Additionally, rate of speech as measured by number of words per minute was calculated.

Content Analysis

Variables pertaining to content analysis included the following:

1. Amount of information as measured by a priori propositions, with a proposition defined as one predicate plus one or more arguments (The original set of a priori propositions was derived by an analysis of the stimulus material, i.e., Cat Story, Wallet Story, procedures. In a previous article on procedural discourse [Ulatowska, Doyel, et al., 1983], the category of a priori propositions was divided into two categories: essential steps and target steps.)
2. Elaboration (i.e., propositions giving additional relevant information beyond that which was established as a priori)
3. Irrelevant propositions (i.e., propositions not related to the task or not adding new information, such as personal comments, digressions, and redundancies)
4. Incorrect propositions (In the Cat Story, these consisted of propositions that were not consistent with the picture stimuli; in the Wallet Story, these consisted of propositions not included in the original story; and in the procedures, these included steps that would not be a part of the performance of that procedure.)

Discourse Structure Analysis

Narrative tasks were evaluated in terms of discourse grammar characteristics. The following components are considered necessary for a well-developed narrative: setting, complicating action, and resolution. Optional elements include an abstract, coda, and evaluation. (For more detail on the methodology used here, see Ulatowska, Freedman-Stern, et al., [1983].) Each of the three narrative tasks (i.e., Cat Story, Wallet Story, and Memorable Experience) was evaluated along two dimensions: first, according to which components were included, and second, according to the percentage of total propositions accounted for by each component.

Reference Analysis

The following measures were employed in the investigation of reference:

1. Pronoun-to-referent ratio: Defined as the ratio of all pronouns to all occurrences of nouns serving as pronominal referents (This measure was assumed to be more sensitive than the overall pronoun-to-noun ratio in revealing a subject's strategies for using reference.)
2. Reference errors: A reference error was assumed to have occurred under the following conditions:
   a. No clear referent for a pronoun could be found
   b. More than one referent could reasonably be assigned to a pronoun (ambiguous reference)
3. Demonstratives: A category consisting of the terms *this/these, that/those, here,* and *there*
4. Indefinite nouns and pronouns: A category that includes such items as *thing, stuff, someone, something,* and so forth
5. Exophoric reference: Defined as a reference item for which the antecedent does not occur in the speaker's text, but rather in the external context or in a previous speaker's discourse

Ratings of Content and Clarity

In addition to the above objective analyses, a rating system was devised to evaluate the informativity of the discourse produced and the clarity of the language. Three trained speech pathologists were asked to listen to randomly ordered tape recordings of the narratives and procedures for both subject groups. For the narratives, the raters were asked to score each text on a 3-point scale for informativity, clarity of language, and relevance. For the procedures, raters were asked to score each text on six measures of content and clarity, using a 3- or 4-point scale.

Results

Standardized Language Tests

Table 4.3 summarizes the language profiles obtained from selected subtests of the Boston Diagnostic Aphasia Examination (BDAE) administered to the 10 DAT subjects. In addition to lower scores on the Severity Rating Scale Profile, four of the five subjects classified as moderate also experienced difficulties on the comprehension of complex material and animal-naming subtests. These same four subjects also performed less well on the reading comprehension of sentences and

TABLE 4.3. DAT subjects' performance on Boston Diagnostic Aphasia Examination.

Test	Possible points	Mean	Range	*SD*
Severity rating	5	4.4	2.5–5.0	0.9
Boston total score	320	296.6	211–320	31.6
Auditory comprehension (total score)	99	91.9	58–99	12.3
Complex ideational material	12	8.9	4–12	2.6
Oral expression (total score)	184	170.7	131–184	15.0
Animal naming	19	11.3	4–19	5.6
Understanding written language (total score)	20	17.6	8–20	3.7
Reading sentences/ paragraphs	10	8.3	5–10	1.9
Writing (total score)	17	16.5	14–17	1.0

Note. $N = 10$.

paragraphs. Within this moderate group, one subject consistently received markedly reduced scores on all subtests with the exception of responsive naming and written confrontation naming.

There was a trend ($p < .1$) toward better performance by the normals on the Verbal Fluency Test (see Table 4.5). Additionally, the results of an analysis of errors made on the Boston Naming Test are included in Table 4.4. The error rate of DAT subjects is significantly higher. The distribution of error types is similar for both populations in that semantically associated errors constitute the most frequent error type and the subtype of "same category" errors is most frequent for both populations.

TABLE 4.4. Naming errors in percentages on Boston Naming Test.

Categories of classifiable errors	DAT	Normal
Unrelated responses	3	0
Visually similar	16	13
Semantically associated		
Same category	55.4	61.9
Superordinate	21.5	4.8
Function	9.2	28.6
Context	7.7	4.8
Part of whole	3.1	0
Attribute	3.1	0
Total	80	87

Note. The naming error rate was 24.4 for DAT subjects and 14.1 for normal subjects with a significance of $p < .001$ on the chi-square test. The naming error rate was derived from the percentage of errors out of the total number of responses obtained for the population.

Cognitive Tasks

Table 4.5 describes the performance of the DAT subjects and the normal subjects on the cognitive tests. The normal patients performed significantly better on the Mini-Mental Status Exam, the Block Design and Symbol Digit (modified) subtests of the Wechsler Adult Intelligence Scale (WAIS), and the Buschke Selective Reminding Test. There was a trend ($p < .1$) toward better performance by the normals on the Symbol Digit Recall Test.

Linguistic Tasks

Success and Failure on Tasks

Nine DAT subjects succeeded in producing the Cat Story while only three were successful at producing the Cat Summary. Four DAT subjects produced a retelling instead of a summary and three failed completely (e.g., by focusing on trivial or irrelevant information). All of the normal subjects succeeded on the Cat Story and nine produced summaries. Only one normal subject produced a retelling instead of a summary. On the Wallet Story, eight DAT subjects completed the task, although one subject had a large number of additions to the story and a different ending than that of the original story. All controls succeeded on the task. On the Memorable Experience, both populations of subjects succeeded on the task. All DAT subjects and all normal subjects succeeded in producing the three procedures.

Sentential Analysis

Table 4.6 summarizes and compares the sentence level characteristics of the narrative and procedural discourses produced by the DAT and normal subjects. They reveal that there was no statistically significant difference between the populations on the amount of language produced as measured by the number of T-units or by the length of T-units and clauses (in number of words). There was also no

Table 4.5. Performance on cognitive tests and Verbal Fluency Test.

	DAT		Normal		
Test (raw score)	Mean	*SD*	Mean	*SD*	Significance
Mini-Mental Status	22.0	5.5	28.7	1.1	$p<.01$
Raven Coloured Progressive Matrices	13.0	6.5	18.1	4.5	
Block Design	17.5	15.0	34.9	9.5	$p<.05$
Symbol Digit (total)	18.2	14.7	39.3	10.4	$p<.01$
Symbol Digit Recall	1.8	2.4	3.4	1.8	
Buschke Memory (total)	5.2	2.2	7.8	0.9	$p<.01$
Buschke Memory (recognition)	16.7	3.5	19.5	1.0	$p<.05$
Verbal Fluency	9.6	5.5	14.6	4.7	

TABLE 4.6. Comparison of DAT and normal subjects on selected sentential measures derived from analysis of narrative and procedural discourse.

Measure	DAT Mean	DAT *SD*	Normal Mean	Normal *SD*	Significance
Number of T-units					
Narratives	47.0	18.9	41.9	9.7	
Procedures	35.4	11.1	34.8	4.9	
Words per T-unit					
Narratives	10.9	1.8	10.7	1.8	
Procedures	10.0	1.5	9.0	1.9	
Clauses per T-unit					
Narratives	1.8	0.3	1.9	0.6	
Procedures	1.6	0.2	1.5	0.3	
Words per dependent clause					
Narratives	6.6	0.6	6.3	0.8	
Procedures	6.7	1.1	6.1	0.9	
Words per minute					
Narratives	131.3	24.7	148.3	21.1	
Procedures	128.1	13.4	140.7	32.0	
Incorrect sentences					
All tasks	1.8	2.1	1.5	1.0	
Incomplete sentences					
All tasks	3.4	2.2	1.5	1.1	$p < .05$

difference in the complexity of language as measured by the number of clauses per T-unit. Finally, there was no significant difference in rate of speech as measured by number of words per minute on either narrative or procedural tasks.

Additional analyses of various types of disruptions of language as manifested by incomplete sentences and incorrect sentences revealed that DAT subjects produced significantly more incomplete sentences on all tasks combined. There was no significant difference on number of incorrect sentences for all tasks combined.

Content Analysis

Table 4.7 summarizes the performance on content measures for DAT and normal subjects. There were significant differences between the populations on the number of a priori propositions on the Wallet Story and on the combined procedures, with DAT subjects producing less information. DAT subjects also produced more incorrect and irrelevant propositions on the combined procedures, and more irrelevant propositions on the Memorable Experience. On the Cat Story, DAT subjects produced more elaborations.

TABLE 4.7. Comparison of DAT and normal subjects on measures of content.

Measure	DAT Mean	DAT *SD*	Normal Mean	Normal *SD*	Significance
A priori propositions					
Cat Story	11.1	2.2	10.2	1.9	
Wallet Story	8.3	2.8	10.0	1.1	$p<.05$
Procedures	12.6	1.2	15.1	1.1	$p<.01$
Elaborations					
Cat Story	5.6	2.7	2.8	1.9	
Wallet Story	0.9	1.1	1.0	0.8	
Procedures	12.0	6.3	17.5	6.4	
Irrelevant/incorrect propositions					
Cat Story	1.8	2.0	1.5	2.2	
Wallet Story	3.1	3.5	1.0	1.6	
Memorable Experience[a]	12.3	15.4	1.3	1.4	$p<.01$
Procedures	11.8	8.1	2.2	3.0	$p<.01$

[a] For the Memorable Experience, only irrelevant propositions were coded.

Discourse Structure Analysis

The results of the analysis of discourse structure of the narrative tasks of the DAT subjects, summarized in Table 4.8, revealed the preservation of narrative superstructure as manifested by the following:

1. All subjects' narratives of the Cat Story and the Wallet Story contained all of the essential elements of the superstructure (i.e., setting, complicating action, and resolution).
2. Six out of seven Memorable Experiences recounting narrative episodes contained resolutions.
3. Some narratives contained the optional elements of evaluations, abstracts, and codas.
4. All DAT subjects who were able to complete the task showed preservation of the chronological sequence on the Cat Story and Wallet Story. Eight subjects showed preservation of chronology on the Memorable Experience.
5. In the Wallet Story and Memorable Experience, the relative length of each element of the narrative superstructure as measured by the proportion of total propositions was not significantly different in the DAT subjects as compared to normals. However, in the Cat Story, the DAT subjects produced a higher proportion of setting propositions at the beginning of the stories and after the resolution, whereas normal subjects produced a higher proportion of resolution propositions.

Performance on Cat Morals

Responses given by the subjects on the moral-giving task were subclassified according to their semantic content and form into the following categories:

TABLE 4.8. Comparison of DAT and normal subjects on mean percentages of propositions in each element of narrative superstructure.

	Cat Story		Wallet Story		Memorable Experience	
Measure	DAT	*N*	DAT	*N*	DAT	*N*
Setting	38.8	22.0*	14.2	13.5	28.1	36.3
Action	33.9	46.0	52.4	55.9	37.4	33.3
Resolution	10.7	16.2*	30.8	30.6	9.1	5.8
Evaluation	16.6	15.8	1.6	0.0	22.5	15.9

*$p < .05$.

moral/proverb, advice, summary, and failure. (See Ulatowska et al. [1981] for more detail on this analysis.) Two normals produced morals; seven produced some kind of advice; and one failed. None of the DAT subjects gave morals; four produced advice; two produced summaries; and four failed. Comparison of the performance of the two populations indicates considerable impairment of DAT subjects on this task.

Reference

Table 4.9 summarizes the performance of DAT and normal subjects on measures of linguistic reference. DAT subjects produced a significantly higher pronoun-to-referent ratio on the combined procedures. DAT subjects produced significantly more reference errors on the combined narrative tasks and on the combined procedures. Also, DAT subjects produced more demonstratives on the narrative tasks. This last effect was due primarily to the greater use of demonstrative adverbs by the DAT subjects, with significant differences being found on the combined narratives and on the combined procedures.

Statistical comparisons for number of indefinite nouns and pronouns and instances of exophoric reference were calculated only for all tasks combined. Compared to normals, the DAT subjects produced significantly more indefinite nouns and pronouns. There was a trend ($p < .06$) for the DAT subjects to produce more exophoric references.

INTERVIEW AND QUESTIONNAIRE

Because of the small sample size, the data from family members who were interviewed and who answered the questionnaire were tallied, but no further statistical analysis was attempted. Data were available for 8 of the 10 subjects. The following is a summary of the results that describe, on a daily basis, the communicative functioning of the DAT subjects.

Social skills were relatively well preserved to the extent that 50% of the subjects frequently shook hands and touched others appropriately. All of the subjects

TABLE 4.9. Comparison of DAT and normal subjects on measures of linguistic reference.

	DAT		Normal		
Measure	Mean	*SD*	Mean	*SD*	Significance
Pronoun/referent ratio					
Narratives	0.73	0.07	0.67	0.08	
Procedures	0.66	0.14	0.50	0.15	$p<.05$
Reference errors					
Narratives	4.2	3.9	2.2	4.0	$p<.05$
Procedures	8.2	9.6	2.2	4.0	$p<.05$
Total demonstratives					
Narratives	11.2	6.0	6.0	3.2	$p<.05$
Procedures	7.6	6.0	3.3	3.3	
Demonstrative adverbs					
Narratives	5.2	3.8	1.7	1.8	$p<.05$
Procedures	3.6	2.8	0.6	1.0	$p<.01$
Indefinite nouns/pronouns (all tasks)	7.8	3.8	2.3	2.0	$p<.01$
Exophoric reference (all tasks)	4.1	3.2	1.8	2.0	

maintained eye contact while speaking, and 75% of the subjects spoke with facial expressiveness and took turns in speaking with others.

All of the subjects conversed with other persons on at least 75% of the days in the reporting period. Twenty-five percent of the subjects were reported to have difficulty with staying on the topic. The majority of subjects (63%) were reported to display memory deficits in their conversation, reflected by often repeating what they had said shortly before, by repeatedly asking another for the same information, or by requiring instructions from others over and over again. To some family members, these repetitions represented the earliest, most salient changes in conversation.

Within the 2-week reporting period, all but one subject talked about matters pertaining to the larger world on at least half the days, 75% recounted a memorable personal experience, and 50% told a joke or said something intended to be funny. None of the subjects used procedural discourse (i.e., gave step-by-step directions about how to do a task).

RATINGS OF CONTENT AND CLARITY

Because the interrater reliabilities were unacceptably low, results of the ratings will not be presented in detail. Generally, the raters were unable to reliably discriminate between DAT and normal subjects on the Cat Story, Wallet Story, Light Procedure, and Memorable Experience. For the Sandwich Procedure, two of the three raters scored the DAT subjects significantly lower than the normals. For the

Cat Summary and Letter Procedure, all three raters gave the DAT subjects significantly lower scores than the normals. The authors feel that the raters' inability to discriminate between groups on several of the tasks reflected a real lack of obvious group differences between the DAT subjects and normals on those tasks. The raters were only allowed to listen to each text one time; more subtle differences in the language performance of the two groups, which emerged in our linguistic analyses, may not have been apparent from a single listening.

Discussion

In this section, the results of this study are summarized. Then the important findings of this study are discussed, and possible explanations for the performance of the DAT subjects are offered. This section of the discussion focuses especially on the impairments of content and reference, which the authors feel to be the most significant findings of the study. Finally, the authors compare and contrast the language performance of DAT, aphasic, and old elderly subjects (ages 77 to 92).

Several significant results emerged from this research. Our group of 10 mild to moderately impaired DAT subjects showed areas of relatively impaired performance and other areas of relatively intact performance. Subjects showed preservation of sentential level and discourse level linguistic structures, as evidenced by the absence of significant differences between DAT and normal subjects either in the amount or complexity of language, or in the manipulation of narrative superstructure. The DAT subjects did show marked deficits in their ability to produce a summary and moral for the Cat Story. Also, DAT subjects showed deficits in both content and reference. Analysis of content revealed that subjects produced a reduced number of a priori propositions and an increased number of incorrect and irrelevant propositions. In the area of reference, subjects showed an increase in reference errors and a greater use of pronouns and deictic terms. (Examples of some of these characteristics of the language of DAT subjects are provided in Appendix 4.A).

The most obvious disruption in the subjects occurred at the level of content, an area in which relatively little formal research has been conducted. Although DAT subjects produced as much language as normals, their language conveyed fewer a priori propositions. Instead, DAT subjects produced a greater amount of irrelevant or incorrect information, particularly on the more difficult tasks (i.e., Memorable Experience and procedures). A significant reduction in a priori propositions was found in the Wallet Story and in the combined procedures. In the Wallet Story, a simple retelling task, the reduction most likely reflected a memory deficit. It is possible that deficits in auditory comprehension, indicated by depressed scores on the Complex Ideational Materials subtest of the BDAE, may have contributed to the reduction in a priori propositions. However, the fact that most subjects were able to correctly reproduce the superstructure of the story suggests that their comprehension of it was relatively unimpaired. Another possible explanation involves attentional deficits: The lowered performance of

DAT subjects may have resulted from a failure to encode some of the information components of the story, rather than an inability to retrieve those components. Our data does not allow us to distinguish between these possibilities.

The reduction of a priori propositions in the combined procedures may reflect more extensive deficits. The procedural tasks were presumably more difficult than the Cat Story and Wallet Story, which were structured, stimulus-bound tasks not requiring recall and organization of information from long-term storage. The procedures, in contrast, do require recall and organization of ideas. (Even though the *performance* of the procedures may be routine, subjects probably seldom have reason to verbally explain how to perform these tasks.) Disruption in procedural discourse could, therefore, occur at a number of points. The reduction of a priori propositions could reflect: (a) memory deficits, since the subject must draw from memory the steps involved in the procedure; (b) an inability to effectively organize one's thoughts, resulting in a simplification of the procedure; or (c) an inappropriate response to the task demands, with subjects assuming that it was unnecessary to relate certain steps of the procedure. It is likely that all three factors contributed to some extent to the reduction of a priori propositions. With respect to organization of thoughts, however, it should be noted that most of the DAT subjects did preserve the correct sequence of steps, even if some steps were omitted.

In addition to the reduction in a priori propositions, there was an increase in irrelevant and incorrect propositions in the discourse of the DAT subjects, with marginally significant differences being found on the Wallet Story, and significant differences on the Memorable Experience and combined procedures. In the Wallet Story, several subjects included incorrect propositions, which were likely attributable to memory deficits. Irrelevant propositions, which were infrequent, were usually of a metalinguistic nature, in which the subject commented on the process of their retelling of the narrative. In the Memorable Experience, irrelevant propositions fell into two main categories: digressions and redundancies. Digressions, indicative of a subject's inability to remain focused on the topic of the narrative or the demands of the task, may reflect a failure to monitor the relationship of current language output to previous output. Both digressions and redundancies may also result from memory deficits, since, in the production of connected discourse, one must maintain a "trace" of what one has previously said. Data from the interviews and questionnaires completed by family members support the finding of frequent repetition in the discourse of DAT subjects: five of eight subjects for whom data were available were reported to show memory deficits manifested in part by a tendency for the subject to repeat himself or herself. In the procedures, incorrect propositions were occasionally produced; digressions were somewhat more frequent. Digressions generally consisted of comments related to but not part of the procedure.

In addition to the possible underlying factors mentioned previously, the production of irrelevant information may result from pragmatic violations. Grice's (1975) principles of conversational discourse (which apply to any type of discourse uttered with communicative intent), dictate that speakers should: (a) provide information that is relevant to the topic, (b) provide neither too much nor too little information, and (c) present their information in a clear manner. DAT subjects violate all three principles, perhaps as a result of failure to recognize the needs of their listeners. As is discussed below, pragmatic violations may also contribute to the disruption of reference seen in DAT subjects.

It is also possible that subjects' production of irrelevant information is related to their inability to produce adequate summaries for the Cat Story. The intrusion of irrelevant propositions into the procedures or narratives reflects a difficulty in differentiating between information that is necessary for the task and information that is not. Similarly, and to an even greater extent, summarizing requires that the subjects differentiate between more important and less important information. An inability to do so would result in a summary that contains either trivial information or, at an even more disrupted level, information not related to the task at all. Both types of inappropriate response occurred in the summaries of DAT subjects.

An unexpected finding that emerged from the analysis of content was the significantly higher number of elaborations, suggestive of a greater level of detail, produced by the DAT subjects in the Cat Story. As mentioned earlier, elaborations consisted of correct units of information beyond what were established as a priori propositions. The authors feel that the greater level of detail given by the DAT subjects for this task was the result of two factors. First, the Cat Story was the easiest of the tasks, since it was prompted by a series of pictures and therefore made fewer demands on memory and organization of thought. Second, it appeared that the DAT subjects may have taken the task more seriously than the normals, some of whom produced terse, abbreviated narratives. On the procedures, which were more difficult tasks, results were in the expected direction: There was a trend for the DAT subjects to produce fewer elaborations.

While our analysis of content measured the amount and type of information conveyed, analysis of narrative superstructure measured the organization of information. Contrary to our expectations, the DAT subjects showed preservation of superstructure elements in the narrative tasks (Cat Story, Wallet Story, and Memorable Experience). Although it is possible that these results indicate that subjects' knowledge of narrative superstructure is resistant to disruption, the authors feel that preservation of superstructure in the present study more likely reflects the relative simplicity of the tasks. In the Cat Story and Wallet Story, the structure is provided, in one case (Cat Story) by a sequence of pictures, and in the other case (Wallet Story) by the narrative stimulus itself. The Memorable Experiences, while more complex, were likely to have been narratives that subjects recounted frequently, so that their structure was in a sense overlearned. The only suggestion of disrupted superstructure among our subjects may have been their tendency to produce longer settings (and proportionately shorter complicating actions and resolutions) in the Cat Story. In this task, setting propositions were generally descriptive statements that contributed relatively little to the narrative. A subject who overuses setting propositions in this type of task is, to some extent, simply producing a picture description, not a narrative. The DAT subjects also produced more setting clauses after the resolution of the story. In a well-formed narrative, setting clauses generally should appear at the beginning. The intrusion of setting propositions into later sections of a narrative may reflect some degree of disruption in knowledge of or ability to manipulate narrative superstructure.

Another area of disruption in DAT subjects was the use of reference. Nicholas et al. (1985) found that presumed DAT subjects showed some disruption of linguistic reference, characterized by greater use of deictic terms (*this, that, here, there*) and by an increased frequency of pronouns without antecedents. Our results replicate these findings, but additionally we have analyzed the disruption of reference in more detail. In particular, we were interested in: (a) possible explanations for the disruption of reference, and (b) the manner in which disrupted reference can contribute to the low informativity or "emptiness" of language, which is often characteristic of the discourse of DAT subjects.

There were significant group differences in the pronoun-to-referent ratio, with DAT subjects producing a higher proportion of pronouns. It should be noted that a high pronoun-to-referent ratio is not in itself an indicator of pathology. Given that use of pronouns is often optional in English, a high proportion of pronouns may in some cases represent a stylistic preference. These measures of pronoun usage are indicators of pathology only when pronouns are being used inappropriately in place of nouns. In our study, there were several examples of DAT subjects producing a text with a high proportion of pronouns, but which was still clear and coherent.

However, as a group, the DAT subjects produced significantly more reference errors than the normals, indicating that they were not only using more pronouns, but were often using them inappropriately. The majority of errors in both groups involved use of pronouns without an explicit antecedent, although in many of these cases the referent could be determined by inference. Another group of errors involved ambiguous reference, which often resulted from inappropriately using a pronoun instead of a noun to reintroduce a referent after a topic shift. There were no differences between DAT and normal subjects in average distance between pronouns and their referents. Thus, the primary factor underlying disruption of reference in DAT subjects does not appear to involve simply a tendency to use pronouns that are relatively far apart from their referents.

At least three explanations can be offered for the higher proportion of pronouns and increased frequency of errors in the DAT subjects: 1) naming difficulties, 2) failure to take into account the pragmatic demands of communication, and 3) memory deficits. For most of the DAT subjects in our sample, the high pronoun-to-referent ratio did not seem to reflect a naming difficulty. The production of an excessive number of pronouns often seemed to reflect a failure to renominalize a noun referent that had already been produced, rather than a simple inability to produce that noun.

However, pragmatic factors (e.g., knowing the listener's needs) do appear to play a role in the disruption of reference seen in DAT subjects. Successful use of pronouns in discourse requires that the listener be able to recover the antecedent for the pronoun without undue effort. Generally speaking, reference items should only be used to refer to the current topic of discourse. If a previous topic is to be reintroduced, a noun, not a pronoun, should be used. It is possible, though necessarily speculative at this time, that DAT subjects have suffered a breakdown in pragmatic knowledge, rendering them less able to take into account their listener's needs.

Memory deficits may also play a role in disruption of reference. Production of discourse requires the speaker to maintain in memory some trace of what he or she has already said. Deficits at this level of processing could manifest themselves as reference errors. However, many reference errors involved pronouns that were relatively near their (presumed) referents. Thus, while memory deficits may help to account for some of the errors made by the DAT subjects, other factors must have contributed as well.

Two classes of reference items particularly contributed to reduced informativity in the language of DAT subjects: demonstratives and indefinite pronouns. Compared to normals, DAT subjects produced significantly more demonstratives, an effect primarily due to a greater use of the demonstrative adverb *there*. In most cases, the DAT subjects used demonstratives appropriately. However, the increased frequency of demonstrative adverbs in these subjects seemed to reflect a lack of specificity: *there* was often used in place of a prepositional phrase to refer to a location (e.g., "He's up there" as opposed to "He is in the tree"). DAT subjects also produced more indefinite pronouns. Some of these pronouns were produced in stereotypic expressions devoid of semantic content (e.g., "So she walked up to her door and *everything*, and someone walked up the driveway, and they had her wallet"). In other cases, indefinite pronouns were indicative of a failure to identify a referent or of a naming problem.

There was a trend for the DAT subjects to use more exophoric reference than the normals. Exophoric reference frequently involved use of demonstratives (e.g., "If a light goes out in *this* ceiling fixture, you have to get a stepladder"). Exophoric reference is not in itself inappropriate, but in the DAT subjects it may have reflected a tendency toward greater context dependence, especially in the Cat Story and procedures.

Disruption at a semantic level in DAT subjects was an expected finding, based on previous research. Problems at the semantic level were evident in a relatively low-level task (i.e., the Boston Naming Test), on which the DAT subjects made more errors than normals. However, the pattern of errors was similar to that for controls. Most of the errors (87%) were semantically related to the target, more suggestive of a word-finding problem than an actual breakdown in semantic structure. In their discourse, DAT subjects occasionally showed evidence of word-finding problems, characterized by a pause followed by an inappropriate lexical item (see Appendix 4.A for examples). It is possible that deficits in naming may be related to the subjects' tendencies to use a higher proportion of pronouns in general and indefinite pronouns in particular. However, it should be noted that on a simple measure of lexical diversity (ratio of different nouns to total nouns), there were no group differences between DAT patients and controls.

In more severely involved subjects, semantic structure may be more vulnerable (for example, a patient studied by Schwartz et al. [1979] showed a loss of certain semantic features, e.g., those distinguishing "dog" from "cat").

Our findings of relatively preserved syntax but disrupted content in DAT subjects is also congruent with previous research (Bayles, 1985; Bayles & Boone, 1982; Obler, 1983; Schwartz et al., 1979), which has suggested that lower level functions of language (phonology, morphology, and syntax) are more resistant to disruption than higher level language functions, such as semantics and pragmatics.

At least three explanations can be offered for the preservation of syntax in DAT subjects. First, it may be that the syntactic components of language are overlearned or automatic, and therefore resistant to disruption. Schwartz et al. (1979), for example, found that even a severely demented patient showed preservation of some aspects of syntax. A second explanation may relate to the relative simplicity of language tasks used in our study. Had we used more difficult types of language tasks, which required subjects to produce more complex syntactic structures, it is possible that disruption at this level may have become evident. On an unstructured, simple language task, it is possible that mildly impaired subjects may intuitively avoid attempting to produce complex syntactic structures. It is worth noting that DAT subjects occasionally did produce marked grammatical errors when attempting to formulate more complex sentences. A third explanation for our finding of preserved syntax may relate to the severity level of the patients. Most of the subjects were in the mildly impaired range. It is possible that more severely involved subjects would show syntactic deficits on the types of tasks presented. However, the small sample size in our study prohibited a reliable analysis of any potential relationship between severity of dementia and degree of syntactic disruption.

One of the surprising findings of this study was the relatively intact performance of the DAT subjects on the Written Cat Story. DAT and normal subjects did not differ significantly on any parameters. Writing is generally assumed to be more difficult than oral expression, and there is some evidence from earlier studies (Kirshner, Webb, Kelly, & Wells, 1984) that writing is disrupted early in the course of dementia. The lack of group differences in the present study may reflect the relatively easy nature of the task or a lack of effort by the normal subjects (for which there was some evidence). We cannot, however, exclude the possibility that writing is preserved relative to oral expression. In particular, it must be kept in mind that writing makes fewer time demands on the subject, since in a writing task the subject can proceed at his or her own pace, and fewer memory demands.

Some interesting results emerged from our rating procedures, even though the interrater reliability was somewhat low. Most importantly, the raters consistently scored the Cat Story summaries of the DAT subjects as being lower than those of the normals on a measure of content, clarity, and relevance. Also, the raters were able to reliably discriminate between groups for the Letter Procedure, which was considered the most complex of the procedures in terms of number of a priori propositions. These rating data, while they reflect methodological problems, provide at least some support for the notion that even mildly impaired DAT subjects do show communicative deficits, not merely linguistic deficits only detectable by formal analysis.

There is a tendency among some researchers to consider the language deficits in DAT patients as a form of aphasia. However, there appear to be a number of important differences between the language impairment of DAT subjects and that of aphasics. (For data on the performance of aphasics on similar tasks, see Ulatowska, Doyel, et al. [1983] and Ulatowska, Freedman-Stern, et al. [1983].) First, DAT subjects do not show a marked disruption of syntax, as do aphasics. Second, DAT subjects, at least in mild stage, show no reduction in the amount of verbal output on the types of tasks presented here. Aphasics do show a reduction in language on similar tasks. Third, compared to aphasics, DAT subjects produce much more irrelevant and incorrect information in the types of tasks presented in this study. Fourth, DAT subjects, compared to aphasics, are often less cooperative and less responsive to task demands, making it more difficult to evaluate objectively their linguistic competence. However, there are also similarities between the language of aphasics and that of DAT subjects on these types of language tasks. Both groups show: (a) preservation of narrative superstructure, (b) reduction of specificity of language in the procedures, and (c) impairment in the ability to produce summaries and morals in narrative discourse.

When DAT subjects are compared to old elderly subjects (ages 77 to 92) (Ulatowska, Hayashi, Cannito, & Fleming, 1986), a number of similarities also emerge. Both groups show: (a) a preservation of syntax, (b) a disruption of reference, (c) a tendency to digress in narrative tasks, and (d) difficulty in producing adequate summaries and morals in narrative discourse. The primary difference between old elderly and DAT subjects appears to be one of degree, with DAT subjects showing more severe deficits. However, comparisons between the two groups should be made cautiously, since the populations were studied under somewhat different conditions.

The apparent similarities in language function between old elderly and DAT subjects raises the possibility that some of the deficits seen in DAT subjects may be partly the effect of normal aging. It would be useful to separate out the effects of normal aging from the effects of the disease process, so as to determine if there are some deficits that are pathognomic for DAT. The design of our study did not allow us to confront this issue directly: to do so would require the use of a wider age range (16 of our 20 subjects were between 61 and 75) and a larger sample, so as to allow grouping by age. Nevertheless, the question of age effects was examined in a preliminary manner by dividing each group by age (younger versus older subjects) and comparing the age groups on the parameters that discriminated normal and DAT subjects. None of these parameters significantly discriminated younger from older subjects in both normal and DAT groups. Thus, we did not find evidence for a relation between age and linguistic deficits within our sample. This apparent lack of a relationship should be interpreted cautiously, due to the narrow age range and small size of our sample. (However, it should be noted that Appell et al. [1982] also failed to find age effects in a larger sample of dementia patients of comparable age to those in the present study.)

This study points to some directions for future research. Mildly impaired dementia subjects need to be tested on more difficult narrative tasks. The Cat Story and Wallet Story used in the present study may make too few linguistic demands on subjects to identify areas of deficient linguistic processing, which might characterize mildly impaired dementia patients. More structured types of linguistic tasks that force the subject to respond in a particular manner may also reveal subtle deficits not apparent in spontaneous discourse. Spontaneous language tasks, while more naturalistic, may serve to mask a patient's deficits by allowing the patient the opportunity to select what he or she will say.

Clinical impressions of mildly impaired dementia patients suggest that the language of these patients is not markedly impaired. The results of our interview and questionnaire, provided by family members for each of the subjects, largely confirm these clinical impressions. Generally, subjects were reported to have an interest in communicating, to participate appropriately in conversation, and to be able to produce a range of discourse styles (e.g., expository, narrative, humorous). This relative preservation of language and communication in everyday functioning underscores the importance of testing dementia patients under experimental conditions, where subtle but unmistakable deficits do emerge. These deficits warrant further study.

Acknowledgments. The authors wish to express their appreciation to Miss Josephine Simonson and Dr. Alan Naarden for their help in selecting patients for this study. Thanks are due to the members of the Dallas Chapter of the National Alzheimer's Association for their encouragement and support throughout our investigation, and to speech-language pathologists Tricia Kraus, Cathy Conner, Corliss Kaiser, Maxine Maxfield, Klaran Warner, and Belinda Reyes for their assistance in rating language samples. Thanks are also due to the spouses of our subjects, whose insight and sensitivity proved invaluable.

References

Appell, J., Kertesz, A., & Fisman, M. (1982). A study of language functioning in Alzheimer patients. *Brain and Language, 17*, 73–91.

Bayles, K.A. (1982). Language function in senile dementia. *Brain and Language, 16*, 265–280.

Bayles, K.A. (1985). Communication in dementia. In H. Ulatowska (Ed.), *The Aging Brain*. San Diego: College-Hill Press.

Bayles, K.A., & Boone, D.R. (1982). The potential of language tasks for identifying senile dementia. *Journal of Speech and Hearing Disorders, 47*, 210–217.

Bayles, K.A., & Tomoeda, C.K. (1983). Confrontation naming impairment in dementia. *Brain and Language, 19*, 98–114.

Bayles, K.A., Tomoeda, C.K., Kaszniak, A.W., Stern, L.Z., & Eagans, K.K. (1985). Verbal perseveration of dementia patients. *Brain and Language, 25*, 102–116.

Buschke, H. (1973). Selective reminding for analysis of memory and learning. *Journal of Verbal Learning and Verbal Behavior, 12*, 543–550.

Grice, P. (1975). Logic and conversation. In P. Cole & J. Morgan (Eds.), *Syntax and semantics* (Vol. 3). New York: Academic Press.

Hier, D.B., Hagenlocker, K., & Shindler, A.G. (1985). Language disintegration in dementia: Effects of etiology and severity. *Brain and Language, 25*, 117–133.

Huff, F.J., Corkin, S., & Growdon, J.H. (1986). Semantic impairment and anomia in Alzheimer's disease. *Brain and Language, 28*, 235–249.

Hunt, K.W. (1965). Grammatical structures written at three grade levels (Research Report No. 5). Champaign, IL: National Council of Teachers of English.

Kirshner, H.S., Webb, W.G., Kelly, M.P., & Wells, C.E. (1984). Language disturbance: An initial symptom of cortical degenerations and dementia. *Archives of Neurology, 41*, 491–496.

LeDoux, J.F., Blum, C., & Hirst, W. (1983). Inferential processing of context: Studies of cognitively impaired subjects. *Brain and Language, 19*, 216–224.

Martin, A., & Fedio, P. (1983). Word production and comprehension in Alzheimer's disease: The breakdown of semantic knowledge. *Brain and Language, 19*, 124–141.

Nicholas, M., Obler, L.K., Albert, M.L., & Helm-Estabrooks, N. (1985). Empty speech in Alzheimer's disease and fluent aphasia. *Journal of Speech and Hearing Research, 28*, 405–410.

Obler, L.K. (1983). Language and brain dysfunction in dementia. In S. Segalowitz (Ed.), *Language functions and brain organization*. New York: Academic Press.

Schwartz, M.F., Marin, O.S.M., & Saffran, E.M. (1979). Dissociations of language function in dementia: A case study. *Brain and Language, 7*, 277–306.

Ulatowska, H.K., North, A.J., & Macaluso-Haynes, S. (1981). Production of narrative and procedural discourse in aphasia. *Brain and Language, 13*, 345–371.

Ulatowska, H.K., Doyel, A.W., Freedman-Stern, R., Macaluso-Haynes, S., & North, A.J. (1983). Production of procedural discourse in aphasia. *Brain and Language, 18*, 315–341.

Ulatowska, H.K., Freedman-Stern, R., Doyel, A.W., Macaluso-Haynes, S., & North, A.J. (1983). Production of narrative discourse in aphasia. *Brain and Language, 19*, 317–334.

Ulatowska, H.K., Hayashi, M.M., Cannito, M.P., & Fleming, S.G. (1986). Disruption of reference in aging. *Brain and Language, 28*, 24–41.

Appendix 4.A. Language Samples from DAT Patients

Sample of Cat Story of DAT Subject

Alright—a cat climbed up the tree out of reach of the man whose *children*	Incorrect proposition: "children" (should be "child")
are having a *cat-fit* on the ground	Inappropriate lexical item: "cat-fit"
because she is—because they are afraid that the cat will not be able to get down, but the—and the little girl particularly had difficulty.	
It turned her head in two directions—anatomic readjusts-ments.	Confabulation

Appendix 4.A (*Continued*)

Sample of Cat Story of DAT Subject (*Continued*)	
The man tried to let her up.	Incorrect proposition
The man crawled up in the tree and the cat jumped off. The little girl looked up and she looks pretty happy about the whole thing.	
And Daddy went to–running to get–this is a *sequential boo-boo* from my viewpoint–	Inappropriate lexical item: "sequential boo-boo"
and got a fireman to come and get the cat down–	Incorrect proposition
the little girl crying all the way–	
the cat sitting there in the last sequence, licking his chops	Inappropriate lexical item: "chops"
and feeling very glad at *discomboborating* everybody in the family and all the neighbors.	Paraphasia: discomboborating

Sample of Memorable Experience of DAT Subject

Well, I went to Lima, Peru with my husband. Well, we– we had a friend there and she lives here now, that took me out shopping. I didn't buy much of the gold or anything that I really liked they had, you know.	
And then my husband and I went to Lima, Peru.	Repetition
I've got a list here in the–in my peignoir about all the places I've been. Would you like to see it?	Digression
And, let me see, we went to Lima, Peru, and one of the women there had married an American and she took me out to shop for jewelry. I didn't buy anything though.	Repetition
And I didn't get to go to England. My husband was sick. And I went to Europe. I went to Rome, and went to Italy, and I saw the Pope. He came out. It's been so long ago, I can't remember it now.	Introduction of new topic

Excerpt from Light Procedure of DAT Subject

Well, first thing, *it's*–it's high enough that–that I couldn't reach *it* from the floor,	Indefinite reference: "it"
but I do have a beautiful stand at the end of the bed and–	
and I have on this stand–I have a red velvet that I–my wife loves me to put it on the bed, and so we put that– It's folded up so I have to take this red velvet off of the bed–off of the stand and put it on the bed.	Digression
Then I step up on that stand and then I can reach up and–and unscrew the *thing* from the glass.	Indefinite reference: "thing"
Now I did one in the kitchen and *it* had a *thing* that long.	Digression Indefinite reference: "it" and "thing"
It was in a case like, so I don't know whether *this* would be the same or not.	Indefinite reference: "it" and "this"

5 Neuropsychological Assessment and Treatment of Head Trauma Patients

CHARLES J. LONG and J. MICHAEL WILLIAMS

The Problem

Head trauma has undoubtedly been a significant problem since the beginning of man, but it's incidence, in our fast-based technological society, has reached staggering proportions. Caveness (1977) estimated that in 1976 there were nearly 10 million head injuries in the United States. Over 8 million were superficial or minor, but nearly 1.5 million were classified as major, including 613,000 concussions, 133,000 skull fractures, and 633,000 intracranial injuries. It is estimated that there are 25 deaths per 100,000 head injuries in the United States. Two thirds of these deaths result from motor vehicle accidents. This number alone is more than the total number killed in the Vietnam War (Rimel, 1980). Current statistics suggest that although less than 5% of head injuries are fatal, head injuries are the leading cause of death in children and young adults, with 90% of the head injuries occurring in individuals under 45 years of age (see Table 5.1). Head trauma remains the third leading cause of death in the United States and is two thirds more common in males.

Advances in medical care have decreased early mortality and resulted in more survivors. Increasing survival from severe head injury results in more patients with chronic deficits, and these cases are a serious challenge to rehabilitation personnel, their families, and community resources. They most often are young adults who were attempting to achieve independence before injury, and families are often confronted with the task of rearing their children anew, this time with greater difficulty and greater frustration.

Until recently, there were no specialized resources available for severely head-injured individuals. Often they were treated in traditional rehabilitation facilities in much the same manner as elderly stroke victims. Later, in the 1970s, numerous specialized head trauma treatment facilities were developed and began offering comprehensive rehabilitative services for severely impaired head injury victims. While more resources of this type are needed, most of these programs are designed for the minority of patients with the most severe injuries and consequently with the poorest prognosis for regaining independent functioning.

Few resources are available for the large number of individuals suffering from the so-called "minor" head injuries each year. It is often assumed that these individuals will recover to normal functioning without significant problems and without the need for assistance. Recent research and clinical observation, however, do not support this contention. Recovery of more obvious physical deficits may be rapid, but data suggest that recovery from more subtle cognitive deficits is protracted (Gulbrandsen, 1983; Walker & Erculei, 1969) and permanent residual damage may remain. In the majority of patients, recovery appears to be near maximum at 2 years, with little change from 2 to 7 years (Oddy, Coughlan, Tyerman, & Jenkins, 1985). Klonoff and associates, in an extensive study with children suffering mild head injury, found that 50% were impaired on over 30% of the tasks presented at 2 years posttrauma (Klonoff & Low, 1974; Klonoff, Low, & Clark, 1977). In addition to cognitive deficits, mildly injured patients often suffer serious emotional problems.

Unlike the severely injured patient who typically has obvious neurological symptoms, the mild to moderately injured patient presents with more subtle impairments in cognitive functioning and impaired stress management. Often the head-injured person and others around them neither expect nor understand these subtle cognitive and emotional effects of the head injury.

Neuropsychological assessment provides an important method for evaluating these subtle effects of head injury, since the focus is upon the behavioral consequences of neurological injury. In fact, neuropsychological assessment is often the only evaluation strategy available to provide information needed to treat these patients effectively. Computed tomography (CT) scans, EEGs, and so forth are of value during the early acute phase of management, but they are not sensitive to the functional consequences of trauma on behavior (Long & Gouvier, 1982). These behavioral changes are often the most disabling consequences of head trauma and may persist for many months or years during the chronic phase of recovery. It is clearly established that a mental handicap contributes more significantly to overall social disability than neurological deficits (Dikmen, Reitan, & Temkin, 1983; Jennett, Snoek, Bond, & Brooks, 1981).

For these reasons, the primary emphasis of this chapter is on the role of neuropsychology in evaluating, educating, and treating patients suffering from mild to moderate head injury. These patients constitute the majority of head injury victims. They also have the best prognosis for recovery, yet often receive the least treatment, and are the most misunderstood. In addition, their recovery is often limited by emotional and situational influences—influences that can be minimized with early diagnosis and intervention.

Organic Factors

The early consequences of head injury are highly variable with more severe injuries requiring immediate medical attention. This early treatment is directed at minimizing the primary impact damage and preventing or treating secondary

TABLE 5.1. Head injury deaths by age group.

Age group (years)	Percent of deaths
0–9	8
10–19	34
20–29	28
30–39	12
40–49	8
50–59	2
60–69	2
70+	2

injuries. There may be initial focal signs of injury that change to more generalized signs due to edema. Focal damage can result from subdural bleeding or from polar damage to the frontal and/or temporal cortices due to impact of the brain against the bony ridges of the skull. There may also be secondary effects due to arterial hypoxemia, raised intracranial pressure, hydrocephalus, and/or posttraumatic epilepsy. In addition, there are usually signs of diffuse generalized damage in patients suffering from closed head injury.

Concussion is a characteristic feature of more severe closed head trauma and represents a transient loss of consciousness produced by a blow to the head. It reflects disruption of brain activity particularly in the brain stem reticular system. Associated changes occur, causing fluctuations in arterial blood pressure, irregular respiration, EEG changes, and increased intracranial pressure.

The possibility has been raised that the basic mechanism of concussion is the bending and stretching of the neck (Friede, 1961). Analysis of the effects of closed head injury relate to the structural design of the head and neck. Head mobility is important (Denny-Brown & Russell, 1941) as the head is almost always unrestrained and may be thrown in motion with the pivot point at the neck. Rapid acceleration and deceleration causes significant pressure changes and rotational sheer forces (Russell & Schiller, 1959) that cause tearing of nerve fibers around long fiber tracts and vessels throughout the central nervous system (CNS) (Strich, 1961). This finding may support the validity of the posttrauma cognitive complaints frequently reported by whiplash victims.

Diffuse pathology has been confirmed in victims of mild head injuries. Strich (1956, 1969) described the presence of retraction balls (myelin breakdown and resorption) confined mainly to white matter in the corpus callosum and long tracts. He also reported the presence of vascular hemorrhages throughout the brain. These forces result in degeneration of white matter and are attributed to cognitive sequelae following head injury (Levin, Handel, Goldman, Eisenberg, & Guinto, 1985). In addition, there is evidence that metabolic disturbances are present following trauma (Ishii, 1966). Cerebral blood flow is suppressed for over 1 year after head injury and appears related to the presence of the chronic head injury syndrome (Barclay, Zemcov, Reichert, & Blass, 1985). Contusion or direct bruising of the brain tissue may occur, but this is less likely in closed head trauma. Penetrating head injuries cause contusion, but are less likely to cause concussion. Here the effects are often focal and penetration of the dura greatly increases the possibility of infection, thereby increasing the likelihood of post-traumatic seizures.

Ommaya and Gennarelli (1974) present an interesting paradigm for head injury mechanics based on the structural design of the head and neck. Their studies show that, when the head is set in motion by a blow, maximum forces occur at the cortex due to its distance from the neck and its proximity to the skull. Furthermore, they conclude that concussion is caused by centripetal sequence of disruptive effects. The effects always begin at the surface of the brain (cortex) and extend inward (centripetally). As the force exerted on the head increases, it may extend into the diencephalon and cause disruption of memory. If severe enough, it may extend further, involving the mesencephalic core and reticular activating system and producing unconsciousness.

Even with damage that is insufficient to cause coma, there may be impaired cortical functioning and decreased cognitive abilities (Dikmen et al., 1983; Rimel, Giordani, Barth, & Jane, 1981, 1982). In cases of concussion, damage to axons emanating from neurons located in the cortex is well documented, and cortical dysfunction may last well beyond recovery of consciousness (Strich, 1969). Such structural damage to the brain has been noted at autopsy in patients with only mild head injuries. In spite of clear documentation that neuronal damage exists after mild head injury, the focus of most patient treatment is directed either toward acute care or emotional sequelae with little treatment or investigation of significant cognitive dysfunction due to cerebral damage.

During the process of recovery, the least damaged systems apparently recover first (Ommaya & Gennarelli, 1974). The brain stem is generally involved to a lesser extent and is first to recover, leading to consciousness. The diencephalon and higher systems may remain impaired. Thus, the patient suffers from post-traumatic amnesia. This refers to the patient's inability to consolidate new information. The patient may recognize significant others and retain remote memories but cannot recall events and facts from day to day or even within a day. As the diencephalon recovers, basic memory consolidation returns. However, this recovery is slow and memory problems usually persist throughout the process of recovery. In addition, there remains persistent cortical damage resulting in other cognitive dysfunction that may be long lasting. Cortical damage will often be the last to recover, may be the most subtle in effect, and produces cognitive dysfunction or weakness that can lead to significant emotional and social problems, particularly when its effects are unrecognized.

This process of damage and resulting recovery can be radically altered when vessels are damaged, producing large subdural or epidural hematomas, or when temporal or frontal poles are damaged by the rough surfaces of the skull. Otherwise, there is a generalized effect with nonfocal consequences. The effect is diffuse, greater at the cortex and decreasing in severity toward the brain stem.

Estimating Severity and Predicting Outcome

Often the relationship between the extent of physical damage and underlying neurological damage is low. Severe neurological damage can be present in individuals with no visible signs of injury. The damage may be primary (e.g., tearing of axons) or secondary, such as that due to brain edema or extracranial factors such as blood loss, arterial hypotension, and pulmonary complications.

Perhaps the most pressing question posed by families of head-injured patients is that of outcome. They often want to know when the patient will recover to preinjury status. Such predictions are difficult and are often complicated by other factors. Family members fail to understand qualified explanations or selectively attend to only the more optimistic parts. When families are questioned later regarding problems that they confronted in the management of their injured family member, they often complain that the staff were inconsistent in their outcome prediction. They often report hearing both extremes by different staff at the same time. This leads to further confusion and frustration and creates doubts and questions of staff competency.

Outcome is always expressed as a probability statement. It is important to communicate this to the family. Traditionally, outcome prediction has been based upon more organically related factors such as the nature of the injury, the duration of coma, and the duration of hospitalization. Coma of greater than 13 weeks generally ends in death or vegetative state (Reyes, Battacharyya, & Heller, 1981). Duration of coma of less than 18 days leads to good recovery (Levin, Grossman, Rose, & Teasdale, 1979). It has been argued that it is not the duration but the course of coma that is important (Teasdale, Knill-Jones, & Van Der Sande, 1978). Both age and duration of hospital stay have been found to offer a somewhat better indication of outcome than coma duration (Reyes et al., 1981). Coma duration and level correlate with recovery of intelligence (Ruesch, 1944; Williams, Gomes, Drudge, & Kessler, 1984), and is thought by some to be a good predictor of outcome (Stanczak et al., 1984; Teasdale et al., 1978). Others point out that coma duration is usually brief, is infrequently measured, and therefore, correlation with outcome is usually poor (Brooks, Aughton, Bond, Jones, & Rizvi, 1980). Thus, it has been recommended that posttraumatic amnesia (PTA) is a better predictor of outcome (Levin, Benton, & Grossman, 1979; Russell, 1932; Steadman & Graham, 1970).

Carlsson, Von Essen, and Lofgren (1968) found good outcome in children with PTA of less than 2 months, but in middle-age patients, there were persistent mental symptoms with PTA of less than 1 week. Russell's widely accepted measure has been criticized by Bond (1983) as overclassifying severe cases. He offers the following modifications that would appear to be of value in more accurately classifying severely injured individuals, whereas Russell's measure is adequate in less severe cases. These adjustments are consistent with the findings of Van Zomeren and Van Den Burg (1985) that PTA of 13 days best discriminates between severe and very severe head injury.

	Russell (1932)	Bond (1983)
Mild	<1 hour	<1 day
Moderate	1–24 hours	1–7 days
Severe	1–7 days	7–28 days
Very severe	>7 days	>28 days

Patients with even relatively brief coma and PTA may suffer from impaired cognitive functions. Subtle damage to the brain is more likely to involve the cortex or the white matter immediately underlying the cortex. In view of the fact that coma relates primarily to damage of the brain stem and PTA relates primarily to damage of the diencephalon, neither measure may be particularly useful in predicting outcome of mildly to moderately impaired patients. A second factor regarding coma and/or PTA and outcome relates to time since injury or time to final outcome. Coma is of shorter duration and is furthest removed from the period of final recovery. PTA may be a better predictor due to the fact that it is of longer duration and closer to the final level of recovery. This reasoning clearly supports the notion that neuropsychological testing should afford the best measure of outcome, as such testing generally occurs closer to the end point of recovery, measures functions that are of longer duration, and assesses the effects of impaired cortical systems where the damage is likely to be greatest and recovery is slowest. Neuropsychological assessment at 2 months posttrauma provides data that correlate higher with final outcome than does coma duration (Klove & Cleeland, 1972; Reynell, 1944). Therefore, where questions of degree and nature of recovery are concerned, neuropsychological assessment should be undertaken at 6 to 12 months. However, when neuropsychological data are to be used in treatment planning, the assessment should be initiated earlier.

There are other critical factors, however, that influence outcome. Symonds (1939), emphasized the premorbid status of the individual in his oft-quoted statement, "It is not only the kind of injury that matters but the kind of head that is injured that determines recovery of function." Clearly this statement reflects the fact that one has to look beyond the injury characteristics to better understand the effects of trauma and the nature and extent of recovery. The pretrauma level of functioning is an important determinant of outcome (Williams et al., 1984). Individuals who are of higher IQ and socioeconomic status, are younger, and come from a stable home environment have a greater likelihood of favorable outcome. Miller (1983) has argued for a broader investigation of factors influencing outcome. He concludes that head trauma outcome is determined by three sets of factors: 1) preinjury status, 2) damage to the brain, and 3) cumulative effects of secondary insults. His view, however, remains firmly seated in organic factors. Historically, both prediction of outcome and rehabilitation strategies have tended to ignore cognitive and social factors that manifest during the period of recovery (Bond, 1976). Many patients recover from apparent physical problems but fail to live up to expectations. They appear normal on routine neurological exam but have impaired concentration, memory, emotional adjustment, and attention

(Ford, 1976). Dikmen et al. (1983) report that complex functions are most sensitive to head injury. Cognitive and intellectual deficits are most common and more disabling socially and vocationally than are physical factors.

Assessment of cognitive functions have been found to be the sensitive measures of patient's ability to function. Information-processing ability has been found strongly related to the patients' ability to function on the job (Gronwall & Wrightson, 1974), and the selective reminding test has been found to be the best predictor of a child's ability to cope with school (Levin & Eisenberg, 1979). These findings and others suggest that Miller's factors can be extended to include: 4) level of posttrauma cognitive functioning, 5) social support system, and 6) vocational ability (Long, 1985).

The Recovery Model

Recovery after head trauma is determined by many factors. As previously discussed, research suggests that there are at least six major factors: 1) preinjury status of the individual; 2) damage to the brain and cumulative effects of secondary insult; 3) effects of brain damage on cognitive functioning; 4) emotional adjustment; 5) socioenvironmental factors; and 6) vocational ability (Long, Gouvier, & Cole, 1984). Preinjury status and the cognitive effects of brain damage have been discussed at length by others (Levin, Benton, Grossman, et al., 1979).

Emotional factors following head trauma are poorly understood. Often there is an inverse correlation between severity and postconcussion symptoms (PCS) as well as estimates of delay in their onset. Numerous postconcussion symptoms, such as irritability and depression, are common following head trauma. Such problems in emotional adjustment may reflect residual impairment of cognitive functioning or lowered self-esteem. The effect of head injury is to impair coping while at the same time increasing stress demands on the individual. Thus, it is not surprising that emotional problems are present in many head trauma victims. Left untreated, emotional distress can lead to disability in individuals with only minor neurological damage and good premorbid functioning (Long & Webb, 1983; Novack, Daniel, & Long, 1984).

Finally, socioenvironmental and vocational factors play a dramatic role in fostering or limiting recovery. Family support, social support, and vocational demands are often involved when individuals fail to recover or recover less than would be expected, based upon degree of brain injury alone.

Effective assessment and treatment of head-injured individuals require an understanding of these six areas. While all undoubtedly work in concert to determine outcome, one or more may represent special barriers to favorable outcome in a given case. Thus, each should receive careful attention in evaluating head-injured patients. This chapter discusses the consequences of and the recovery from head trauma focusing upon these six areas.

Another method to aid in understanding the recovery process following head trauma is to consider cognitive functioning over time. As can be seen from Figure 5.1, the patient may initially be rendered comatose by the trauma. Recovery

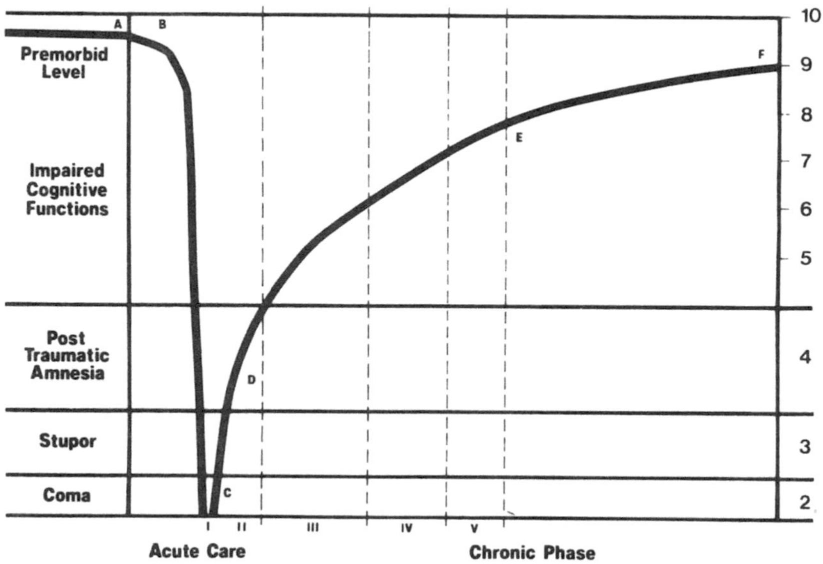

FIGURE 5.1. *Top*: Diagrammatic representation of level of cortical functioning as a function of time since head trauma (A = premorbid level, B = retrograde amnesia, C = coma and/or stupor, D = post-traumatic amnesia, E = impaired cortical functions, and F = level of recovery). *Bottom*: Assessment procedures designed to assess patient's progress through each level (I = coma scale, II = amnesia assessment, III = neuropsychological evaluation, IV = short-term intervention, and V = vocational assessment).

from coma frequently has no clear end point. Rather, the patient has increasing frequent lucid periods and/or gradually lengthening period(s) of awareness. This is followed by a period of posttraumatic amnesia (PTA). This period is longer than coma and is characterized primarily by impaired memory consolidation. Again, recovery from PTA is gradual and is assumed to represent the time from the injury to the point in time when the patient has consistent memory. The important aspect of Figure 5.1 is that at this point the patient is far from recovered. While, in all likelihood, they have normal CT scans and EEGs and certainly are medically stable, as can be seen from Figure 5.1, they may be functioning 40% to 60% below their premorbid level. It is during this time and at this level of recovery that they are most vulnerable. Furthermore, it is at this time that neuropsychological assessment can play an important role in determining the overall level of functioning and in identifying primary areas of weakness. Such information is necessary in aiding the patient and family in understanding the problems following head injury, and in assisting in formulating an effective treatment plan.

Recovery of function viewed in this light suggests that most recovery occurs early with less dramatic evidence of recovery as the patient approaches asymptote. Serial assessment of patients following head trauma is generally consistent with this process of recovery (Drudge, Williams, Gomes, & Kessler, 1984; Long & Haban, 1985). These findings further highlight the importance of considering time since injury, as well as estimates of severity of injury, when administering neuropsychological evaluations.

Preinjury Factors

Preinjury factors such as genetic predisposition, early experience, personality characteristics, educational background, and occupational history are related to recovery from head injury. The individual who is functioning effectively before trauma has more resources available and more reserves. The presence of a low-stress environment is likely to produce less stress following trauma. An individual functioning above average before trauma may have a decline in function, but may still function at an average level after trauma, whereas a person functioning at a borderline level before injury may be reduced to an impaired level after trauma.

Constitutional and brain damage factors influence outcome following head injury, with a greater mortality rate in older patients (Slater, 1962). Other factors related to preinjury status (physical, cognitive, and emotional) are important in predicting recovery, but they are difficult to assess and more variable in their apparent effects (Dikmen & Reitan, 1976; Lishman, 1978).

Support for the importance of preinjury factors was reported by Denckler (1958, 1960) in studies with identical twins. While the head-injured twin was inferior to the noninjured control, the defects were subtle and postconcussion symptoms were found to relate more to genetics than to the occurrence of head injury.

Personality factors prior to trauma are also related to outcome. Family history of character disorder, retardation, or psychosis is related to psychosocial adjustment after injury (Lishman, 1978). Postconcussion symptoms are more likely in such patients. In fact, postconcussion symptoms are most likely to occur in patients who experience high stress or who have ineffective coping skills (Long & Novack, 1985; Wood, Novack, & Long, 1984).

Kozol (1946) found that less egocentric, more responsible, socially minded individuals prior to trauma recover best, even though they may have substantial neurotic characteristics, suggesting that brain injury may precipitate the expression of preexisting behavioral aberrations.

While brain injury may cause more impulsivity and poor judgment, such tendencies are likely to have been present prior to trauma, as evidenced by the higher incidence of head injury in young males, of low IQ, low social and occupational status, with poor social responsibility (Miller, 1961a, 1961b).

Thus, preinjury factors not only play a significant role in the occurrence of head injury, but contribute to the extent of impairment and limit the degree of recovery. Such factors must be investigated and considered in evaluating head-injured patients, in formulating treatment plans, and in developing realistic rehabilitation outcome goals.

Cognitive Dysfunction

Recovery from head injury involves a gradual improvement in cognitive functions (see Figure 5.1). Recovery begins during coma (in the severely impaired), progresses through resolution of posttraumatic amnesia, and may continue for months. The process of recovery clearly reflects neurological damage revealed behaviorally as impaired consciousness, memory dysfunction, and attenuated cognitive functions (Long & Gouvier, 1982). The question remains, however, as to the nature and relationship between cognitive dysfunction and the degree of tissue damage.

Memory

In some cases, posttraumatic amnesia appears to end abruptly, however, careful measurement reveals it to be gradual with islands of memory for emotionally significant events. Patients generally complain of memory deficits long after posttraumatic amnesia has abated. Memory weakness is one of the most common postconcussion symptoms. Tooth (1947) found that marked learning deficits often persisted long after the injury. Brooks et al. (1980) found a deficit on delayed recall 2 years after injury. Brooks (1983) investigated the nature of memory deficit following head trauma and found that one of the reasons for persistent memory deficits was poor attention. Brooks found impairment on digit span with severe but not mild head trauma, and further obtained data suggesting storage and retrieval problems. Lezak (1979) found memory recovery varies with the nature of the function, task complexity, and severity of injury. Furthermore, she found evidence of memory impairment after 3 years in over half of the patients studied. The majority of the data suggest that recovery, of at least the more subtle aspects of memory, lags behind other cognitive measures following head trauma.

Memory deficits are more subtle with less severe injury or with a longer period of recovery. Patients are more impaired in continuous recognition tasks and generally adopt a more cautious response style (Richardson, 1979). Retrieval cueing improves functioning by encouraging focused search and memory (Crovitz, 1979). These findings suggest that the primary deficit may remain in higher cortical functions rather than simply memory consolidation.

Intelligence

The assessment of intellectual functions and information processing also yields consistent data suggesting impairment in IQ following head injury. Fodor (1972) found that IQ impairment was more closely associated with severity of injury than with memory function. The data generally suggest that verbal IQ usually recovers to near asymptote within the 1st year, whereas performance IQ may be delayed 3 years or more in recovery (Landsell & Smith, 1975; Mandleberg & Brooks, 1975; Miller, 1979). Miller (1979) found that even severe head trauma patients can have a good recovery. However, there is more to the nature of head trauma than measured intelligence, and Miller is careful to point out that it is wrong to conclude that because the patient's IQ score increases, he or she has also recovered cognitively.

Intellectual impairment appears to correlate well with neurological findings regarding severity of injury, with .85 to .90 correlations found between intellectual measures and measures derived from CT scans (Uzzell, Zimmerman, Dolinksas, & Obrist, 1970). IQ also correlates higher with cortical than ventricular atrophy (Willanger, Thygesen, Nietsen, & Peteroon, 1968). One of the difficulties in using intellectual assessment as a measure of recovery relates to the varying premorbid level of functioning, which can only be roughly estimated (Wilson et al., 1978; Wilson, Rosenbaum, & Brown, 1979). It is difficult to determine whether a patient who has recovered to a normal level of intelligence was, in fact, functioning at a normal level prior to trauma or at a higher level.

Attempts at developing a formula for calculating premorbid IQ (Wilson et al., 1978) have limited application with head-injured patients (Bolter, Gouvier, Veneklasen, & Long, 1982; Gouvier, Bolter, Veneklasen, & Long, 1983; Williams et al., 1984). Thus, the clinician is generally left to his own best judgment. This judgment is augmented by obtaining appropriate historical data and evaluating intertest scatter.

Ruesch and Moore (1943) found that the serial sevens procedure was sensitive to the cognitive dysfunction caused by head trauma. In studying this procedure, they found that the major loss was related to the inability to maintain a sustained effort. These observations are supported by numerous studies reporting that patients are most impaired on the Digit Symbol subtest of the Wechsler Adult Intelligence Scale (WAIS) (Mandleberg & Brooks, 1975).

Higher Cortical Functions

Attention and speed of perception are impaired following brain injury, and slowness of thought, fatigue, and poor memory are found to be primary features following head trauma (Denckler & Lofving, 1958; Levin, O'Donnell, & Grossman, 1979; Ruesch, 1944). The nature of cognitive dysfunction following head trauma suggests that brain-injured patients are limited in their ability to process a number of items at one time, that is, they have reduced channel capacity (Gronwall & Wrightson, 1974). Using this assessment, Gronwall and Wrightson found that even when patients felt well enough to return to work and scored in the average range on intelligence tests, they may remain impaired on the Paced Auditory Serial Addition Test (PASAT). This test is apparently sensitive to the more subtle aspects of cognitive function and has been employed by them in measuring the individual's ability to resume vocational or educational pursuits. Most jobs require attention and effort and the patient tends to tire rapidly (Gronwall & Wrightson, 1974). With fatigue, stress mounts along with headaches and irritability. This state of affairs further attenuates cognitive function and limits the patient's ability to manage work or educational demands.

Increased reaction time, slow decision making, and impaired information-processing abilities have been found to reflect the consequences of brain injury

(Van Zormeren & Deelman, 1980). In fact, research has suggested that the discriminative power of reaction time in brain disease is equivalent to more sophisticated and complex psychological tests (Elsass, 1986). Miller (1970) states that slow response resembles the aging brain and reflects delayed information capacity. The overall effect of neurological trauma on reaction time is interpreted as due to the negative effect that the neuron loss has on signal-to-noise ratio (Wellford, 1962), which results in increased central processing time (Gronwall & Wrightson, 1974). Miller (1970) found a deficit in choice reaction time due to a central deficit disorder.

The majority of the research demonstrates that head trauma impairs memory, intelligence, and higher cortical functions. Much of the research evaluating these factors indicates that subtle deficits in higher cortical functions persist after apparent physical recovery and that those deficits limit the patients' ability to cope with their environment. Dikmen and Reitan (1976) found impairment in higher cortical functions as measured by the Halstead-Reitan Neuropsychological Battery. They found recovery greatest during the 1st year, with greatest recovery in patients with the greatest deficits. A comparison of performance on the Halstead-Reitan Battery (HRB) to EEG and CT scans found the HRB to be far superior in detecting deficits in mild and moderately impaired patients (CT scan, 28%; EEG, 25%; HRB, 84%); however, all were nearly equivalent with severely injured patients (Long & Gouvier, 1982). Even with these findings, the data suggest that neuropsychological assessment, while far superior to other medical assessment devices in investigating the effects of brain-impaired individuals, only touches on the problem of the overall behavioral disturbance following head trauma.

Symonds in 1939 stated that the dysfunction following head trauma appears to be due to slowness of perception, inability to see the picture as a whole, imprecise figure formation, and perseveration. The deficits revealed by neuropsychological assessment may be due to numerous persistent factors such as attention deficit (Miller & Cruzat, 1981), poor memory, and impaired information processing (Gronwall, 1977).

Goldstein and Ruthven (1983) described a disinhibition that resulted in increased threshold for excitation, sustained overreaction to stimuli, defective perception, and perseveration, language problems, and slowness in perception as factors accounting for changes in behavior following head injury.

The overall research findings suggest that while head injury impairs a broad range of cognitive functions, impairment is a function of severity of the injury, the patient's premorbid level of functioning, and time since injury. While the general neuropsychological assessment provides a more sensitive measure of impairments in cognitive function than more traditional psychometric tests, such as intellectual or memory assessment, there remains the question as to the extent to which neuropsychological assessment effectively assays the underlying problems. Considerable research suggests that neuropsychological assessment may, in fact, be rather insensitive to some subtle cognitive deficits (Dikmen & Reitan, 1976). On the other hand, it may be that behavior reflects, in addition to cognitive dysfunction, the emotional and situational factors that have been undoubtedly modified by the trauma and serve to influence the patient's behavior. Certainly, the common characteristics of head-injured individuals are similar to those of other individuals with frontal lobe damage. It may be this frontal lobe damage that results in poor social judgment, impaired motivation, and many of the other symptoms that account for the subtle but pervasive long-term effects of head injury.

Emotional Factors

One of the most persistent disabling consequences of head injury is poor emotional adjustment. In fact, it is estimated that in excess of 38% of trauma patients are significantly impaired by emotional factors. Fahy, Irving, and Millac (1967) found that only 5 of 22 patients studied were free of emotional complications, but only 2 patients actually sought psychiatric assistance. Of further interest is the fact that emotional factors are likely to augment focal cognitive deficits (Fogel & Sparadeo, 1985).

Families and friends of patients are likely to describe personality changes in the head injury victim. They usually describe changes in temperament, including depression, anxiety, obsessional characteristics, and persistent irritability. These changes appear to reflect an attenuation in coping skills and, in all probability, is secondary to cognitive dysfunction resulting from the injury. The effects of injury appear greater in lower socioeconomic groups who might be expected to have more stressful problems both before and after trauma. The general lack of understanding of the effects of brain injury on cognitive functions might be interpreted as a major factor in the subsequent emotional problems. Finally, reduced stamina, irritability, and lower impulse control lead to behavioral problems that further complicate the patient's posttrauma adjustment. In effect, the patient is less able to cope at a time when the stress demands are greatest. The emotional consequences of head injury might best be understood by considering emotional manifestations at three levels of severity: postconcussion symptoms, posttraumatic neurosis, and posttraumatic psychosis.

Postconcussion Symptoms

Postconcussion symptoms are the most commonly reported consequence of head injury and are reported by 40% to 60% of head injury patients. They represent the most frequent reason for medical referral (Klonoff & Thompson, 1969). Yet, in spite of their high frequency and similar characteristics across individuals, there remains considerable misunderstanding with regard to the significance of postconcussion symptoms in the patient's recovery and emotional adjustment. Symonds (1962) concluded that it is fruitless to attempt to resolve the issues of whether such symptoms are functional or organic as they must always be both. Certainly, postconcussion symptoms are similar to symptoms of psychological stress, but this does not suggest that they are without a physical basis.

The consistency of postconcussion symptoms has led to the concept of postconcussion syndrome; however, research has demonstrated that the consistency is not sufficient to document the presence of a syndrome (Lidvall, Linderoth, & Norlin, 1974). What is referred to as PCS is merely a collection of symptoms (e.g., headaches, dizziness, fatigue, irritability, language disturbance, visual problems, tinnitus, alcohol intolerance). While there may be a correlation between concentration and memory weakness, there is no other clear-cut symptom cluster and, thus, the concept of postconcussion syndrome would appear misleading (Rutherford, Merritt, & McDonald, 1977).

In part, the misunderstanding about postconcussion symptoms relates to the inconsistent manner in which they are evaluated, and lack of understanding of the relationship between postconcussion symptoms and the organic basis for injury. The development and exacerbation of symptoms weeks or months after mild to moderate head injury is difficult to explain from an organic perspective alone (Lidvall et al., 1974). The longer postconcussion symptoms persist, the less likely they are to be organic (Ruesch & Bowman, 1945). Some of the symptoms that develop and persist, such as anxiety and depression, are not easily attributed to brain injury. Finally, if PCS are a direct reflection of brain injury, a positive relation with injurity severity would be expected. Unfortunately, postconcussion symptoms are considered to be psychological in nature as no organic abnormality can be easily detected by routine medical tests. It is true that PCS overlaps with symptoms experienced by individuals suffering neurotic disorders. Thus, such symptoms could reflect emotional factors arising from or predating the head injury (Adler, 1945; Elia, 1972; Guthkelch, 1979; Kozol, 1945). Elia (1972), however, stated that postconcussion symptoms reflect not only the result of brain damage, but the patient's emotional response as well. There is a correlation between symptoms and age (Elia, 1972; Rutherford et al., 1977), but both physiological and psychological factors appear important.

Research investigating the characteristics of head-injured patients and the relationship between neurological damage, premorbid level of functioning, and situational factors reveals that postconcussion symptoms reflect an interaction between neurological damage and these other factors. Professionals have postconcussion symptoms but they are less disruptive (Taylor, 1967). It has been observed that severely injured patients generally report fewer postconcussion symptoms; however, such reports are made in individuals who have less situational demands placed on them. They generally are not attempting to return to work or school. In contrast, less severely impaired patients with less extensive neurological damage report considerably more postconcussion symptoms that are of greater magnitude. However, their symptoms can often be correlated with changes in their environment. Postconcussion symptoms are seen most frequently in impaired individuals who are attempting to resume their premorbid social role (Wood et al., 1984). Perhaps it is for this reason that postconcussion symptoms may first develop or worsen many months after head injury, for that is when the patient is most likely to attempt the resumption of their normal duties. Based on this assumption, it has been hypothesized that postconcussion symptoms are a valuable source of information to the treating professional because they give insight into the net effect of neurological and situational factors and the extent to which the patient can effectively cope (Gronwall & Wrightson, 1974; Long & Novack, 1985). Taylor (1967) concludes that "patients who have minor difficulties in concentration and performance which irritate them and make them act unusual are not 'neurotic,' they are 'cerebrally disorganized' and for good organic reasons" (p. 70).

Posttraumatic Neurosis

The expression *posttraumatic neurosis* was originally used over 100 years ago by Oppenheim to describe an organic, neurological condition due to changes in the nervous system (Bloch & Bloch, 1972). It was only later that this was interpreted as an emotional reaction. While posttraumatic neurosis obviously includes postconcussion symptoms, the difference generally relates to the severity or disruptive effects of the symptoms. Postconcussion symptoms are frequently seen in individuals resuming normal duties, whereas posttraumatic neurosis represents a more severe state where patients are unable to meet the demands of their environment. Such a neurosis is seen as a process neurosis (Bloch & Bloch, 1972) caused by trauma, either psychological or organic (Thompson, 1965). The onset of posttraumatic neurosis is delayed in a similar manner to postconcussion symptoms and is also found to be inversely related to severity. Thus, posttraumatic neurosis, like postconcussion symptoms, reflects an interaction between the consequences of the trauma on the nervous system functioning and situational and premorbid factors.

In addition to postconcussion symptoms, personality changes often reflect a tendency in the individual toward more stereotyped, cautious, and defensive modes of functioning (Lishman, 1978). There is evidence of perseverative thinking, and episodes of disorientation and confusion (Montanky & Zaks, 1971). Later adaptation leads to constriction of emotions, simplification of the environment, and denial of ambiguity. The patient, thus, develops a rigid defensive posture as a mode of coping with the experienced changes. Obsessive-compulsive neurosis may be an exaggerated form of this rigid defensive posture and is frequently observed in patients suffering head trauma (McKeon, McGuffin, & Robinson, 1984).

While there is clearly a relationship between impaired cognitive function and attenuated coping skills, there remains an element of trauma associated with both the primary and secondary effects of neurological injury. Such trauma can be augmented in individuals with loss of family members or friends or in situations where negligence appears to be a primary contributing factor. Certainly, the injury can serve as a focal point for all of life's other problems (Berger, 1975; Foster, 1964), or the trauma may simply be an added stress that leads to the development of anxiety, representing an alarm reaction that is unwarranted by the situation (McKay, 1960), and may be further aggravated by feelings of inadequacy or vulnerability before or after the accident. Patients who experience severe tension often have persistent fears that they will lose control (Pathak, Renjhen, Mallick, & Chawla, 1974).

Litigation and Secondary Gain

Miller (1961a, 1961b) has claimed that postconcussion symptoms are related to compensation. The majority of his articles focused on the intent of the patient to extract his or her just rewards from insurance companies. He described many cases of malingering. Considerable data are available to the contrary, however, which support Strauss and Savitsky's (1934) view that there was too much emphasis upon "neuropaths taking advantage of insurance companies." Furthermore, they felt that the problem relates to failure to distinguish between malingering and neurosis.

While there is still a general feeling among many health care professionals that patients involved in litigation will exaggerate their symptoms, many now see these factors in a somewhat different light. Miller and Cartlidge (1972) report that malingerers need help as much as hysterics and can, in fact, be helped.

The majority of the research indicates that the emphasis on litigation and secondary gain has been excessive (Strauss & Savitski, 1934; Thompson, 1965). Braverman (1977) studied ski and work-related injuries in Austria where the individual receives 6 months disability regardless of the cause. He found that 82% returned to work after 6 months and there were no significant differences between the two groups. In both groups, the patients who had the greatest problems in recovery were those less prepared for the eventuality of an accident. He further concluded that compensation/litigation has psychological effects but does not cause posttraumatic reaction. There appear to be individuals who are predisposed to disability (disability neurosis) due to early deprivation, unmet dependency needs, and/or early responsibility (Ford, 1976, 1977–1978). While litigation does not appear to be the overwhelmingly significant factor as once believed, the process of litigation can augment the patient's fears and concerns. Litigation is most likely to occur in situations where negligence is alleged. It may be the anger and hostility over negligence rather than strong desires for secondary gain that contribute to the emotional factors in patients undergoing litigation. Patients are subjected to a great deal of uncertainty until damages are awarded. The award or decision for no award might be considered much like the exam for the student. There is considerable tension and anxiety due to this uncertainty and once decided, one way or the other, there is considerable relief. Certainly, litigation does not cause the symptoms, but can augment the patient's response.

Posttraumatic Psychosis

Psychosis is not a common consequence of head injury. When it does occur, there is generally some evidence of a constitutional predisposition or premorbid maladjustment. Acute posttraumatic psychosis is usually short-lived and present at the time when the patient is in a period of maximum confusion. Even psychosis developing later may have an organic basis. The neuronal damage may impair the patient's coping style, disrupt effective input, and thus interact with any predisposing factors. Achte and Halberg (1969) conducted one of the most comprehensive studies of psychotic illness after head trauma. They found that only 2.6% of the head trauma population studied developed psychosis resembling schizophrenia. However, this was well above the incidence in the normal population. Only 0.84% developed primary schizophrenia, the remainder being schizoform or borderline. More patients with mild injuries developed schizophrenia than did those with severe injuries. No significant correlations were found between psychotic state and hemisphere or region of the brain injured. Shapiro (1939) studied patients exhibiting schizophrenia following head injury. The majority of the patients either demonstrated evidence of persistent neurological damage or had evidence of a constitutional predisposition for schizophrenia. Seven of 21, however, had well-integrated premorbid personalities. Hillbom (1951) argued for an organic etiology to schizophrenia based upon his finding that the majority of his patients with schizophrenia-like symptoms (especially paranoia) had sustained damage to the temporal lobes. In spite of these findings, it is doubtful that it is the physical damage to the brain alone that causes psychosis.

Research and clinical experience on the emotional consequences of head trauma clearly document that changes in emotional behavior when studied alone can be very misleading and do not provide the entire picture. Nevertheless, these symptoms may be employed as an effective assessment of the patient's overall level of functioning. Increases in postconcussion symptoms may provide insights into the individual's ability to cope with the stress. As symptoms increase in number and/or severity, adjustments to situational demands can be recommended and psychotherapeutic assistance can be implemented to avoid the development of more severe emotional problems. Difficulties in cognitive and emotional adjustment in head-injured persons place considerable stress on their caregivers and impair their emotional recovery. McKinlay and Brooks (1984) estimate that over 70% of close relatives report high stress, and many need professional assistance.

Social and Vocational Factors

Head trauma has traditionally been viewed as primarily a neurosurgical problem; however, research over the past 10 years has revealed that the recovery from head trauma is greatly influenced by nonorganic factors. Attention has been directed to the premorbid functioning of the individual, cognitive impairment, and emotional adjustment. However, there remains an area that may bear the greatest influence on recovery and one that can be significantly modified. This area involves the social support system and the vocational role of the individual following trauma.

Head trauma patients may demonstrate poor social judgment, which leads to social disability. Family members are often embarrassed by the patient's lack of inhibition and, in response, tend to restrict their activities and the activities of the patient accordingly. Numerous authors have found that such psychosocial disabilities account for more of the overall disability than neurological deficits (Bond, 1976; Heaton & Pendleton, 1981; Jennett, Snoek, Bond, & Brooks, 1981; Newcombe, 1982; Gore, 1981). Head injury patients are less able to cope with their jobs, have decreased interest in avocational pursuits, frequently complain of boredom, and have decreased social contacts (Weddell, Oddy, & Jenkins, 1980).

While social/vocational variables encompass a broad range of the patient's environment, recent research findings have emphasized the importance of social support during recovery from head trauma (Cassel, 1974, 1976; Gottlieb, 1981; Wagner, Long, & Williams, 1985). The adequacy of social support systems has been found to be associated with speed and level of recovery as well as with the patients' ability to cope with their illness (DiMatteo & Hays, 1981; Gore, 1981; La Rocco, House, & French, 1980; Wagner et al., 1985). Social support buffers or reduces the impact of environmental stress factors on the patient and facilitates recovery; unfortunately, the role of social support is often ignored in rehabilitation (Bond, 1976).

Family

Perhaps nowhere are social influences greater than in the family. Rosenthal and Muir (1983) emphasize the significance of the family role by stating that the best neurosurgical intervention may be of no value if the patient is significantly impaired in their quality of life. They emphasize the importance of knowing how the family and patient handle stress and point out the need for identifying high-risk families in formulating effective family intervention techniques. These intervention techniques involve education, counseling, or therapy, depending on the severity of the problem.

Family members' personalities have been found to influence the patient's experience of stress. McKinlay and Brooks (1984) found that high neuroticism within the family was related to patient difficulties. Lezak (1978) has also considered the influence of family dynamics during recovery from head trauma, but she emphasizes characterological deficits of the patient that disrupt family interactions. Patients have poor social perceptions and impaired control and self-regulation, resulting in impulsivity, restlessness, and impatience. They often exhibit stimulus-bound behavior resulting in social dependency, and they generally demonstrate an inability to profit from experience. However, the characterological changes contribute most to family stress. Lezak has found that even minor changes in irritability or reduced drive can have stressful effects on the family. Family members frequently feel isolated. This is attributed to being embarrassed by the patient's behavior in public or when having friends to the home. Many family members suffer from emotional turmoil of their own and are in need of supportive counseling. Stress on the family is worse at 1 month and levels off at 6 months with no further decline in families of severely impaired individuals (Oddy, Humphrey, & Uttley, 1978). In fact, Oddy et al. (1978) found that two thirds of the relatives of head trauma patients needed counseling and often medication. Their role is critical in determining the patients' perceptions of their environment and in influencing changes in their behavior. Thus, supportive counseling or education serves as a vital mechanism for aiding patients in recovery. Counseling goals should be directed toward readjusting expectations, giving practical advice on management, and should serve to alert family members to their own needs (Lezak, 1978). Initial advice may fall on deaf ears, but with time the family becomes all too aware of the problems. With proper education and counseling, the family can be assisted to function more effectively and thus to provide better support.

In spite of the importance of the family's role in rehabilitation, they are often given vague and sometimes contradictory outcome expectations and little support, and they rarely receive training in terms of more effective procedures for facilitating patient recovery (Livingston, Brooks, & Bond, 1985; Livingston, 1986; Novack, Bergquist, Bennett, & Hartley, 1987; Oddy et al., 1978).

Demographics show that most head injury victims are young males with low socioeconomic status who have poor social support. In many cases, their failure to recover appears related to inadequate family support. Families need to be educated with regard to their role as "a facilitator and not a doer," and to establish methods of interaction that minimize the patient's stress as well as their own, while fostering independence rather than reacting in ways that serve to sustain dependency. The ideal role of the family is to aid the patient by structuring programs of activity, encouraging or insisting on patient participation, but realizing the patient's limitations. Family members need to know when and how to decrease support and foster independence. They need to work toward providing social contacts outside of the family situation and appropriate external stimulation.

Head trauma patients, their families, and significant others will all benefit if they are educated as to the facts of head trauma and strategies for aiding recovery and reasonable recovery expectations. Education should be directed at patient and family understanding of their present level of functioning. They need some guidelines as to probable level of recovery, although emphasis should always be placed on the fact that no one can set fixed limits. Patients and family members should be educated as to the relationship between postconcussion symptoms and stress. By properly educating family members, recovery may far exceed expectation based on duration of coma or posttraumatic amnesia.

Vocational Factors

Effective social support systems, particularly the family, clearly play a vital role in influencing the recovery of the head injured patient. However, even the most supportive family can be overtaxed unless the patient can obtain some type of employment. For without employment, they generally have no source of funds and thus remain dependent. The patient who makes a good recovery up to this point but either fails to find or fails to maintain some type of employment remains dependent upon the family and/or society. They progress to the level of near-independence but can't manage to sustain true independence. This undoubtedly frustrates the patient as well as the family and all frequently worry about what will happen when the parents or caregivers are not longer around. Both families and patients become caught up in this unsatisfactory situation where undesired behavior patterns (i.e., dependency) are established and unwittingly maintained.

Many rehabilitative programs are now specifying vocational or educational goals in the final stages of rehabilitation (Jellinek & Harvey, 1982). Obviously such goals must be set with regard to the patient's abilities (e.g., ambulation, upper limb use, nonverbal abstract reasoning) (Weisbroth, Esibill, & Zuger, 1971). So proper assessment of patients' abilities is a must. Prevocational work adjustment can deal with attentional problems, visual scanning, visuospatial abilities, and problem solving (Bolger, 1983).

The importance of vocation in recovery is reported in anecdotal case studies demonstrating that among patients who returned to work there is likely to be continued improvement in functions such as intelligence and memory, whereas recovery among nonemployed head trauma patients tends to level off at approximately 2 years.

Our own experience with head trauma patients indicates outcome can frequently be predicted based on measures of severity of trauma and premorbid level of functioning. The exceptions, of which there are many, generally are individuals who either have exceptionally good or exceptionally poor social support systems. Certainly, knowledge is limited with regard to the specifics of such a complex interaction; however, sufficient data are available to suggest that further studies may offer significant insights into effective intervention strategies in augmenting recovery from neurological trauma.

Rehabilitation

The process of recovery after head injury is poorly understood and may relate to reorganization of the brain, actual recovery of function, or substitution that involves the development of compensatory skills. Whatever the case may be, it is known that nonorganic factors play a significant role in recovery and some psychological and social factors can be manipulated to the benefit of the patient.

Rehabilitation planning must take into account neural, medical, psychiatric, and environmental factors. Although head injury is often characterized in terms of the patient's cognitive weaknesses, the patient's competencies and skill strengths must also be determined (Anthony, 1980). Consequently, intervention begins with a comprehensive neuropsychological assessment including a detailed social history and an inventory of postconcussion symptoms (Diller & Gordon, 1981; Long & Gouvier, 1982; Williams, 1987).

The patient and family must be brought to understanding the patient's current level of functioning, taught how to identify barriers to recovery, and be given strategies for managing such barriers.

Barriers change as recovery progresses. Initially, attentional deficits may be most prominent. Later, memory weakness, not attributable to poor concentration, may be shown. Learning difficulties and information-processing inefficiency resolve slowly and exert a persistent and often subtle influence on the patient's behavior. Finally, emotional factors must be reckoned with as they are usually the most protracted and can be the most devastating.

The treatment and the treatment setting should vary as a function of the needs of the patient. Unfortunately, many patients receive assistance from good resources for a time, only to be released to their families with no continuation of treatment. Severely impaired patients may need rehabilitation that focuses upon physical resources. In such cases, physical, occupational, and speech therapists play a primary role. The effects of a physically oriented program will eventually reach their limits and other treatment orientations are needed. Generally, behaviorally oriented approaches are most effective at this point, for here the emphasis is directed toward memory and information processing with assistance in stress management. This approach also reaches its limits and emphasis should be shifted toward daily life behaviors, preferably in the situation where the patient will function. Ultimately, the needs of the patient shift to vocational/educational problems.

Rehabilitation planning, therefore, involves the following considerations:

1. Severity of injury
2. Time since injury
3. Level of cognitive functioning
4. Emotional adjustment
5. Deviation from premorbid level
6. Level of CNS involvement
7. Specific weaknesses and strengths
8. Intrapersonal or environmental factors
9. Family and social support systems
10. Vocational and/or educational status

Treatment for these problems follows three main principles: patient and family education, treatment for stress reactions, and family support. Interventions in these areas are all designed to prevent psychosocial complications of mild injury in the same sense that the neurosurgeon attempts to prevent physical complications in the acute phase of treatment.

Patient and Family Education

Self-appraisal, recovery expectations, and the cognitive demands of a patient's environment are very important since postconcussion symptoms may develop or be exacerbated by premature resumption of premorbid vocational/educational activities. This is a common problem after mild (to moderate) head injury—especially for patients whose work requires a high level of cognitive efficiency. Often such patients appear to rapidly recover. Since they function normally in casual/social interactions, they typically feel ready for work. Upon returning to work, however, they discover that they are unable to function at a normal efficiency level. They may be irritable and distractable and may be plagued by headaches. In addition, subtle cognitive weaknesses (e.g., memory) may become obvious to the patient and others. Probably the greatest service the neuropsychologist can provide is educating the mildly injured patient about the cognitive and emotional consequences of the brain injury. The patient and family must be told, in simple terms, that the consequences of mild injuries are not always trivial and a gradual resumption of premorbid activities must be followed to allow full cognitive recovery and to avoid developing stress-related problems. Some professionals are reluctant to provide such information for fear of suggesting postconcussion symptoms (Miller, 1961a, 1961b, 1979). This is a reasonable concern. Suggestible or somatisizing patients may in fact develop symptoms per suggestion or at least suffer by ruminating on the possibility of cognitive symptoms that may never develop. To avoid this possibility, the patient must be educated in general terms using only the patient's current symptoms (or common symptoms such as headache) in explaining the role of stress.

Stress Reactions and Treatment

Usually, neuropsychologists first see mild head injury patients after they have had difficulty resuming their vocational/educational activities. By that time they are likely to be depressed, anxious, and worried. In general, their symptoms and complaints are like those attributed to stress reactions, such as fatigue, irritability, and headaches. In cases of more severe head injury, however, those symptoms reflect, in part, reduced ability to concentrate and efficiently process information, and the patient's emotional reaction to those problems.

These stress-related symptoms can be managed with stress reduction techniques (Sena, 1985). Biofeedback monitoring and relaxation training can be used to alleviate anxiety and muscle tension associated with headache and irritability. In some cases, antidepressant medications may be used if the reactions are severe or if the patient becomes significantly depressed; however, caution is advised since such drugs may temporarily reduce the patient's overall cognitive ability.

Stress can also be reduced by modifying the work environment. This can range from reducing time and/or responsibility in the patient's current job to temporary reassignment to a less demanding job. In any case, the employer's understanding and cooperating must be developed by the psychologist. As a general rule of thumb, the supervisors and employers are less tolerant of the patient's special needs in the smaller company. In contrast, many larger corporations have a special commitment to disabled workers.

Most mildly injured patients succeed by simply easing back into their former employment with counseling to monitor stress reactions and to devise strategies to manage problems as they arise (Diller & Gordon, 1981). Such counseling is important in all cases of head injury. Often all that is necessary is problem-oriented counseling to head off difficulties and prevent psychosocial complications.

Family Support

The nature and degree of family/social support influence recovery after head injury (Wagner et al., 1985), if for no other reason than the fact that most rehabilitation in the outpatient setting is mediated by the family and social network of the patient. If a patient needs outpatient physical therapy or cognitive retraining, it is often a family member who seeks out and arranges such services. Family members also provide problem-oriented counseling and perhaps even alternative job opportunities for patients who cannot adjust to their old employment.

Outpatient treatment programs should marshal the resources of the family at the earliest possible moment. Any rehabilitation program will benefit from a coordinated program involving the rehabilitation counselor, patient, and family members (Wright, 1980). The family should receive the same education about head injury as the patient receives. This will head off misinterpretations of the patient's behavior and provide a context for the role of family members in the patient's progress toward occupational adjustment. The family can be trained to deal with the patient's symptoms rather than react to them in a debilitating manner. If significant family members are involved in the patient's ongoing struggles, then they should become part of the counseling process and should be invited to sessions with the patient. Family dynamics will influence the patient's manifestation of symptoms and occupational adjustment. These family problems should be addressed in family therapy or counseling. Often such influences on rehabilitation from head injury are neglected, but they may be just as influential as any other part of the rehabilitation intervention.

While almost any approach to rehabilitation can aid in improving recovery to some extent, the effectiveness of any program depends upon the identification of problems or barriers to recovery and their removal. Goldstein and Ruthven (1983) reviewed rehabilitation strategies and identified four models of rehabilitation: 1) physical, 2) psychiatric, 3) behavioral, and 4) neuropsychological. They pointed out that chance rather than need is often the big factor in determining not only outcome but institutionalization. Goldstein and Ruthven (1983) and Caplan (1982) have argued for rational rehabilitation, that is the application of resources based upon the patient's needs rather than the availability of staff and other resources.

Vocational/educational goals and accomplishments represent the final and perhaps most important step in the rehabilitation process. If the patient cannot obtain employment, he or she remains dependent on the family or social agencies and may never reach true independence or full recovery. In cases of severe injury, the options may be limited, but even work in a sheltered work environment may have a significant impact on the patient's self-concept and eventual recovery. Unfortunately, there is and has always been a significant gap between acute care and vocational rehabilitation (Lewin, 1968).

In summary, rehabilitation of mild injuries is an extremely complex process that often involves occupational adjustment and emotional adjustment to a greater extent than rehabilitation of more severe injuries. Rehabilitation of mild injuries is carried out in the outpatient setting and requires the coordination of community agents, such as family and employers, to facilitate and complement the patient's efforts. This is accomplished through the use of patient, family, and employer education, management of the patient's stress reactions, and the building of family and social support. Through the coordinated action of all of these components, comprehensive rehabilitation efforts can be effective.

References

Achte, K.A.E., & Halberg, V. (1969). Psychoses following war brain injuries. *Acta Psychiatrica Scandinavica, 45*, 1–18.

Adler, A. (1945). Mental symptoms following head injury. *Archives of Neurology and Psychiatry, 53*, 34–43.

Anthony, W. (1980). Psychological rehabilitation: A concept in need of a method. *American Psychologist, 32*, 658–662.

Barclay, L., Zemcov, A., Reichert, W., & Blass, J.P. (1985). Cerebral blood flow decrements in chronic head injury syndrome. *Biological Psychiatry, 20*, 146–157.

Berger, J.C. (1975). Some psychological aspects of industrial injury. *Illinois Medical Journal, 147*, 364–365.

Bloch, G.R., & Bloch, N.H. (1972). Traumatic and post-traumatic neurosis. *Industrial Medicine, 41*, 5–8.

Bolter, J.F., Gouvier, W.D., Veneklasen, J.A., & Long, C.J. (1982). Using demographic information to predict premorbid IQ: A test of clinical validity with head trauma patients. *Clinical Neuropsychology, 4*, 171, 174.

Bolger, J.P. (1983). Educational and vocational deficits. In M. Rosenthal, E. Griffith, M. Bond, & J. Miller (Eds.), *Rehabilitation of the head injured adult*, (pp. 219–225. Philadelphia: Davis.

Bond, M.R. (1976). Assessment of the psychosocial outcome of severe head injury. *Acta Neurochirurgica, 34*, 57–70.

Bond, M.R. (1983). Standardized methods of assessing and predicting outcome. In M. Rosenthal, E. Griffith, M. Bond, & J. Miller (Eds.), *Rehabilitation of the head injured adult*, (pp. 97–113). Philadelphia: Davis.

Braverman, M. (1977). Validity of psychotraumatic reactions. *Journal of Forensic Science, 22*(3), 654–662.

Brooks, D.N. (1983). Disorders of memory. In M. Rosenthal, E. Griffith, M. Bond, & J. Miller (Eds.), *Rehabilitation of the head injured adult*, (pp. 185–196). Philadelphia: Davis.

Brooks, D.N., Aughton, M.E., Bond, M.R., Jones, P., & Rizvi, S. (1980). Cognitive sequelae in relationship to early indices of severity of brain damage after severe blunt head injury. *Journal of Neurology, Neurosurgery and Psychiatry, 43*, 529–534.

Caplan, B. (1982). Neuropsychology in rehabilitation: Its role in evaluation and intervention. *Archives of Physical Medicine and Rehabilitation, 63*, 362–366.

Carlsson, C.A., Von Essen, C., & Lofgren, J. (1968). Factors affecting the clinical course of patients with severe head injuries. *Journal of Neurosurgery, 29*, 242–251.

Cassel, J. (1974). Psychosocial processes and "stress": Theoretical formulations. *International Journal of Health Services, 6*, 471–482.

Cassel, J. (1976). The contribution of the social environment to host resistance. *American Journal of Epidemiology, 104*, 107–123.
Caveness, W. (1977). Epidemiologic studies of head injury. *Trauma, 18*(6), 61–66.
Crovitz, H.F. (1979). Memory retraining in brain damaged patients: The airplane list. *Cortex, 16*, 131–134.
Denckler, S.J. (1960). Closed head injury in twins. *Arch General Psychiatry, 20*, 569–574.
Denckler, S.J. (1958). A follow-up study of 128 closed head injuries in twins using co-twins as controls. *Acta Psychiatrica et Neurologica Scandinavica, 33*(Suppl. 123), 1–125.
Denckler, S.J., & Lofving, B.A. (1958). A psychometric study of identical twins discordant for closed head injury. *Acta Psychiatrica et Neurologica Scandinavica, 33*(Suppl. 122), 119–126.
Denny-Brown, D., & Russell, W.R. (1941). Experimental cerebral concussion. *Brain, 64*, 93–164.
Dikmen, S., & Reitan, R.M. (1976). Psychological deficits and recovery of function after head injury. *Transactions of the American Neurological Association, 101*, 72–77.
Dikmen, S.A., Reitan, R.M., & Temkin, N.R. (1983). Neuropsychological recovery in head injury. *Archives of Neurology, 40*, 303–338.
Diller, L., & Gordon, W.A. (1981). Rehabilitation and clinical neuropsychology. In S. Filskov & T. Boll (Eds.), *Handbook of Clinical Neuropsychology*, New York: Wiley.
DiMatteo, M.R., & Hays, R. (1981). Social support and serious illness. In B.H. Gottlieb (Ed.), *Social networks and social support*. Beverly Hills: Sage Publications.
Drudge, O., Williams, J.M., Gomes, F., & Kessler, M. (1984). Recovery from closed head injuries: Repeat testings with the Halstead-Reitan Neuropsychological Battery. *Journal of Clinical Psychology, 40*, 259–265.
Elsass, P. (1986). Continuous reaction time in cerebral dysfunction. *Acta Neurologica Scandinavica, 73*, 225–246.
Elia, J.C. (1972). The post concussion syndrome. *Industrial Medicine, 41*, 23–31.
Fahy, T.D., Irving, M.H., & Millac, P. (1967). Severe head injuries: A six year follow-up. *Lancet, ii*, 475–479.
Fodor, I.E. (1972). Impairment of memory functions after acute head injury. *Journal of Neurology, Neurosurgery and Psychiatry, 35*, 818–824.
Fogel, B.S., & Sparadeo, F.R. (1985). Focal cognitive deficits accentuated by depression. *Journal of Nervous and Mental Diseases, 173*, 120–124.
Ford, B. (1976). Head injuries: What happens to survivors. *Medical Journal of Australia, 1*, 603–605.
Ford, C.V. (1977–1978). A type of disability neurosis: The Humpty Dumpty Syndrome. *International Tour of Psychiatry in Medicine, 8*(3), 285–294.
Foster, M.W. (1964). Neurosis and trauma. *Clinical Orthopsychiatry, 32*, 54–59.
Friede, R.L. (1961). Experimental concussion acceleration: Pathology and mechanics. *Archives of Neurology, 4*, 449–462.
Goldstein, G., & Ruthven, L. (1983). *Rehabilitation of the brain-damaged adult*. New York: Plenum Press.
Gore, S. (1981). The effect of social support in moderating the health consequences of unemployment. *Journal of Health and Social Behavior, 17*, 157–165.
Gottlieb, B.H. (Ed.). (1981). *Social networks and social support*. Beverly Hills: Sage Publications.
Gouvier, W.D., Bolter, J.F., Veneklasen, J.A., & Long, C.J. (1983). Predicting verbal and performance IQ from demographic data: Further findings with head trauma patients. *Clinical Neuropsychology, 5*, 119–121.

Gronwall, D.M.A. (1977). Paced auditory serial-addition task: A measure of recovery from concussion. *Perceptual and Motor Skills, 44*, 367–373.
Gronwall, D., & Wrightson, P. (1974). Delayed recovery of intellectual function after minor head injury. *Lancet, ii*, 605–609.
Gulbrandsen, G.B. (1983). Neuropsychological sequelae of light head injuries in older children 6 months after trauma. *Journal of Clinical Neuropsychology, 6*, 257–268.
Guthkelch, A.N., II. (1979). Assessment of outcome: Post-traumatic amnesia, post-concussional symptoms, and accident neurosis. *Acta Neurochirurgica* (Suppl. 28), 120–133.
Heaton, R.K., & Pendleton, M.G. (1981). Use of neuropsychological tests to predict adult patients' everyday functioning. *Journal of Consulting and Clinical Psychology, 49*(6), 807–821.
Hillbom, E. (1951). Schizophrenic-like psychoses after brain trauma. *Acta Psychiatrica et Neurologica Scandinavica* (Suppl. 60), 36–47.
Ishii, S. (1966). Brain swelling: Studies of structural, physiologic, and biochemical alterations. In W. Caveness & A.E. Walker (Eds.), *Head injury conference proceedings* (pp. 276–299). Philadelphia: Lippincott.
Jellinek, H.M., & Harvey, R.F. (1982). Vocational/educational services in a medical rehabilitation facility: Outcomes in spinal cord and brain injured patients. *Archives of Physical Medicine and Rehabilitation, 63*, 87–88.
Jennett, B., Snoek, J., Bond, M.R., & Brooks, M. (1981). Disability after severe head injury: Observations on the use of the Glascow Outcome Scale. *Journal of Neurology, Neurosurgery and Psychiatry, 44*, 285–293.
Klonoff, H., & Low, M.D. (1974). Disordered brain function in young children and early adolescents: Neuropsychological and electroencephalographic correlates. In R.M. Reitan & H.A. Davison (Eds.), *Clinical neuropsychology: Current status and applications*. New York: Wiley.
Klonoff, H., Low, M.D., & Clark, C. (1977). Head injuries in children: A prospective five year follow-up. *Journal of Neurology, Neurosurgery and Psychiatry, 40*, 1211–1219.
Klonoff, H., & Thompson, G.B. (1969). Epidemiology of head injuries in adults: A pilot study. *Canadian Medical Association Journal, 100*, 235–241.
Klove, H., & Cleeland, D.S. (1972). The relationship of neuropsychological impairment to other indices of severity of head injury. *Scandinavian Journal of Rehabilitation Medicine, 4*, 55–60.
Kozol, H.L. (1945). Pretraumatic personality and sequelae of head injury. *Archives of Neurology and Psychiatry, 53*, 358–364.
Kozol, H.L. (1946). Pretraumatic personality and psychiatric sequelae of head injury. *Archives of Neurology and Psychiatry, 56*, 245–275.
Landsell, H., & Smith, P.J. (1975). Asymmetrical cerebral function for two WAIS factors and their recovery after brain injury. *Journal of Consulting and Clinical Psychology, 43*(6), 923.
LaRocco, J.M., House, J.S., & French, J.R., Jr. (1980). Social support, occupational stress, and health. *Journal of Health and Social Behavior, 21*, 202–218.
Levin, H.S., Benton, A., & Grossman, R.G. (1979). *Neurobehavioral consequences of closed head injuries*. New York: Oxford University Press.
Levin, H.S., & Eisenberg, H.M. (1979). Neuropsychological outcome of closed head injury in children and adolescents. *Child's Brain, 5*, 281–292.
Levin, H.S., Grossman, R.G., Rose, J.E., & Teasdale, G. (1979). Long-term neuropsychological outcome of closed head injury. *Journal of Neurosurgery, 50*, 412–422.

Levin, H.S., Handel, S.F., Goldman, A.M., Eisenberg, H.M., & Guinto, F.C. (1985). Magnetic resonance imaging after 'diffuse' nonmissile head injury. *Archives of Neurology, 42*, 963–968.

Levin, H.S., O'Donnell, V.M., & Grossman, R.B. (1979). The Galveston orientation and amnesia test: A practical scale to assess cognition after head injury. *Journal of Nervous and Mental Disease, 167*, 675–684.

Lewin, W. (1968). Rehabilitation after head injury. *British Medical Journal, 1*, 465–470.

Lezak, M.D. (1978). Living with the characterologically altered brain injured patient. *Journal of Clinical Psychiatry, 39*(7), 592–598.

Lezak, M.D. (1979). Recovery of memory and learning functions following traumatic brain injury. *Cortex, 15*(1), 63–72.

Lidvall, H., Linderoth, B., & Norlin, B. (1974). Recovery from head injury. *Acta Neurologica Scandinavica, 50* (Suppl).

Lishman, W.A. (1973). The psychiatric sequelae of head injury: A review. *Psychological Medicine, 3*, 304–318.

Lishman, W.A. (1978). Head injury. In *Organic psychiatry* (Ch. 5, pp. 192–261). London: Blackwell.

Livingston, M.G. (1986). Assessment of need for coordinated approach in families with victims of head injury. *British Medical Journal, 293*(20), 742–744.

Livingston, M.G., Brooks, D.N., & Bond, M.R. (1985). Patient outcome in the year following severe injury and relatives' psychiatric and social functioning. *Journal of Neurology, Neurosurgery and Psychiatry, 48*, 876–881.

Long, C.J. (1985). Neuropsychology in private practice: Its changing focus. *Psychotherapy in Private Practice, 3*, 45–55.

Long, C.J., & Gouvier, W.D. (1982). Neuropsychological assessment of outcome following closed head injury. In R.N. Malatesha & L.C. Hartlage (Eds.), *Neuropsychology and cognition* (Vol. II) (pp. 116–128). The Hague: Martinus Nijhoff Publishers.

Long, C.J., Gouvier, W.D., & Cole, J.C. (1984). A model of recovery for the total rehabilitation of individuals with head trauma. *Journal of Rehabilitation, 50*(1), 39–45.

Long, C.J., & Haban, G. (1985, August). *Treatment planning and intervention with head trauma patients*. Paper presented at American Psychological Association Meeting, Los Angeles.

Long, C.J., & Novack, T. (1985). Interpretation and treatment of post-concussion symptoms following head trauma: Interpretation and treatment. *Southern Medical Journal, 79*, 728–732.

Long, C.J., & Webb, W. (1983). Psychological sequelae of head trauma. In P.C.W. Hall Ed.), *Psychiatric Medicine* (pp. 35–77). New York: S.P. Medical and Scientific Books.

Mackay, R.P. (1960). Post traumatic neuroses. *Industrial Medicine and Surgery*, 200–203.

Mandleberg, I.A., & Brooks, D.N. (1975). Cognitive recovery after severe head injury: 1. serial on the WAIS. *Journal of Neurology, Neurosurgery and Psychiatry, 38*, 1121–1126.

McKeon, J., McGuffin, P., & Robinson, P. (1984). Obsessive-compulsive neurosis following head injury: A report of four cases. *British Journal of Psychiatry, 144*, 190–192.

McKinlay, W.W., & Brooks, D.N. (1984). Methodological problems in assessing psychosocial recovery following severe head injury. *Journal of Clinical Neuropsychology, 61*(1), 87–99.

Miller, E. (1970). Simple and choice reaction time following severe head injury. *Cortex, 77*, 121–129.

Miller, E. (1979). The long term consequences of head injury: A discussion of the evidence with special reference to the preparation of legal reports. *British Journal of Social and Clinical Psychology, 18*, 87–98.

Miller, E., & Cruzat. (1981). A note on the effects of irrelevant information on task performance after mild and severe head injury. *British Journal of Clinical Psychology, 20*, 61–70.

Miller, H. (1961a). Accident neurosis I. *British Medical Journal. April 1*, 919–925.

Miller, H. (1961b). Accident neurosis II. *British Medical Journal, April 8*, 992–998.

Miller, H., & Cartlidge, N. (1972). Simulation and malingering after injuries to the brain and spinal cord. *Lancet, March 11*, 580–585.

Miller, J.D. (1983). Early evaluation and management. In M. Rosenthal, E. Griffith, M. Bond, & J. Miller (Eds.), *Rehabilitation of the head injured adult* (pp. 37–73). Philadelphia: Davis.

Montanky, G.V., & Zaks, M.S. (1971). Psychological changes following brain damage with autopsy confirmation of the lesion. *International Review of Applied Psychology, 20*, 89–99.

Newcombe, F. (1982). The psychological consequences of closed head injury: Assessment and rehabilitation. *Injury, 14*, 111–136.

Novack, T.A., Bergquist, T.F., Bennett, G., & Hartley, D. (1987). Cognitive stimulation in the home environment. In J.M. Williams & C.J. Long (Eds.), *The rehabilitation of cognitive disabilities* (pp. 149–169). New York: Plenum Press.

Novack, T.A., Daniel, M.S., & Long, C.J. (1984). Factors related to emotional adjustment following head injury. *International Journal of Clinical Neuropsychology, 6*, 139–142.

Oddy, M., Coughlan, T., Tyerman, A., & Jenkins, D. (1985). Social adjustment after closed head injury: A further follow-up seven years after injury. *Journal of Neurology, Neurosurgery and Psychiatry, 48*, 564–568.

Oddy, M., Hymphrey, M., & Uttley, D. (1978). Subjective impairment and social recovery after closed head injury. *Journal of Neurology, Neurosurgery and Psychiatry, 41*, 611–616.

Ommaya, A., & Gennarelli, T. (1974). Cerebral concussion and traumatic unconsciousness. *Brain, 97*, 633–654.

Pathak, L.R., Renjhen, R.C., Mallick, S.C., & Chawla, S. (1974). Neurosis following head injury. *Neurology India, 22*, 147–151.

Reyes, R.L., Battacharyya, A.K., & Heller, D. (1981). Traumatic head injury: Restlessness and agitation as prognosticators of physical and psychological improvement in patients. *Archives of Physical Medicine and Rehabilitation, 62*, 20–23.

Reynell, W.R. (1944). A psychometric method of determining intellectual loss following head injury. *Journal of Mental Science, 90*, 710.

Richardson, J.T.E. (1979). Signal detection theory and the effects of severe head injury upon recognition memory. *Cortex, 15*, 145–148.

Rimel, R. (1980). *Epidemiology and recovery following head injury.* Presented at Brain Injury '80—Accent on Treatment, Fisherville, VA.

Rimel, R.W., Giordani, B., Barth, J.T., & Jane, J.A. (1981). Disability caused by minor head injury. *Neurosurgery, 9*, 221–228.

Rimel, R.W., Giordani, B., Barth, J.T., & Jane, J.A. (1982). Moderate head injury: Completing the clinical spectrum of brain trauma. *Neurosurgery, 11*, 344–351.

Rosenthal, M., & Muir, C.A. (1983). Methods of family intervention. In M. Rosenthal, E.R. Griffith, M.R. Bond, & J.D. Miller (Eds.), *Rehabilitation of the head injured adult* (pp. 407–418). Philadelphia: Davis.

Ruesch, J. (1944). Intellectual impairment in head injuries. *American Journal of Psychiatry, 100*, 480-496.
Ruesch, J., & Bowman, K.M. (1945). Prolonged post-traumatic syndromes following head injury. *American Journal of Psychiatry, 102*, 145-163.
Ruesch, J., & Moore, B. (1943). Measurement of intellectual functions in the acute stage of head injury. *Archives of Neurology and Psychiatry, 50*, 165-170.
Russell, W.R. (1932). Cerebral involvement in head injury: A study based on the examination of 200 cases. *Brain, 35*, 549-603.
Russell, W.R., & Schiller, F. (1959). Crushing injuries to the skull: Experimental observations. *Journal of Neurology, Neurosurgery and Psychiatry, 12*, 52-60.
Rutherford, W.H., Merritt, J.D., & McDonald, J.R. (1977). Symptoms at one year following concussion from minor head injuries. *Injury, 10*(3), 225-230.
Sena, D. (1985). *Outpatient cognitive retraining in the private practice clinic.* Paper presented at the annual convention of the American Psychological Association. Los Angeles.
Shapiro, L.B. (1939). Schizophrenic-like psychoses following head injury. *Illinois Medical Journal, 76*, 250-254.
Slater, E. (1962). Psychological aspects. In *Modern views on 'stroke' illness.* Tavistock Square, London: The Chest and Heart Association.
Stanczak, D.E., White, J.G., Gouvier, W.D., Moehle, K.A., Daniel, M., Novack, T., & Long, C.J. (1984). Assessment of level of consciousness following severe neurological insult: A comparison of the psychometric qualities of the Glasgow Coma Scale and the Comprehensive Level of Consciousness Scale. *Journal of Neurosurgery, 60*, 955-960.
Steadman, J.H., & Graham, J.G. (1970). Rehabilitation of the brain impaired. *Proceedings of Royal Society of Medicine, 63*, 23-28.
Strauss, I., & Savitsky, N. (1934). The sequelae of head injury. *American Journal of Psychiatry, 91*, 189-202.
Strich, S.J. (1956). Diffuse degeneration of the cerebral white matter in severe dementia following head injury. *Journal of Neurology, Neurosurgery and Psychiatry, 19*, 163-185.
Strich, S.J. (1961). Shearing of nerve fibers as a cause of brain damage due to head injury. *Lancet, 2*, 443-448.
Strich, S.J. (1969). The pathology of brain damage due to blunt head injuries. In A. Wolker, W. Caveness, & M. Critchley (Eds.), *The late effects of head injury* (pp. 501-529). Springfield, IL: Thomas.
Symonds, C. (1962). Concussion and its sequelae. *Lancet*, 1-5.
Symonds, C.P. (1939). Mental disorder following head injury. *Proceedings of the Royal Society of Medicine, 30*, 1081-1094.
Taylor, A.R. (1967). Post-concussional sequelae. *British Medical Journal, 3*, 67-71.
Teasdale, G., Knill-Jones, R., & Van Der Sande, J. (1978). Observer variability in assessing impaired consciousness and coma. *Journal of Neurology, Neurosurgery and Psychiatry, 41*, 603-610.
Thompson, G.N. (1965). Post-traumatic psychoneurosis: A statistical survey. *American Journal of Psychiatry, 121*, 1043-1048.
Tooth, G. (1947). On the use of mental tests for the measurement of disability after head injury. *Journal of Neurology, Neurosurgery and Psychiatry, 10*, 1-11.
Uzzell, B.P., Zimmerman, R.A., Dolinksas, C.A., & Obrist, W.D. (1970). Lateralized psychological impairment associated with CT lesions in head injury patients. *Cortex, 15*, 391-401.
Van Zomeren, A.H., & Deelman, B.G. (1980). Differential effects of simple and choice reaction time after closed head injury. *Clinical Neurology and Neurosurgery, 79*, 81-90.

Van Zomeren, A.H., & Van Den Burg, N. (1985). Residual complaints of patients two years after severe head injury. *Journal of Neurology, Neurosurgery and Psychiatry, 48*, 21–48.

Wagner, M., Long, C.J., & Williams, J.M. (1985). *Perceived outcome following head injury as related to social network support*. Paper presented at the National Academy of Neuropsychology Convention, Philadelphia.

Walker, A.E., & Erculei, F. (1969). *Head injured men fifteen years later*. Springfield, IL: Thomas.

Weddell, R., Oddy, M., & Jenkins, D. (1980). Social adjustment after rehabilitation: A two year follow-up of patients with severe head injury. *Psychological Medicine, 10*, 257.

Weisbroth, S., Esibill, N., & Zuger, R.R. (1971). Factors in the vocational success of hemiplegic patients. *Archives of Physical Medicine and Rehabilitation, October*, 441–446.

Wellford, A.T. (1962). On changes of performance with age. *Lancet, 1*, 335–339.

Willanger, R., Thygesen, P., Nietsen, R., & Peteroon, O. (1968). Intellectual impairment and cerebral atrophy. *Danish Medical Bulletin, 15*, 65–93.

Williams, J.M. (1987). The role of cognitive retraining in comprehensive rehabilitation. In J.M. Williams & C.J. Long (Eds.), *The rehabilitation of cognitive disabilities* (pp. 43–55). New York: Plenum Press.

Williams J.M., Gomes, F., Drudge, O., & Kessler, M. (1984). Predicting outcome from closed head injury by early assessment of trauma severity. *Journal of Neurosurgery, 61*, 581–585.

Wilson, R., Rosenbaum, G., & Brown, G. (1979). The problems of premorbid intelligence in neuropsychological assessment. *Journal of Clinical Neuropsychology, 1*, 49–53.

Wilson, R., Rosenbaum, G., Brown, G., Rourke, D., Whitman, D., & Grisell, J. (1978). An index of premorbid intelligence. *Journal of Consulting and Clinical Psychology, 46*, 1544–1555.

Wood, F., Novack, T., & Long, C.J. (1984). Post-concussion symptoms: Cognitive, emotional and environmental aspects. *International Journal of Psychiatry in Medicine, 14*, 277–283.

Wright, R. (1980). *Total rehabilitation*. New York: Little, Brown.

6
Automatic Processing of Frequency Information in Survivors of Severe Closed Head Injury

FELICIA C. GOLDSTEIN and HARVEY S. LEVIN

Several information processing theories have proposed that individuals possess limited capacity for engaging in activities and that performance on various tasks depends, in part, upon the quantity and type of resources required (Hasher & Zacks, 1979; Kahneman, 1973; Navon & Gopher, 1979; Posner & Snyder, 1975; Shiffrin & Schneider, 1977). The notion of capacity refers to the basic amount of information that can be stored, transmitted, and processed. Individual difference variables such as age or intelligence have been posited to affect the amount of basic processing resources available for efficient performance. With increasing age, for example, less capacity may be available for performance on memory tasks that ordinarily place a heavy load on this limited pool. On the other hand, task variables such as difficulty or prior experience can also determine the ease of processing. Tasks that are relatively unfamiliar may require more resources than others.

Considerable controversy exists regarding the definition and measurement of "capacity" as well as delineation of these subject/task variables. However, there are several useful neuropsychological applications for the ideas that there may be individual variation in processing resources and that tasks may differ in their demands on the system. First, characterization of cognitive operations along an "automatic/volitional" continuum allows us to ask how various neurological conditions affect the attentional system. Given an a priori distinction between tasks that minimally draw from the capacity pool (i.e., require no active processing strategies) versus those that require sustained attention and effort, one can begin to explore whether conditions such as depression or progressive degenerative dementia selectively impair one type of processing over the other or result in a global deficit. Such questions can be of use in clinical diagnosis, pinpointing specific deficits, and evaluating the effects of treatment such as clinical drug trials. In addition, attempts to separate processing tasks along attentional demands can help, within a given clinical population, to document the degree and pattern of cognitive deterioration at various stages of the illness, as in senile dementia (Jorm, 1986; Whitehouse, 1986). For example, is dementia characterized by an initial loss of efficiency on effort-demanding tasks followed by generalized decrements in basic attentional processes? This strategy of investigating cognitive impairment can also be used to depict recovery curves for various functions after stroke or traumatic brain injury. Finally, one can define the skills that need to be addressed during rehabilitation, given a distinction in memory operations among those that are essentially strategy dependent (e.g., prose recall) versus those that require intactness of a core attentional system (monitoring frequency of events).

In this chapter, we examine an influential capacity theory of memory (Hasher & Zacks, 1979, 1984). After describing the automatic-versus-effortful processing framework proposed by Hasher and Zacks and reviewing the evidence supporting or refuting their position, we summarize findings obtained in the elderly and various neurological and psychiatric conditions. We also present two experiments conducted in our laboratory and discuss implications for the possible mechanisms underlying memory disorder after closed head injury.

Automatic/Effortful Framework

Hasher and Zacks (1979, 1984) propose that encoding operations in memory vary in terms of their demands on the attentional system. Certain features of to-be-remembered material are registered continuously without active intention, deliberate learning, or draining of this central capacity pool. These so-called "automatic processes" consist of the storage of such attributes as frequency information (the number of times various activities occur), temporal location (the order in which events occur), and spatial location (the relative position of events). For example, after attending a lecture, the listener is aware of whether many or few slides were presented, the order in which the material was presented, and the position of various objects in the room (slide projector, blackboard, etc.) without having actively encoded this information. In contrast, "effortful processes" (e.g., remembering a list of words) are capacity limited and require deliberate strategies. In order to remember the lecture for future recall, one must have organized, rehearsed, and elaborated the material. Such processes drain capacity and are susceptible to individual differences in performance such as age (Attig & Hasher, 1980; Zacks, Hasher, & Sanft, 1982).

The notion that individuals are sensitive to certain features of the environment without deliberate strategies or expenditure of effort has importance in terms of memory functioning. Hasher and Zacks argue that encoding includes storage not only of the basic material but also of certain attributes such as its position in time and space as well as its meaning. The fact that we can encode numerous features of to-be-remembered information with minimal effort allows us to operate more efficiently in terms of leaving capacity available for the target material. In addition, the results of automatically encoded information can aid in future recall. For example, sensitivity to relative frequencies of naturally occurring names in the English language can aid in trying to remember a person's name (was it familiar or nonfamiliar), whereas the ability to encode temporal features can aid in reconstructive memory (to find my keys, I need to retrace the steps I took in leaving the house this morning) (Hasher & Zacks, 1979). With respect to frequency processing, Hasher and Zacks (1984) cite numerous studies showing that individuals are sensitive to the natural occurrences of real-world events, such as letters, syllables, words, and reasons for mortality, without having deliberately encoded these features. The ability to encode repetitive qualities of events may serve a variety of functions in everyday memory activities (e.g., cueing oneself that there are more items on a grocery list).

The distinction made between automatic and effortful processing rests on the prediction of differential responsiveness to certain features. First, automatic processing does not require active intention. For example, one is sensitive to whether or not a name is common, whereas trying to remember the name necessitates strategies such as rehearsal, imagery, and association (effortful processing). Second, automatic processing is unaffected by task variables such as practice and feedback or individual differences including age and education. Hasher and Zacks suggest that certain abilities are innately programmed or established at a young age and therefore will show limited developmental trends. Finally, automatic processes are hypothesized to remain intact despite reductions of capacity caused by stress and arousal. These processes are assumed to drain minimal energy from the attentional system. Therefore, taking away capacity by imposing extra demands on the individual such as an additional task will not affect processing of frequency, temporal, or spatial attributes.

Not all studies have been supportive of the separation between automatic and effortful abilities. In fact, there is current debate regarding whether task and individual difference variables are unimportant to performance for temporal (Zacks, Hasher, Alba, Sanft, & Rose, 1984), spatial (Cooper & Marshall, 1985; Puglisi, Park, Smith, & Hill, 1985), and frequency encoding. In the following section, we review the evidence for the "automaticity" of frequency processing, the focus of our studies with head-injured patients.

Frequency Processing in Neurologically Intact Populations

Experimental studies of frequency processing typically expose individuals to examples of real-world events (letters, disease states, categories) or experimenter-contrived situations (words or pictures presented at various repetitions). Tests for sensitivity to frequency involve asking the subject to make actual estimates, forced-choice discriminations, or rank-orderings of the events. As shown in Table 6.1, three major predictions of the Hasher and Zacks framework on the alleged "automaticity" of such processing have received mixed support. These criteria include intentionality to encode frequency information, the effects of strategies and practice on performance, and whether reductions in capacity decrease the efficiency of frequency monitoring.

INTENTIONALITY

One criterion for assuming that an attribute is automatically encoded is the lack of benefit in warning subjects that they will be asked to make frequency decisions. With respect to intentional versus incidental instructions, several early studies (e.g., Flexser & Bower, 1975; Hasher & Chromiak, 1977; Howell, 1973; Zacks et al., 1982) appeared to demonstrate that informing subjects about an upcoming test of frequency versus an unspecified memory test for the items did not significantly influence the accuracy of frequency judgments. For example, Flexser and Bower (1975) and Hasher and Chromiak (1977, Experiment 1) told subjects either that they would be asked to estimate the number of times words were presented (informed condition) or that they would be asked to remember the words (uninformed condition). Flexser and Bower found that initial instructions produced no significant impact on sensitivity to frequency changes (correlation coefficient between estimated versus actual frequency: $r = .78$ for informed subjects; $r = .75$ for uninstructed subjects). Hasher and Chromiak (1977) did report greater accuracy for an informed group but only for items occurring at higher frequencies (e.g., words presented three or four times each). Moreover, there was no differential benefit of instructions for subjects at various educational levels (second, fourth, and sixth graders and college students), thus supporting the notion that automatic processing should show developmental invariance in contrast to "effortful" processes such as free recall.

More recently, the incidental paradigm used to assess the "automaticity" of frequency processing has been criticized as a weak and inappropriate manipulation (Fisk, 1986). First, it has been argued that the incidental versus intentional conditions are not very different. For example, informed and uninformed subjects are both told to expect some type of test and to process the stimuli, and therefore the groups are actually performing under *intentional* conditions. Second, studies typically do not control or take into account the strategies that subjects may be adopting. Failure to find differences in frequency estimations between informed and uninformed (e.g., to expect a memory test) groups could occur because: (a) the "memory" group adopted a strategy of registering frequency information to aid their future anticipated recall; or (b) the "frequency" group did not have an appropriate strategy and therefore performed at the level of the "memory" group (Greene, 1984).

It has been suggested that a stronger test of instructional variables would be to include a condition in which subjects are given no indications to process stimuli in any particular manner, either in preparation for recall or for frequency. If frequency processing is automatically encoded, then these subjects should be as accurate as those who try to process the stimuli (e.g., to remember them). Effects of the benefits of intentionality to learn material on frequency estimations have been found when such a truly incidental condition is used. Greene (1984) employed a paradigm in which a series of five digits appeared on a computer screen followed by a word that the subject repeated outloud as a distractor task

TABLE 6.1. Research examining the automaticity of frequency of occurrence processing.

	Intentional vs. incidental learning	Strategies and practice	Competing task demands
Prediction	Frequency processing should be unaffected by intentional vs. incidental instructions	Frequency processing should be insensitive to strategies and practice	Frequency processing should be unaffected by reductions in capacity
Studies supportive of prediction	Alba et al., 1980 (Exp. 2); Flexser & Bower, 1975; Hasher & Chromiak, 1977 (Exp. 1); Howell, 1973; Kausler & Puckett, 1980; Zacks et al., 1982 (Exp. 3)	Alba et al., 1980 (Exp. 2); Hasher & Chromiak, 1977 (Exp. 2); Straub et al., 1985; Zacks et al., 1982 (Exp. 1 & 2)	Zacks et al., 1982 (Exp. 3)
Studies unsupportive of prediction	Greene, 1984; Greene, 1986 (Exp. 1 & 2); Naveh-Benjamin & Jonides, 1986 (Exp. 3)	Greene, 1984 (Exp. 2); Greene, 1986 (Exp. 3); Maki & Ostby, 1987 (Exp. 1 & 2); Naveh-Benjamin & Jonides, 1986 (Exp. 2); Rose & Rowe, 1976	Kausler, Wright, & Hakami, 1981; Maki & Ostby, 1987 (Exp. 3); Naveh-Benjamin & Jonides, 1986 (Exp. 1)

before recalling the digits. There were 96 trials in which 32 words occurred once and 32 words occurred twice (presented on nonconsecutive trials). One group (intentional learning) was told that their memory (but not frequency judgment) for the words would be tested at the end of the experiment (the importance of remembering words was emphasized), while another group (incidental) was told that they would not be tested on memory for the words. This latter condition fits the definition of a truly incidental manipulation since subjects supposedly are not trying to process the words. There were significant differences in accuracy on the unexpected test of deciding whether word pairs were presented once or twice (mean proportion correct: intentional group = .85; incidental group = .69) as well as in correlations between estimated and actual frequency ($r = .71$ for intentional group; $r = .41$ for incidental group). Greene also showed in a second experiment the advantages of either warning subjects of memory for words or an upcoming frequency test in contrast to a no-instruction group. Subjects in the latter condition performed poorly in judging frequencies.

Greene (1986) demonstrated the importance of the emphasis of instructions given to subjects in processing stimuli and helped to clarify the differences between his earlier results and those reported by Kausler, Lichty, and Hakami (1984). Kausler et al. used the same three groups as in Greene's second experiment, but yet found no discrepancies in accuracy of frequency judgments. Employing a similar digit distractor task as in his original study, Greene (1986) used an incidental group (no mention made of a memory test for distractor words), a weak intentional group (told that they would be tested on the frequency of the words but that performance on the digit-recall task was equally important), and a strong intentional group (similar to the latter group but the frequency task was emphasized as more important than digit recall). While the incidental (mean proportion correct = .69) and weak-intentional groups (mean proportion correct = .72) made similar frequency judgments, the strong-intentional group was clearly more accurate (mean proportion correct = .85). Additionally, performance on the digit-recall task showed opposite trends, with the strong-intentional group performing the poorest. In opposition to an automaticity notion, it appears that the cover task provided to subjects, as well as the emphasis placed on the importance of processing particular types of information, can play a role in accuracy of frequency judgments.

Strategies and Practice

Two other variables that have received mixed support in the Hasher and Zacks framework concern the effects of strategies and practice on frequency judgments. An automatic process is assumed to be insensitive to techniques applied by an individual to help performance or to extended repetitions and feedback. In support of the predictions of the theory, instructions to use a counting strategy (Greene, 1986; Straub, Marshall, & Valencia, 1985) or conditions that make it easy to keep track of frequencies (e.g., to keep counts) (Alba, Chromiak, Hasher, & Attig, 1980) generally do not improve accuracy. Alba et al. (Experiment 2) asked subjects to judge the number of items occurring within various categories. There were nine categories with each of three categories containing three, six, or nine instances. In an easy version, all of the words belonging to a category were presented contiguously, while in a more difficult condition, exemplars of categories were placed in a random fashion. It was found that subjects produced comparable accuracy judgments in both conditions.

In contrast, studies that have induced subjects to adopt various strategies using a levels-of-processing framework have found differential effects on frequency judgments (Maki & Ostby, 1987; Naveh-Benjamin & Jonides, 1986; Rose & Rowe, 1976). The levels of processing paradigm (Craik & Lockhart, 1972) entails asking subjects questions of to-be-remembered material according to certain features such as semantic (is it a toy?), physical (does it begin with a capital letter?) or phonemic (does it rhyme with fall?). In terms of memory recall (an effortful process), semantic analysis generally has been found to improve performance relative to the other conditions. There should be no differential effect of type of processing on the ability to encode frequency information, however, if such encoding is immune to strategies. Naveh-Benjamin and Jonides (1986) presented words to subjects and asked them to either generate as many semantic or acoustic associates as they could think of. Words were presented at frequencies of one to six times. After this task, subjects were required to estimate the number of times each word occurred. Semantic analysis led to greater sensitivity to changes among presented frequencies. Maki and Ostby (1987) showed that increases in estimated frequency with actual frequency were greatest for words processed semantically (whether they were easy or difficult to imagine) versus structurally (whether they were short or long).

Zacks, Hasher, and Hock (1986) have argued that different orienting tasks produce changes in the amount of covert rehearsals that items receive, and therefore they do not see these results as a challenge to their theory. For example, physical analysis (e.g., to count the number of letters in a word) tends to promote isolated rehearsal, whereas semantic analysis (e.g., to rate the pleasantness of words) tends to encourage the subject to compare ratings of previous words. As a result, semantic analysis should lead to higher frequency ratings. Consistent with this viewpoint, Rose and Rowe (1976) observed that overall frequency judgments were lowest in physical (M = 3.07) versus rhyming (M = 3.93) or semantic (M = 4.13) groups. Maki and Ostby (1987) have recently challenged the covert rehearsal explanation of Hasher and Zacks by demonstrating that conditions designed to promote greater covert rehearsals (e.g., words that are more familiar and therefore easier to rehearse) do not necessarily produce better discriminability between estimated and actual frequency. They suggest that the levels of processing manipulation alters frequency judgments through its effect on attention rather than on rehearsal, per se. Finally, while it is plausible that semantic analysis could lead to higher estimates than other types of processing based on more rehearsal of items, it is unclear why semantic processing also produces better discriminability (Naveh-Benjamin & Jonides, 1986).

The effects of practice on frequency processing have been explored, but to a lesser extent than the previously discussed variables. According to Hasher and

Zacks, repeated exposure to frequency information produces no improvement in accuracy. In contrast, repeated presentation of memory items on effortful tasks improves performance by facilitating the use of active strategies (e.g., rehearsal). Hasher and Chromiak (1977, Experiment 2) investigated the joint effects of feedback and practice on estimations. Subjects heard lists of words at various occurrences and were asked to estimate their frequencies. After this task, they were shown the actual frequencies of the words that they had rated and then received another frequency test with new words. The researchers did not observe any practice effects in terms of sensitivity (as measured by the slope) or accuracy of frequency estimation. Similar results have also been reported by Zacks et al. (1982) who found no improvement in accuracy of frequency estimation after practice on three prior lists. However, effects have been reported in an experiment that used multiple trials over 12 sessions (Hockley, 1984). Zacks et al. (1986) argue that their definition of automaticity differs from other investigators (e.g., Fisk & Schneider, 1984) who typically use hundreds of trials before a process is viewed as automatic.

Competing Task Demands

Finally, a third assumption of the Hasher and Zacks framework is that reductions in capacity, which impair processing on effortful cognitive tasks, are inconsequential for sensitivity to frequency information. Since automatic encoding requires minimal capacity, taking away resources from the attentional system should not hinder performance. This prediction has received preliminary support (Zacks, et al., 1982) in a study that warned subjects of either a future frequency test, a recall test, or both a frequency and recall test. This latter group was viewed as placing competing demands on capacity and was expected to show no disadvantage in automatic processing. Consistent with the automaticity notion, subjects in all three instructional groups were comparable in frequency accuracy (85% correct). In contrast, recall performance was poorest under the dual-instruction versus the single-instruction conditions.

This early study has been criticized because of the possibility that frequency judgments and memory performance may not be independent (e.g., frequency judgments may have been employed to aid the future recall of the memory group; the dual task group similarly may have been using frequency information to access memory traces). Therefore, one might not expect to find differences in frequency accuracy. In addition, there is a lack of information on the *amount* of cognitive demands that competing task loads impose and their interaction with frequency processing. Dual-task methodology requires the subject to engage in two concurrent activities and examines the effects of manipulating the capacity demands of one task on performance of a second task. Two recent studies (Maki & Ostby, 1987; Naveh-Benjamin & Jonides, 1986) used dual-task paradigms that manipulated the cognitive effort demanded by a secondary task (varying the difficulty of a concurrent arithmetic task). Both studies found clear effects on discriminability among frequencies, with greatest task demands producing the poorest performance.

SUMMARY

In summary, considerable controversy and research have been generated from the automatic/effortful distinction. Hasher and Zacks (1979) initially stated that *all* manipulations (e.g., practice, individual differences such as age, orienting instructions) must produce null effects in order to satisfy the criteria that a process is "automatic." However, Zacks et al. (1984) have more recently noted that automatic processes may range in degree from relative insensitivity to task and subject variables (e.g., frequency processing) to those that are more vulnerable to disruptive effects (e.g., temporal processing). A review of the literature reveals that individuals are sensitive to frequency information even if manipulations alter the slope of the judgments. Perhaps the application of dual-task methodology to the measurement of capacity demands will be useful in classifying processes along an attentional continuum. Moreover, there has been a tendency to dichotomize automatic/effortful processes rather than to characterize them as ranging from low to high attentional demands. Recent evidence (Maki & Ostby, 1987) suggests that attention may be important only in the initial (early) stages of processing frequency information. Therefore, a major difference that may emerge between automatic and effortful processing could be the degree of sustained attention required from individuals.

In the following section, we review the findings obtained in the application of the automatic/effortful framework to the elderly and neurological/psychiatric populations.

Studies of Frequency Processing in the Aged and Psychiatric/Neurological Groups

Attempts to classify tasks along an automatic/effortful dimension and to study the impact of various conditions such as aging or depression on performance have perhaps been most vigorously applied to the distinction between episodic and semantic memory (Tulving, 1972). Recently, however, investigators have begun to examine frequency sensitivity as an example of a process that poses minimal demands on the attentional system. In their review of the frequency of occurrence literature, Hasher and Zacks (1984) cited data indicating that certain sources of capacity reduction, such as stress, disease, aging, or depression, would be expected to adversely affect performance on effortful tasks that require the use of active strategies and problem-solving abilities. On the other hand, neurological conditions, such as Alzheimer's disease, could impair frequency judgments as well. There have been a number of studies examining the automatic/effortful distinction in subpopulations that have attempted to dissociate a core encoding problem from a capacity deficit. The general findings are summarized in Table 6.2. The effects of variables such as orienting instructions and competing task loads on frequency processing have not yet been explored systematically. Although the research is sparse, there is some support for the role of differential mechanisms underlying memory difficulties in various groups who are most likely to be referred for neuropsychological evaluation.

Studies conducted with the elderly have generally indicated performance decrements on tasks requiring the use of active strategies (e.g., effortful processing) but a relative preservation of sensitivity to frequency information (automatic processing) (Attig & Hasher, 1980; Hasher & Zacks, 1979; Kausler et al., 1984; Kausler & Puckett, 1980). Hasher and Zacks (1979, Experiment 2) compared the abilities of college undergraduates and senior citizens (ages 56 to 80) in making frequency estimates of words presented under intentional versus incidental (e.g., to prepare for a memory task) instructions. While the estimates made by the elderly increased at a slower rate with increments in actual frequency, both groups showed sensitivity to the differences in occurrence of the words. Similarly, Kausler and Puckett (1980) demonstrated that relative frequency judgments (e.g., selecting the member of a word pair that occurred more often) were preserved in both an elderly sample and younger adults. However, memory performance on a paired-associate learning task clearly differentiated the groups. While Kausler et al. (1984) did find age differences in frequency processing among young and elderly adults, the researchers noted that instructions and rehearsal strategies were unimportant to performance on this task for both groups. Moreover, in sharp contrast to memory recall, the differences on the automatic processing task were minimal (mean judgment score = 15.81 for young subjects; 14.56 for elderly subjects) with only 8% of the elderly sample performing below the accuracy of younger subjects.

The above cited studies in the elderly are viewed as support for the notion that aging produces a capacity reduction which will be selectively demonstrated on those tasks requiring sustained attention and strategies (effortful tasks). A similar pattern of performance has also been found in depressed patients (Hasher & Zacks, 1979; Roy-Byrne, Weingartner, Bierer, Thompson, & Post, 1986; Weingartner, Cohen, Murphy, Martello, & Gerdt, 1981). Hasher and Zacks (1979, Experiment 3) reported comparable frequency estimation abilities in depressed and nondepressed college students classified according to the Beck Depression Inventory. Roy-Byrne and colleagues (1986) also noted clear differences in free-recall performance but not in frequency monitoring between patients hospitalized for major depression versus healthy controls. Studies with the elderly and depressed patients offer some preliminary support for differences in psychobiological mechanisms underlying automatic and effortful encoding (Weingartner et al., 1981). For example, it has been found that dopamine selectively improves free-recall performance but not frequency processing in the elderly (Newman, Weingartner, Smallberg, & Calne, 1984). Systematic investigation of the role of neurotransmitters in mediating these processes and potential pharmacological interventions appears worthwhile to pursue.

The automatic/effortful framework has recently been applied to various neurological conditions as well. It has been shown that Parkinson's disease produces a selective deficit on effortful but not automatic encoding tasks (Weingartner, Burns, Diebel, & LeWitt, 1984). Weingartner and colleagues tested the ability of

TABLE 6.2. Summary of findings for automatic (frequency of occurrence) versus effortful processing tasks in the aged and psychiatric/neurological patients.

	Elderly	Depression	Parkinson's disease	Korsakoff's syndrome and progressive idiopathic dementia	Focal brain lesions
Comparison group(s)	Three groups of adults (mean age = 22, 43, and 68 yrs.) (Attig & Hasher, 1980); college students (18–24 yrs.) vs. senior citizens (M=67.5 yrs.) (Hasher & Zacks, 1979); college students (M=21.3 yrs.) vs. senior citizens (M=70.6 yrs.) (Kausler & Puckett, 1980); young (M=20.5 yrs.) vs. elderly (M=71.9 yrs.) adults (Kausler et al., 1984)	College students classified as depressed or non-depressed on the Beck Depression Inventory (Hasher & Zacks, 1979); patients hospitalized for major depression vs. matched nondepressed controls (Roy-Byrne et al., 1986)	Patients with idiopathic PD vs. matched unimpaired controls (Weingartner et al., 1984)	Patients with KS, early PID and normal matched controls (Weingartner et al., 1983)	Patients with excisions of the LT, RT, or RF lobes and unimpaired controls (Smith & Milner, 1983)
General finding	Frequency processing comparable; effortful processing (paired associate learning; digit recall) poorer in elderly	Frequency processing comparable; effortful processing (free recall) impaired in depressed patients	Frequency processing comparable; effortful processing (free recall; serial list learning) poorer in PD patients	Frequency and effortful processing impaired in KS and PID patients relative to controls	Frequency processing of verbal material (words) comparable among groups; RF group selectively impaired in frequency estimation of visual material (designs)

Note. PD = Parkinson's disease; KS = Korsakoff's syndrome; PID = progressive idiopathic dementia; LT = left temporal; RT = right temporal; RF = right frontal.

six patients with idiopathic Parkinson's disease to judge the frequencies of words presented from one to seven times. On another task, these subjects were read a similar word list and were required to freely recall the items. Patients were as accurate as controls in judging how often the words occurred, but their recall performance was significantly poorer. In contrast, a study with alcoholic Korsakoff patients and those with progressive idiopathic dementia has indicated a global memory deficit. Weingartner, Grafman, Boutelle, Kaye, & Martin (1983) demonstrated that both patient groups were selectively impaired in judging how often various words had been presented relative to control subjects. This finding indicates a more general cognitive disturbance that transcends limited capacity skills and failure to use mnemonic techniques. Recently, Smith and Milner (1983) tested the ability of patients with right frontal, right temporal, or left temporal lobe excisions to estimate how often various words or pictures had been presented relative to controls. While the groups performed similarly on the verbal task, patients with right frontal lobe lesions in contrast to those with left or right temporal lobe lesions made impaired frequency estimates of visual designs, thus providing evidence for a neuroanatomical correlate of automatic processing.

Automatic and Effortful Processing in Survivors of Severe Closed Head Injury

We sought to extend the automatic versus effortful processing framework to survivors of severe closed head injury (Levin, Goldstein, High & Williams, in press). Under the assumption that closed head injury (CHI) disproportionately reduces attentional capacity and the use of active learning strategies, we predicted that severely head injured patients would exhibit a deficit relative to controls in free recall over multiple trials versus a sparing of automatic processing on a task involving frequency judgments. On the other hand, if CHI produces a more fundamental impairment in the basic encoding system, then we expected a commensurate deficit in automatic processing abilities.

In the first experiment, we studied 15 nonaphasic, long-term survivors of severe CHI with no antecedent history of head injury, substance abuse, or neuropsychiatric disorder. Thirteen patients were enrolled in the Transitional Learning Community, a residential cognitive rehabilitation facility in Galveston, Texas. The remaining two patients were participants in ongoing research to study neuropsychological outcome of head injury. The duration of impaired consciousness was at least 2 weeks for all but one patient who had a right frontoparietal contusion. Fourteen control subjects recruited from hospital personnel were matched to the CHI patients on the basis of age (CHI mean = 26.1 years, *SD* = 4.7) and education (CHI mean = 13.1 years, *SD* = 2.8).

The automatic processing task followed the procedure described by Attig and Hasher (1980) with critical words occurring from zero to seven times. The design is summarized in Table 6.3. Subjects were told that they would hear a taped word list in which some words would be repeated more often than others and that

Table 6.3. Design of experiments.

	Stimuli	Procedure	Test form	Dependent measure(s)
Experiment 1				
Automatic processing	Taped words presented at frequencies of 0–7 (3 words at frequency 0, 4 words at frequency 1, 5 words at frequency 2, 6 words at frequencies 3 and 4, 3 words at frequency 5, 2 words at frequency 6, 1 word at frequency 7) (1 word presented/ 2 seconds)	Before hearing list, subjects told they would be required to circle members of word pairs that occurred more often (Relative Judgment)	15 paired choices representing a combination of three levels of absolute differences between words (1, 2, and 3) with five levels of the less frequent pair member (0, 1, 2, 3, and 4)	Total correct choices out of 15 possible
Effortful processing	Five successive taped word lists of 10 words each (1 word presented/2 seconds)	After hearing a list, subjects told to recall the words in any order (Free Recall)	Examiner recorded order of words recalled on each trial.	Total recall (50 words possible)
Experiment 2				
Automatic processing	Two parallel sets of word lists, consisting of 12 words each at frequencies 0, 2, 4 and 6 (1 word presented/2 seconds)	Subjects served in two conditions: *Relative Judgment*, Same as Experiment 1;	24 paired choices, four at each frequency combination (0–2, 0–4, 0–6, 2–4, 2–6, 4–6).	Total correct choices out of 24 possible
		Absolute Judgment: Before hearing list, subjects told they would be required to estimate the number of times they heard particular words	16 randomly placed words, four at each frequency level (0, 2, 4, and 6).	(1) Mean estimates at each frequency level; (2) correlations between actual and estimated frequency

following presentation of the list, they would be given a typed sheet of word pairs (e.g., *metal-king*) and be asked to circle the member of the pair they thought occurred most frequently. The effortful processing task was a free recall procedure with memory for words assessed after each trial.

Figure 6.1 (*left side*) depicts the mean number of total correct frequency judgments (out of 15 possible) for the automatic processing task. As seen, the CHI patients made an average of 10 (*SD* = 2.10, range = 7–14) correct frequency judgments versus an average of 11.6 (*SD* = 2.31, range = 6–15) for controls. A one-way ANOVA to test the difference between groups approached significance (p = .055). Figure 6.2 shows the variability of performance on this task. Only four patients scored above the control median of 11.5, whereas 13 controls performed above the CHI median of 9.8.

In contrast to judgment of frequency, the results on the recall task indicated clearer differences in favor of controls (Figure 6.1). Controls recalled an average of 32.1 words (*SD* = 5.46, range = 19–39) versus 22.9 (*SD* = 4.85, range = 17–30) for the head-injured patients. Analysis of total free recall over five lists (50 total words possible) confirmed a highly significant effect of group (p < .001). No patient recalled above the control median of 30 words. In addition, as shown in Figure 6.2, the overlap between patient and control performance was greater on the automatic processing task as opposed to the pronounced separation in memory ability.

While the results of our first experiment indicated a clear difference in effortful processing abilities between head-injured patients and controls, the question of whether automatic processing is preserved in the patients remained more ambiguous. Although some patients were quite proficient in frequency judgment, a number had scores that fell below the distribution of the control group.

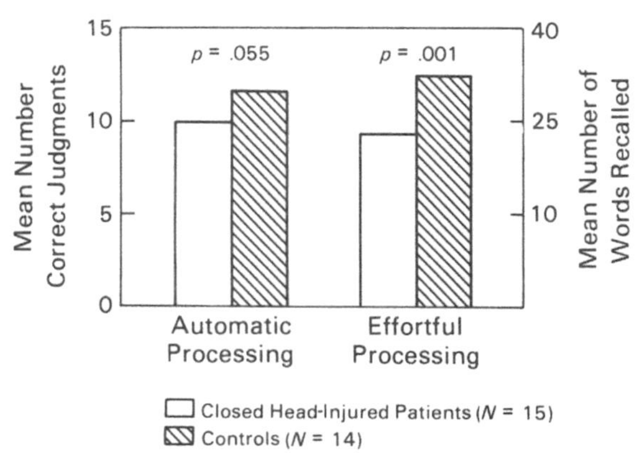

FIGURE 6.1. Experiment 1: Performance on the automatic and effortful processing tasks for head-injured patients and controls. The p values represent the level of significance of the main effect for groups on the frequency judgment and memory recall tasks. (From Levin et al., *Brain and Cognition*, in press.)

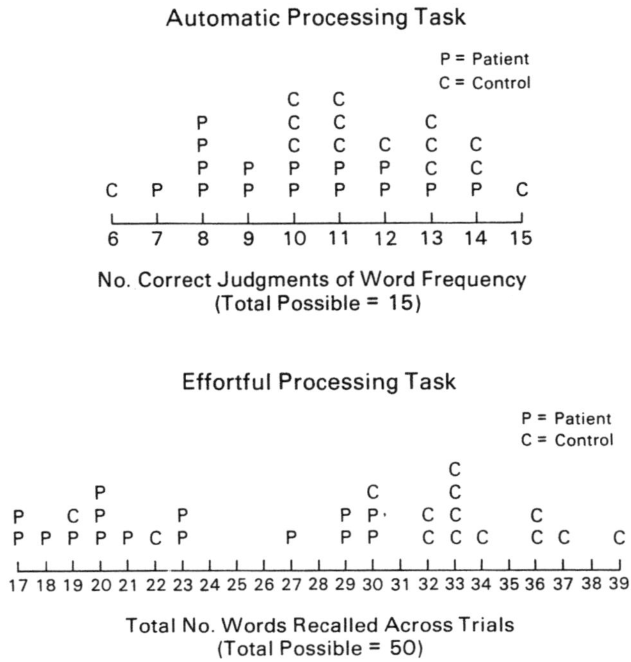

FIGURE 6.2. Experiment 1: Variability of performance on the automatic and effortful processing tasks for head-injured patients and controls. (From Levin et al., *Brain and Cognition*, in press.)

Moreover, the proportion of errors made at every frequency combination was in almost all cases greater for patients versus controls.

We designed a second experiment to provide a stronger test of the hypothesis that frequency of occurrence processing is preserved following CHI. Two types of measures were used. As shown in Table 6.3, subjects were asked to make a relative judgment regarding which of two words occurred most often. In addition, we employed an absolute decision task that required subjects to estimate the number of times a given word was presented.

A new sample of 16 chronic survivors of severe CHI was recruited from the same residential rehabilitation program that provided the patients in the first experiment. Similar to the sample studied in our first investigation, the patients had no previous hospitalization for head injury nor did they have an antecedent history of neuropsychiatric disorder. Sixteen control subjects were matched to the patients on relevant demographic features. The particular set of words used for the relative and absolute judgment procedures was counterbalanced (e.g., half of the subjects heard Set A words and half heard Set B words in the relative judgment condition). All subjects were tested under both absolute and relative judgment conditions.

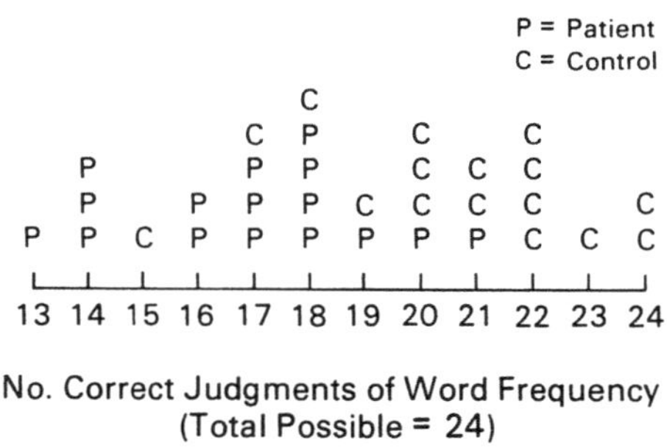

FIGURE 6.3. Experiment 2: Variability of performance on the relative judgment task for head-injured patients and controls. (From Levin et al., *Brain and Cognition*, in press.)

The results for the relative judgment procedure provided more compelling evidence for differences in automatic processing abilities between patients and controls. The head-injured patients had an average of 17 correct choices of the most frequently presented member of the word pairs (SD = 2.28, range = 13–21) versus 21 correct judgments for controls (SD = 2.47, range = 15–24). A one-way ANOVA on total correct judgments (out of 24 possible) indicated a significant group difference in favor of controls ($p < .001$). Inspection of individual performance on the relative frequency judgment task (Figure 6.3). shows that only one patient performed at the level of the control median of 21. In contrast, 15 of the 16 controls performed at or above the patient median of 17.

For the absolute judgment task, we observed a closer coupling between estimated and actual frequency of occurrence in the control subject data as compared to the results obtained in head-injured patients. We found a significant interaction of subject group and frequency estimation, which is shown in Figure 6.4.

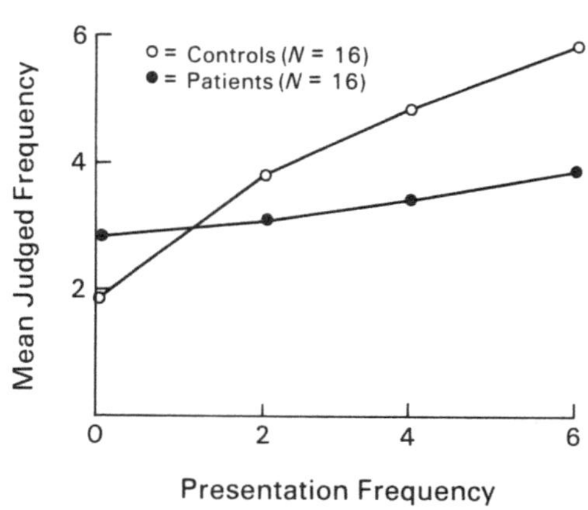

FIGURE 6.4. Experiment 2: Mean judged frequency as a function of presentation frequency for head-injured patients and controls. (From Levin et al., *Brain and Cognition*, in press.)

Although the mean estimates of both groups increased with greater frequency of presentation, controls were more sensitive to actual changes in frequency. The more impressive gains in estimation occurred for controls between presentation frequency 0 to 2 and 2 to 4, whereas the estimates by patients did not significantly vary from one contrast to the next. In addition, we tested whether the slopes for the two groups were different. Consistent with the impression of Figure 6.4, there was a significant interaction of group with linear trend ($p < .001$), indicating that controls were more sensitive than patients to frequency changes.

As a further test of sensitivity to frequency differences, a Pearson Product Moment correlation coefficient was calculated for each subject (Flexser & Bower, 1975). This correlation represents the relationship between actual versus judged presentation frequency for all 24 words used in the paper-and-pencil task. The correlation should be positive and significant to the extent that a subject gives larger estimates commensurate with increases in actual frequency of word presentation, regardless of the accuracy of the estimates. Table 6.4 displays the correlation coefficients for every subject. As seen, only six CHI patients demonstrated a significant positive correlation, whereas 12 controls gave larger

TABLE 6.4. Experiment 2: Pearson Product Moment correlation coefficients between estimated versus actual presentation frequency for patients with closed head injuries and controls.

Head-injured patient correlation coefficient	Matched control correlation coefficient
−.03	.52*
.19	.57*
.51*	.80**
−.55	.79**
.29	.82**
.62**	.84**
.12	.33
.29	.71**
.67**	.70**
.49	.49
−.11	.80**
0.0	.42
.43	.79**
.55*	.70**
.51*	.55*
.59*	.48
Mean=.29, *SD*=.33	Mean=.64, *SD*=.16

Significance of correlations in the Expected Positive Direction
*$p < .05$
**$p < .01$.

estimates of each word as actual frequency increased. The mean correlation coefficients were significantly different ($p < .001$), (patient mean = .29, control mean = .64).

Finally, we administered a cognitive estimation task similar to that described by Shallice and Evans (1978) to 15 of the patients and 15 of the controls to detect subtle deficits in judgment and problem-solving abilities. We felt that our findings could represent a general deficit in estimation by CHI patients as opposed to a specific impairment in monitoring frequency per se. Table 6.5 provides examples of questions asked and the means and ranges of answers given by patients and controls. Separate one-way ANOVAs on the values for each question failed to reveal significant differences between the groups.

In summary, our experiments revealed deficits in both effortful and automatic processing abilities following severe CHI. As expected, patients performed poorly on an effortful memory task requiring them to freely recall a series of word lists over multiple trials. Our finding that chronic survivors of severe CHI also had difficult in monitoring frequency information corroborates the results obtained in head-injured patients by Vakil and Tweedy (1985). Moreover, we found that this deficit was not explained by poorer cognitive estimation skills between the groups. Thus, our results indicate that severe CHI results in a disruption of basic encoding operations rather than a selective impairment on tasks requiring active learning techniques. In the following section, we review general implications of the automatic/effortful distinction for amnesic disturbance and its relevance to memory problems seen after CHI.

TABLE 6.5. Experiment 2: Means and ranges on cognitive estimation questions.

	CHI patients (*N*=15)		Controls (*N*=15)	
Questions	Mean	Range	Mean	Range
Number of TV programs on a TV channel between 6:00 pm and 11:00 pm	7.0	3–17	6.5	4–12
Age of oldest person in America today	103.2	65–140	108.7	100–115
Length of average man's spine (inches)	32.9	11–48	30.3	20–36
Number of slices in a loaf of sandwich bread	29.7	18–64	27.1	15–47
Height of average American woman (inches)	65.2	51–70	65.6	62–70
Weight of average American male	178.9	149–230	174.5	150–205
Length of a dollar bill (inches)	5.9	4–8	6.0	4–10
How fast race horses run (miles per hour)	40.1	15–60	35.6	10–50
Seating capacity of a city bus	47.6	28–80	46.4	22–103
Weight of a full can of Coca Cola (ounces)	13.3	3–32	11.3	4–16

Implications of Automatic Processing Deficits for Amnesia

Memory disturbance is a common source of disability in a wide range of etiologies including closed head injuries, postencephalitic conditions, and ruptured aneurysms (Levin, Benton, & Grossman, 1982; Wilson & Moffat, 1984). A particularly intriguing form of memory disorder is the organic amnesic syndrome, which is characterized by an inability to learn and to retain everyday information (anterograde amnesia), a difficulty in recalling events prior to the illness (retrograde amnesia), and a tendency in some patients to confabulate (e.g., to "fill in" memory gaps with erroneous information). In contrast, amnesics demonstrate average immediate memory (e.g., forward digit span) and relatively preserved intelligence (Signoret, 1985).

It has recently been proposed that amnesia may represent a loss of automatic processing abilities (Hirst, 1982; Kovner, Mattis & Pass, 1985). Hirst (1982) suggests that ordinarily effortless activities now require an inordinate amount of capacity, which imposes constraints on performing other tasks. As a result, contextual cues are either not available at the time of retrieval because they have not been encoded, or conversely, resources have been taken away from remembering target information due to the increased capacity demands of registering cues.

Although these hypotheses have not been rigorously tested, there is some evidence that amnesics have difficulty encoding incidental features of to-be-remembered material and that memorizing requires more "effort." Support for deficits in registering intrinsic/extrinsic context, for example, comes from studies showing preserved learning abilities on supposedly context-free tasks such as motor and perceptual activities (Cohen & Squire, 1980; Corkin, 1968; Parkin, 1982) and improved memory when context is highlighted for amnesics (Winocur & Kinsbourne, 1978). Lack of sensitivity to temporal order information was shown by Hirst and Volpe (1982) who demonstrated that amnesics' ability to recognize news events was as accurate as controls, but their dating of the events was significantly poorer. In addition, it has been found that Korsakoff amnesics are deficient in processing information such as recency and frequency (Huppert & Piercy, 1976, 1978; Meudell, Mayes, Ostergaard, & Pickering, 1985; Squire, 1982). Within a capacity framework, the passive learning strategies of amnesic Korsakoff patients and improvement in their recall produced by intensive memorizing (Hirst, 1982) or structured contextual cues (Kovner et al., 1985) suggest that memorizing may now require more effort.

It is possible that amnesia represents a breakdown in sensitivity to temporal, spatial, and frequency information, but a direct test of this hypothesis within the Hasher and Zacks framework has not been systematically explored. In our previous discussion of findings in neurological populations, it was noted that Weingartner and colleagues (1983) observed that Korsakoff amnesics were impaired in making frequency judgments but not selectively so in relation to patients with progressive idiopathic dementia (generalized intellectual and memory disturbance). Hirst and Volpe (1984) demonstrated that amnesics' sensitivity to spatial attributes was impaired relative to controls. Whereas amnesics' encoding of spatial location information improved under an intentional learning condition, control performance was comparable in both intentional and incidental manipulations. Finally, diPellegrino and Nichelli (1986) contrasted effortful (recognition memory) and automatic (frequency of occurrence) processing abilities in six amnesics of varying etiologies versus young (mean age = 25) and elderly (mean age = 69) controls. The amnesics evidenced poorer performance on both tasks in contrast to the other groups who differed only on the recognition (effortful) task.

Extrapolating to the severely head-injured population who exhibit residual memory problems, events that are ordinarily automatically processed may now require more effort. The common observation of deficits in vigilance and arousal following CHI (Van Zomeren, Brouwer, & Deelman, 1984) indicates a basic impairment in capacity available to the processing system. As Hirst (1982) has noted, encoding is not a unitary process but requires attention to multiple sources of information (e.g., target material plus the context in which it is learned). It is possible that more capacity of the head-injured individual is required for encoding "automatic" contextual features, thus leaving fewer capacity resources for to-be-remembered material. As a result, the patient may be required to divide attention between two sources of information in an already deficient attentional system, resulting in overall poorer memory performance (Hirst, 1982).

An impairment in automatic processing would have repercussions for memory and particularly rehabilitation efforts. Sensitivity to frequency, for example, can determine both the success of initial encoding (e.g., the recognition that there are more items of one category than another) and subsequent retrieval (e.g., that there are more items still to be accessed) (Hasher & Zacks, 1984). Events that are processed with relatively few attentional demands might now require active processing (Salmon & Butters, 1987). While instructions such as "Use a counting strategy" are unimportant to the performance of neurologically intact individuals, it may be that specific training techniques are required with the head-injured population. In addition, since encoding would now be more effortful, it is reasonable to expect that patients might require longer processing times in order to register automatic, contextual features (Salmon & Butters, 1987).

We observed impressive individual differences among the CHI patients in processing frequency of occurrence information. Our sample was small, and therefore performance could not be adequately assessed using clinical indices such as localization of mass lesions. Diffuse axonal injury, which produces cortical-subcortical disconnection (Ommaya & Gennarelli, 1974) and degeneration of the cerebral white matter (Strich, 1956), could conceivably reduce efficiency of information processing, which is most evident under conditions of increasing frequency of occurrence and rate of presentation (Gronwall & Wrightson, 1974). In addition, it is reasonable to posit a role of the frontal lobes in frequency estimation given Smith and Milner's (1983) finding that patients with right frontal lobe excisions are impaired in making frequency judgments of visual designs and studies showing that frontal lobe-damaged patients are deficient on judgments of recency (Lavadas, Umilta, & Provinciali, 1979; Milner, 1973) and self-monitoring of temporally ordered events (Petrides & Milner, 1982).

The automatic/effortful framework is currently undergoing extensive investigation and scrutiny of its assumptions. However, we conclude that the distinction between processes requiring sustained attention versus those that impose minimal demands can be useful in dissociating the types of deficits seen in neuropsychiatric populations with varying degrees of attentional/memory disturbances. Moreover, the idea that certain features of the environment may not be encoded along with target material has relevance to rehabilitative strategies. Future studies should examine the role of task variables (e.g., intentionality, practice) to explore whether a production or mediation deficiency exists and the impact on memory performance. Finally, the suggestions by Weingartner and colleagues (1981; Newman et al., 1984) of separate psychobiological mechanisms underlying automatic/effortful processes may point the way toward potential pharmacological treatments.

Acknowledgments. Preparation of this chapter and research that was completed in Galveston were supported by grants NS 2-1889, Javits Neuroscience Investigator Award, and Moody Foundation Grant 84-152, Magnetic Resonance Imaging After Severe Head Injury: Relationship to Outcome of Rehabilitation (HSL). Walter M. High, Jr., M.A. and David Williams, M.A. were collaborators on the studies completed in Galveston. We thank Liz Zindler for manuscript preparation.

References

Alba, J.W., Chromiak, W., Hasher, L., & Attig, M.S. (1980). Automatic encoding of category size information. *Journal of Experimental Psychology: Human Learning and Memory, 6,* 370–378.

Attig, M.S., & Hasher, L. (1980). The processing of frequency of occurrence information by adults. *Journal of Gerontology, 35,* 66–69.

Brooks, J.E. (1985). Judgments of category frequency. *American Journal of Psychology, 98,* 363–372.

Cohen, N.J., & Squire, L.R. (1980). Preserved learning and retention of pattern analyzing skills in amnesia: Dissociation of knowing how and knowing what. *Science, 210,* 207–210.

Cooper, A., & Marshall, P.H. (1985). Spatial location judgments as a function of intention to learn and mood state: An evaluation of an alleged automatic encoding operation. *American Journal of Psychology, 98,* 261–269.

Corkin, S. (1968). Acquisition of motor skill after bilateral medial temporal-lobe excision. *Neuropsychologia, 6,* 255–265.

Craik, F.I.M., & Lockhart, R.S. (1972). Levels of processing: A framework for memory research. *Journal of Verbal Learning and Verbal Behavior, 11,* 671–684.

diPellegrino, G., & Nichelli, P. (1986). *Is there a trade-off between episodic and automatic memory in amnesia?* Paper presented at the 9th Annual European Convention of the International Neuropsychological Society, Veldhoven, The Netherlands.

Fisk, A.D. (1986). Frequency encoding is not inevitable and is not automatic: A reply to Hasher and Zacks. *American Psychologist, 41*, 215-216.

Fisk, A.D., & Schneider, W. (1984). Memory as a function of attention, level of processing, and automatization. *Journal of Experimental Psychology: Learning, Memory and Cognition, 10*, 181-197.

Flexser, A.J., & Bower, G.H. (1975). Further evidence regarding instructional effects on frequency judgments. *Bulletin of the Psychonomic Society, 6*, 321-324.

Greene, R.L. (1984). Incidental learning of event frequency. *Memory & Cognition, 12*, 90-95.

Greene, R.L. (1986). Effects of intentionality and strategy on memory for frequency. *Journal of Experimental Psychology: Learning, Memory, and Cognition, 12*, 489-495.

Gronwall, D., & Wrightson, P. (1974). Delayed recovery of intellectual function after minor head injury. *Lancet, 2*, 605-609.

Hasher, L., & Chromiak, W. (1977). The processing of frequency information: An automatic mechanism? *Journal of Verbal Learning and Verbal Behavior, 16*, 173-184.

Hasher, L., & Zacks, R.T. (1979). Automatic and effortful processes in memory. *Journal of Experimental Psychology: General, 108*, 356-388.

Hasher, L., & Zacks, R.T. (1984). Automatic processing of fundamental information: The case of frequency of occurrence. *American Psychologist, 39*, 1372-1388.

Hirst, W. (1982). The amnesic syndrome: Descriptions and explanations. *Psychological Bulletin, 91*, 435-460.

Hirst, W., & Volpe, B.T. (1982). Temporal order judgments with amnesia. *Brain and Cognition, 1*, 294-306.

Hirst, W., & Volpe, B.T. (1984). Encoding of spatial relations with amnesia. *Neuropsychologia, 22*, 631-634.

Hockley, W.E. (1984). Retrieval of item frequency information in a continuous memory task. *Memory & Cognition, 12*, 229-242.

Howell, W.C. (1973). Storage of events and event frequency: A comparison of two paradigms in memory. *Journal of Experimental Psychology, 98*, 260-263.

Huppert, F.A., & Piercy, M. (1976). Recognition memory in amnesic patients: Effect of temporal context and familiarity of material. *Cortex, 12*, 3-20.

Huppert, F.A., & Piercy, M. (1978). The role of trace strength in recency and frequency judgments by amnesic and control subjects. *Quarterly Journal of Experimental Psychology, 30*, 347-354.

Jorm, A.F. (1986). Controlled and automatic information processing in senile dementia: A review. *Psychological Medicine, 16*, 77-88.

Kahneman, D. (1973). *Attention and effort.* Englewood Cliffs, NJ: Prentice-Hall.

Kausler, D.H., Lichty, W., & Hakami, M.K. (1984). Frequency judgments for distractor items in a short-term memory task: Instructional variation and adult age differences. *Journal of Verbal Learning and Verbal Behavior, 23*, 660-668.

Kausler, D.H., & Puckett, J.M. (1980). Frequency judgments and correlated cognitive abilities in young and elderly adults. *Journal of Gerontology, 35*, 376-382.

Kausler, D.H., Wright, R.E., & Hakami, M.K. (1981). Variation in task complexity and adult age differences in frequency-of-occurrence judgments. *Bulletin of the Psychonomic Society, 18*, 195-197.

Kovner, R., Mattis, S., & Pass, R. (1985). Some amnesic patients can freely recall large amounts of information in new contexts. *Journal of Clinical and Experimental Neuropsychology, 7*, 395-411.

Lavadas, E., Umilta, C., & Provinciali, L. (1979). Hemisphere-dependent cognitive performances in epileptic patients. *Epilepsia, 20,* 493–502.

Levin, H.S., Benton, A.L., & Grossman, R.G. (1982). *Neurobehavioral consequences of closed head injury.* New York: Oxford University Press.

Levin, H.S., Goldstein, F.C., High, W., Jr., & Williams, D. (in press). Automatic and effortful processing after severe closed head injury. *Brain and Cognition.*

Maki, R.H., & Ostby, R.S. (1987). Effects of level of processing and rehearsal on frequency judgments. *Journal of Experimental Psychology: Learning, Memory, and Cognition, 13,* 151–163.

Meudell, P.R., Mayes, A.R., Ostergaard, A.L., & Pickering, A. (1985). Recency and frequency judgments in alcoholic amnesics and normal people with poor memory. *Cortex, 21,* 487–511.

Milner, B. (1973). Hemispheric specialization: Scope and limits. In F.D. Schmitt & F.G. Worden (Eds.), *The neurosciences: Third study program* (pp. 75–89). Boston: MIT Press.

Naveh-Benjamin, M., & Jonides, J. (1986). On the automaticity of frequency coding: Effects of competing task load, encoding strategy, and intention. *Journal of Experimental Psychology: Learning, Memory and Cognition, 12,* 378–386.

Navon, D., & Gopher, D. (1979). On the economy of the human-processing system. *Psychological Review, 86,* 214–255.

Newman, R.P., Weingartner, H., Smallberg, S.A., & Calne, D.B. (1984). Effortful and automatic memory: Effects of dopamine. *Neurology, 34,* 805–807.

Ommaya, A.K., & Gennarelli, T.A. (1974). Cerebral concussion and traumatic unconsciousness: Correlation of experimental and clinical observations on blunt head injuries. *Brain, 97,* 633–654.

Parkin, A.J. (1982). Residual learning capability in organic amnesia. *Cortex, 18,* 417–440.

Petrides, M., & Milner, B. (1982). Deficits on subject-ordered tasks after frontal- and temporal-lobe lesions in man. *Neuropsychologia, 20,* 249–262.

Posner, M.I., & Snyder, C.R. (1975). Attention and cognitive control. In R.L. Solso (Ed.), *Information processing and cognition: The Loyola symposium.* Hillsdale, NJ: Erlbaum.

Puglisi, J.T., Park, D.C., Smith, A.D., & Hill, G.W. (1985). Memory for two types of spatial location: Effects of instructions, age, and format. *American Journal of Psychology, 98,* 101–118.

Rose, R.J., & Rowe, E.J. (1976). Effects of orienting task and spacing of repetitions on frequency judgments. *Journal of Experimental Psychology: Human Learning and Memory, 2,* 142–152.

Roy-Byrne, P.P., Weingartner, H., Bierer, L.M., Thompson, R.M., & Post, R.M. (1986). Effortful and automatic cognitive processes in depression. *Archives of General Psychiatry, 43,* 265–267.

Salmon, D.P., & Butters, N. (1987). Recent developments in learning and memory: Implications for rehabilitation of the amnesic patient. In M. Meier, A.L. Benton, & L. Diller (Eds.), *Neuropsychological rehabilitation.* New York: Churchill-Livingstone.

Shallice, T., & Evans, M.E. (1978). The involvement of the frontal lobes in cognitive estimation. *Cortex, 14,* 294–303.

Shiffrin, R.M., & Schneider, W. (1977). Controlled and automatic human information processing: II. Perceptual learning, automatic attending and a general theory. *Psychology Review, 84,* 127–190.

Signoret, J.L. (1985). Memory and amnesias. In M. Mesulam (Ed.), *Principles of behavioral neurology* (pp. 169–192). Philadelphia: Davis.

Smith, M.L., & Milner, B. (1983). Effects of focal brain lesions on sensitivity to frequency of occurrence. *Society for Neuroscience Abstracts, 9,* 30.

Squire, L.R. (1982). Comparisons between forms of amnesia: Some deficits are unique to Korsakoff's syndrome. *Journal of Experimental Psychology: Learning, Memory, and Cognition, 8,* 560–571.

Straub, H., Marshall, P.H., & Valencia, R. (1985). *Accuracy of frequency judgments influenced by instructions and presentation rate.* Paper presented at the Southwestern Psychological Association, Austin, Texas.

Strich, S.J. (1956). Diffuse degeneration of the cerebral white matter in severe dementia following head injury. *Journal of Neurology, Neurosurgery, and Psychiatry, 19,* 163–185.

Tulving, E. (1972). Episodic and semantic memory. In E. Tulving & W. Donaldson (Eds.), *Organization of memory* (pp. 381–403). New York: Academic Press.

Vakil, E., & Tweedy, J.R. (1985). *Head injury and automatic encoding of frequency, temporal, and spatial information.* Paper presented at the 13th Annual Convention of the International Neuropsychological Society, San Diego, California.

Van Zomeren, A.H., Brouwer, W.N., & Deelman, B.G. (1984). Attentional deficits: The riddles of selectivity, speed, and alertness. In N. Brooks (Ed.), *Closed head injury: Psychological, social, and family consequences* (pp. 74–107). New York: Oxford University Press.

Weingartner, H., Burns, S., Diebel, R., & LeWitt, P.A. (1984). Cognitive impairments in Parkinson's disease: Distinguishing between effortful and automatic cognitive processes. *Psychiatry Research, 11,* 223–225.

Weingartner, H., Cohen, R.M., Murphy, D.L., Martello, J., & Gerdt, C. (1981). Cognitive processes in depression. *Archives of General Psychiatry, 38,* 42–47.

Weingartner, H., Grafman, J., Jr., Boutelle, W., Kaye, W., & Martin, P.R. (1983). Forms of memory failure. *Science, 221,* 380–382.

Whitehouse, P.J. (1986). The concept of subcortical and cortical dementia: Another look. *Annals of Neurology, 19,* 1–6.

Wilson, B.A., & Moffat, N. (Eds.), (1984). *Clinical management of memory problems.* Rockville, MD: Aspen.

Winocur, G., & Kinsbourne, M. (1978). Contextual cueing as an aid to Korsakoff amnesics. *Neuropsychologia, 16,* 671–682.

Zacks, R.T., Hasher, L., Alba, J.W., Sanft, H., & Rose, K.C. (1984). Is temporal order encoded automatically? *Memory & Cognition, 12,* 387–394.

Zacks, R.T., Hasher, L., & Hock, H.S. (1986). Inevitability and automaticity: A response to Fisk. *American Psychologist, 41,* 216–218.

Zacks, R.T., Hasher, L., & Sanft, H. (1982). Automatic encoding of event frequency: Further findings. *Journal of Experimental Psychology: Learning, Memory, and Cognition, 8,* 106–116.

7
Linguistic Competence and Level of Cognitive Functioning in Adults with Traumatic Closed Head Injury

ELISABETH H. WIIG, ELIZABETH W. ALEXANDER, and WAYNE SECORD

In recent discussions and investigations of language and communication following traumatic head injury, the central issue has been whether (a) categorical linguistic deficits (e.g., aphasia, apraxia) result or (b) language becomes disorganized in a global disorganization process. This research reflects the global disorganization perspective. It was performed to test two hypotheses: first, that language impairments after traumatic closed head injury could be differentiated by measures on a formal test of linguistic competence and metalinguistic ability (Wiig & Secord, 1985); second, that the selected measures of linguistic competence would reflect ratings of level of cognitive functioning (Hagen, 1984).

There is support in the literature for both the categorical linguistic deficit and the global disorganization theories. The categorical linguistic deficit theory is supported by reports that the language impairments after traumatic head injury most closely resemble Wernicke's aphasia (Heilman, Safron, & Geschwind, 1971; Waterhouse & Fein, 1982). It is also supported by observations that the pattern in language recovery associated with severe focal lesions shifts from initial global aphasia to sensory aphasia and finally resolves into amnestic aphasia with anomia (Thomsen, 1976). Sarno (1980, 1984) also identified categorical linguistic deficits after traumatic head injury. She observed three clinical groups: Group 1 with aphasia, Group 2 with subclinical aphasia, and Group 3 with dysarthria and subclinical aphasia. Levin, Grossman, and Kelly (1976) also observed aphasic disorders in patients with traumatic head injury. The reported studies used different tests to delineate the aphasia syndromes. They did not consider the patients' level of recovery of cognitive functioning or compare the performances of patients with traumatic head injury with performances by patients with left hemisphere cerebral vascular accident (CVA) aphasia.

The global disorganization theory is supported in the literature with increasing frequency. Several sources suggest that language after traumatic head injury is disrupted in qualitatively different ways and patterns from the categorical deficits observed in left hemisphere CVA aphasia (Bernstein-Ellis, Wertz, Dronkers, & Milton, 1985; Hagen, 1982, 1984; Holland, 1982; Milton, Prutting, & Binder, 1984; Milton, Turnstall, & Wertz, 1983). One supportive study compared 15 bilaterally brain-damaged patients with traumatic head injury and 15 left CVA patients with aphasia (Bernstein-Ellis et al., 1985). Both groups showed similar score profiles on the Ranked Response Summary of the Porch Index of Communicative Ability (PICA) (Porch, 1981). However, stepwise discriminant analysis identified five subtests that differentiated the groups with 90% overall accuracy and indicated qualitatively different performance patterns. Group comparisons indicated that the patient group with traumatic head injury performed significantly better in the Writing modality and significantly poorer in the Visual modality than the group with left CVA aphasia.

Observations of pragmatic deficits in patients with traumatic head injury also support the global disorganization theory. Holland (1982) observed that patients with traumatic head injury talk better than they communicate, while the reverse holds for patients with left hemisphere CVA aphasia. Milton et al. (1984) observed and rated the pragmatic behaviors of five patients with traumatic head injury, who scored at or above normal on two formal tests, the Communicative Abilities in Daily Living (CADL) inventory (Holland, 1980) and the Western Aphasia Battery (Kertesz, 1981). Three subjects showed inappropriate reciprocal behaviors, which regulate discourse between speakers and listeners (i.e., illocutionary and perlocutionary acts). The authors stated that cognitive abilities are intricately involved in the successful management of conversation, supporting a cognitive deficit perspective.

The strongest support for a global disorganization theory appears to stem from Hagen and his associates. Hagen (1984) observed that in patients with traumatic head injury, impairments are often found in the organization of the linguistic database, rather than of the database itself. Hagen states that "it is conceivable that some of the language variability involved in language formulation and processing. . .is heavily influenced, and in some instances created, by cognitive dysfunction" (p. 249). Hagen also reports that abstract thought and conceptual integration and synthesis of elemental parts of whole perception are impaired in traumatic head injury. Three groups of patients seem to emerge after the initial phases of recovery with diffuse symptomatology. They consist of patients with (a) disorganized language secondary to cognitive disorganization, (b) predominantly specific language disorders with coexisting minimal cognitive impairment, and (c) attentional, retentional, and recent memory impairments without language dysfunction (p. 251). The language disorganization is perceived to result from a breakdown of ability to "structure mental processes volitionally to deal differentially with stimuli, to mentally structure ongoing events, [and] to shift cognitive sets" (p. 253). This description suggested that divergent production (i.e., fluency, flexibility, originality, and/or elaboration) in response to linguistic input, as delineated by Guilford (1967), and planning for linguistic production, as delineated by, among others, Bock (1982), would be impaired after traumatic head injury.

The global disorganization theory has influenced the direction of clinical research of patients with traumatic closed head injury. Hagen and associates investigated the cognitive and behavioral consequences of traumatic head injury and integrated cognitive management concepts into rehabilitation assessment, planning, and management (Hagen, 1982; Hagen, Malkmus, Durham, & Bowman, 1979; Malkmus, 1979, 1983; Malkmus, Booth, & Doyle, 1980). Within this perspective, patients are assessed behaviorally and rated on an ordinal scale, the Rancho Level of Cognitive Functioning. The scale assigns a numerical value to observations of the patient's level of cognitive functioning. Patients are assigned to Level of Cognitive Functioning (LOCF) as follows: 1) I, no response; 2) II, generalized response; 3) III, localized response; 4) IV, confused, agitated; 5) V, confused, inappropriate; 6) VI, confused, appropriate; 7) VII, automatic, appropriate; and 8) VIII, purposeful and appropriate. Table 7.1 presents a more detailed description of the rating scale. The question had not been asked previously whether patients rated at different Rancho Levels of Cognitive Functioning could be differentiated by performances on an independent measure of linguistic competence and metalinguistic ability, designed for adolescents.

Recent literature on the nature of language and learning disabilities in adolescents suggests that "strategic inefficiency," resulting from metacognitive and metalinguistic deficits, is central to delays in acquiring communicative competence and in academic underachievement (Baker, 1982; Meichenbaum, 1977; Reid & Hresko, 1981; Torgesen, 1977; Wiig, 1984; Wiig & Becker-Caplan, 1984). The cognitive-linguistic strategy deficit theory of language-learning disabilities led to the development of the *Test of Language Competence* (Wiig & Secord, 1985). Five areas were identified for developing test formats: 1) interpreting sentence ambiguities, 2) making inferences, 3) planning for and recreating speech acts, 4) interpreting and matching metaphoric expressions, and 5) recalling paired associate words. In these areas, there were theoretical models and/or consistent developmental data. Thus, psycholinguistic research gives evidence of parallel patterns in the acquisition of linguistic competence and metalinguistic ability for, among others, concept formation, interpretation of sentence ambiguity, figurative language, and pragmatics (Allen & Brown, 1977; Alvy, 1973; Anglin, 1977; Delia & Clark, 1977; Winner, Rosenstiel, & Gardner, 1976). Similar patterns have been reported for the acquisition of memory and metamemory strategies (Crowder, 1976; Torgesen, 1977). All developmental data indicated that metalinguistic/metacognitive competence was attained after ages 11 to 13.

The subtests of the Test of Language Competence utilize formats that probe divergent production, cognitive-linguistic flexibility, and planning for production, all hypothesized to be implicated after traumatic head injury. They require: (a) problem solving, (b) planning and decision making, and/or (c) alternative solutions or responses to the same linguistic input. The test was designed for students with suspected or diagnosed language-learning disabilities in the age range from 10 to 21 years. It was not designed for patients with traumatic head injury. Subsequent to standardization, two hypotheses, pertaining to patients with traumatic head injury, were formulated. The first was that language impairments, resulting from traumatic closed head injury, would be reflected differentially by performances on the Test of Language Competence. The second was that measures on the Test of Language Competence would differentiate patients with

TABLE 7.1. Summary of the Rancho Level of Cognitive Functioning Scale and associated behavioral characteristics.

Level	Label	Behavioral characteristics
I	No response	Patient does not respond to external stimuli and appears asleep.
II	Generalized response	Patient reacts to external stimuli in nonspecific, inconsistent, and nonpurposeful manner with stereotypic and limited responses.
III	Localized response	Patient responds specifically and inconsistently with delays to stimuli, but may follow simple commands for motor action.
IV	Confused, agitated	Patient exhibits bizarre, nonpurposeful, incoherent or inappropriate behaviors, has no short-term recall, and attention is short and nonselective.
V	Confused, inappropriate, nonagitated	Patient gives random, fragmented, and nonpurposeful responses to complex or unstructured stimuli. Simple commands are followed consistently, memory and selective attention are impaired, and new information is not retained.
VI	Confused, appropriate	Patient gives context appropriate, goal-directed responses, dependent upon external input for direction. There is carry-over for relearned, but not for new tasks, and recent memory problems persist.
VII	Automatic, appropriate	Patient behaves appropriately in familiar settings, performs daily routines automatically, and shows carry-over for new learning at lower than normal rates. Patient initiates social interactions, but judgment remains impaired.
VIII	Purposeful, appropriate	Patient orients and responds to the environment, but language and abstract reasoning abilities are decreased relative to premorbid levels.

Note. Adapted from Hagen (1984, pp. 257–258).

ratings of cognitive functioning at Rancho Levels VI (confused, appropriate), VII (automatic, appropriate), and/or VIII (purposeful, appropriate).

A third question was also formulated. It concerned memory deficits and prognostic indices for recovery after traumatic head injury. The severity of memory deficits after traumatic head injury is typically predicted by the duration of coma and/or posttraumatic amnesia. Some studies indicate no consistent negative relationship between duration of coma and memory performance (Brooks, 1976, 1980, 1983). A significant negative correlation was, however, found between the duration of posttraumatic amnesia and memory deficits and recovery (Brooks, 1983). The question therefore arose whether performances on the paired associate word recall task of the Test of Language Competence would differentiate patients grouped by Rancho Level of Cognitive Functioning (LOCF) or by duration of coma and amnesia.

In summary, the major objective was to determine whether different Rancho LOCF ratings in adults with traumatic closed head injury would be associated with different levels of performance on a test of linguistic competence and metalinguistic ability. The study evaluated if patients, rated at Rancho Levels VI, VII, and VIII, would be differentiated by the linguistic and/or memory measures of the Test of Language Competence (TLC), when controlling for duration of coma/amnesia and time postinjury.

Method

Subjects

Subjects were 17 adults with traumatic closed head injury in residence at a head trauma rehabilitation program in New England. All were included on the basis of responses to a subject selection checklist. The criteria specified that patients included must: 1) have a primary diagnosis of closed traumatic head injury; 2) function at Rancho Level of Cognitive Functioning VI, VII, or VIII (Hagen et al., 1979); 3) be native speakers of English; 4) be between ages 16 and 50; 5) have a premorbid IQ within normal range; 6) have completed 10th grade; 7) pass a standard audiometric screening test; 8) obtain speech intelligibility scores of 7/8 for the high probability items of Boston Diagnostic Aphasia Examination (BDAE) Subtest IIIE, Oral Expression/Repeating Phrases (Goodglass & Kaplan, 1983); 9) obtain oral comprehension scores of 8/12 on BDAE Subtest IID, Auditory Comprehension/Complex Ideational Material (Goodglass & Kaplan, 1983); 10) obtain oral reading scores of 6/10 on BDAE Subtest IIIL, Oral Expression/Oral Sentence-Reading (Goodglass & Kaplan, 1983); 11) be free of oral apraxia based on BDAE Subtest IIIE, Oral Expression/Repeating Phrases (Goodglass & Kaplan, 1983); 12) be free of a nominal aphasia based on the Boston Naming Test (Kaplan, Goodglass, & Weintraub, 1976); 13) be free of interfering behavior disorders as determined by a clinical neuropsychologist and/or psychologist; and 14) be free of premorbid language deficits.

The patients, who met criteria for inclusion, ranged in age from 17 to 47 years. Duration of coma and amnesia ranged from none to 14 weeks and time postinjury from 2 to 37 months. Patients were rated on the Rancho Level of Cognitive Functioning scale by a minimum of three independent evaluators. This resulted in three groups: 1) Group LOCF VI (n = 5), 2) Group LOCF VII (n = 7), and 3) Group LOCF VIII (n = 5). An overview of biographical information is presented in Table 7.2.

All subjects were administered the Peabody Picture Vocabulary Test-Revised (PPVT-R) (Dunn & Dunn, 1981) in a session prior to the experimental testing. For subjects rated at LOCF VI, the PPVT-R Standard Score (SS) mean was 87.20 (SD = 18.42). For subjects rated at LOCF VII, the mean was 97.57 (SD =

TABLE 7.2. Biographical data for 17 patients with closed traumatic head injury.

LOCF	Age	Gender	Coma/amnesia	Posttrauma	Primary lesion
VI	17	F	7 weeks	12 months	L subdural hematoma
VI	27	F	14 weeks	11 months	Brain stem contusion; occipital laceration
VI	32	F	6 weeks	9 months	Brain stem contusion
VI	39	M	6 weeks	4 months	Intracerebral; R frontal & parietal; L temporal
VI	41	M	5 days	5 months	Intraventricular & subarachnoid hemorrhage
VII	22	M	4 weeks	12 months	Hemorrhagic contusion; R temporal & parietal; L frontal hematoma
VII	27	M	8 weeks	12 months	Intracerebral hematoma; cerebral contusion
VII	27	F	9 weeks	36 months	Bilateral cerebral concussion
VII[a]	28	M	N/A	2 months	Brain stem contusion
VII	31	F	6 days	5 months	L cerebral contusion
VII	37	M	1 week	7 months	R subdural hematoma
VII	47	M	2 weeks	9 months	R frontotemporal-parietal hematoma
VIII	18	M	4 weeks	4 months	Bi-frontal, midbrain contusion
VIII	19	M	5 weeks	37 months	Bi-frontal
VIII	20	M	7 days	22 months	Diffuse cerebral edema
VIII	21	M	N/A	24 months	R frontal epidural hematoma
VIII	22	M	5 days	13 months	Severe cerebral contusion. brain stem

[a] Bilingual (English-Spanish).

11.42), and for subjects rated at LOCF VIII, the mean was 95.20 (SD = 11.77). Simple ANOVA indicated no significant mean SS differences among groups (F = 0.69) on the PPVT-R.

MATERIALS

The Test of Language Competence (Wiig & Secord, 1985) assessed recovery of linguistic competence. It contains four major subtests: 1) Understanding Ambiguous Sentences, 2) Making Inferences, 3) Recreating Sentences, and 4) Understanding Metaphoric Expressions, and a supplemental paired associate word recall task, Remembering Word Pairs. The subtests are described and sample items presented in Appendix 7.A.

The Test of Language Competence was standardized nationally on 1,796 students, ranging from 9 to 18+ years, in regular educational settings. Subtest, Composite (Subtests 1 to 4), and Partial (Subtests 3 and 4) raw scores can be converted to standard scores (Wiig & Secord, 1985). For the standardization sample, factor and discriminant analyses indicated a language competence cluster (Subtests 1 to 4) and a distinct memory cluster (Remembering Word Pairs). Items on each of the four major subtests clustered independently. Diagnostic validity was established for two matched groups of 28 students each with (a) diagnosed language disabilities and academic underachievement and (b) normal language developmental and academic achievement.

Administration and Scoring

The Test of Language Competence was administered individually and the procedures specified in the administration manual were followed. Testing was performed by the second author in the rehabilitation setting in which the subjects were residents. The test was given in one session in the order specified. Responses were recorded and scored by the test authors, using manual directives. Consent forms were obtained from the legally responsible party. All subjects agreed to participate and all completed the test procedure. Subtest, Partial (Subtests 3 and 4), and Composite (Subtests 1 to 4) raw scores provided the data for the statistical analyses.

Results

Subjects were first grouped into three clinical groups based on Rancho LOCF to evaluate the significance of mean differences on the TLC measures. Mean raw scores and standard deviations for each group and measure are shown in Table 7.3. Results of the statistical analyses are presented in Table 7.4.

Analysis of covariance, controlling for time postonset and coma and amnesia duration, indicated significant mean differences among groups on Subtest 4 (Understanding Metaphoric Expressions) ($F\ (2,12) = 6.74$, $p < .05$), and for the Composite (Subtests 1 to 4) ($F\ (2,12) = 4.49$, $p < .05$) and Partial scores (Subtests 3 and 4) ($F\ (2,12) = 8.34$, $p < .01$). There were no other significant mean differences among groups.

Further analysis indicated that 52% of the total variance was explained uniquely by the language measure Interpreting Metaphoric Expressions (Subtest 4), and 58% of the variance was explained uniquely by the Partial score, a measure combining the scores for Subtests 3 (Recreating Sentences) and 4 (Interpreting Metaphoric Expressions). The Composite score, a measure combining the scores for Subtests 1 to 4, uniquely explained 42% of the variance.

TABLE 7.3. Test of Language Competence raw score means and standard deviations by Level of Cognitive Functioning.

Language measure	LOCF VI		LOCF VII		LOCF VIII	
	Mean	*SD*	Mean	*SD*	Mean	*SD*
1. Ambiguous Sentences	27.00	5.22	32.57	3.92	31.40	3.83
2. Inferences	27.80	6.27	30.86	2.99	29.80	4.92
3. Recreating Sentences	65.40	5.78	70.86	5.22	71.40	3.56
4. Metaphors	29.40	4.91	35.14	0.99	32.80	2.40
Remembering Word Pairs	5.33	5.56	6.57	5.37	7.00	3.67
Partial (3, 4)	94.80	7.81	106.00	4.66	104.20	5.88
Composite (1–4)	149.60	14.84	169.43	8.91	165.40	9.66

Note. LOCF = Level of Cognitive Functioning.

TABLE 7.4. Analysis of covariance, controlling for time postinjury and duration of coma and amnesia.

Measure	Source	SS	*df*	Mean square	*F*	*P*
Subtest 1	Groups	108.26	2	54.13	2.26	NS
	Error	287.79	12	23.98		
	Total	396.05	14			
Subtest 2	Groups	16.55	2	8.28	0.27	NS
	Error	374.55	12	31.21		
	Total	391.10	14			
Subtest 3	Groups	198.03	2	99.02	3.52	NS
	Error	337.78	12	28.15		
	Total	535.81	14			
Subtest 4	Groups	119.05	2	59.53	6.74	.05
	Error	105.96	12	8.83		
	Total	225.01	14			
Remembering word pairs	Groups	33.47	2	16.74	0.87	NS
	Error	230.55	12	19.21		
	Total	264.02	14			
Partial (3, 4)	Groups	592.08	2	296.04	8.34	.01
	Error	426.00	12	35.50		
	Total	1018.08	14			
Composite (1–4)	Groups	1404.58	2	702.29	4.49	.05
	Error	1876.38	12	156.37		
	Total	3280.96	14			

Note. NS = not significant.

Tukey's Wholly Significant Difference (WSD) test was performed for Subtest 4, the Partial, and the Composite scores. For Subtest 4 (Interpreting Metaphoric Expressions), the only significant mean difference ($p < .05$) occurred between the groups rated at Levels of Cognitive Functioning VII and VI. For the Partial and Composite scores, the only significant mean difference ($p < .05$) also occurred between these groups (LOCF VII and VI).

Subjects were also grouped on the basis of the relative duration of coma and amnesia. This resulted in two clinical groups: (A) with 0–2-week durations (n = 8), and (B) with 4–14-week durations (n = 9). Analyses of covariance, controlling for time postinjury, indicated no significant mean differences between groups for Subtests 1 ($F = 1.95$), 2 ($F = 1.81$), 3 ($F = 0.01$), or 4 ($F = 1.83$), the paired associate word recall task ($F = 4.37$), the Partial ($F = 0.42$), or the Composite scores ($F = 1.75$). These findings were validated by multiple linear regression analysis with coma duration measured in days, which was also nonsignificant.

Relative to the standard score distribution for the Partial and Composite scores on the Test of Language Competence (mean = 100, *SD* = 15), using the age group from 17 years 10 months to 18 years 10 months for comparison, the Partial SS for group LOCF VI (mean = 86) was within, but at the lower limit, of -1 *SD* of the normative mean. The Composite SS (mean = 84) was slightly below -1 *SD* of the normative mean. The Partial SSs for Groups LOCF VII (mean = 104) and VIII (mean = 102) were slightly above the mean for the normative group. The Composite SSs (mean = 99 and 95, respectively) were slightly below the normative mean, but well within the normal range.

Relative to the standard score distribution for Subtest 4 (Understanding Metaphoric Expressions) (mean = 10, *SD* = 3), using ages 17–10 to 18–11+ for comparison, the SS for Group LOCF VI (mean = 8) was below the average normal, but within the normal range. The SSs for Groups LOCF VII (mean = 13) and VIII (mean = 11) were above the mean.

Discussion

The first question asked was whether patients with traumatic closed head injury, grouped at Rancho Levels of Cognitive Functioning VI, VII, and VIII, would be differentiated by subtests and measures on the Test of Language Competence. Analysis of covariance, controlling for the duration of coma and amnesia and for time postinjury, indicated that patients with ratings at Rancho Level VI performed at significantly lower levels than patients with ratings at Rancho Level VII on Subtest 4 (Understanding Metaphoric Expressions). They also obtained significantly lower Composite (Subtests 1 to 4) and Partial (Subtests 3 and 4) scores. This indicates that the present measure of linguistic competence and metalinguistic ability was able to differentiate between patients at two of the rated levels of recovery of cognitive functioning, Rancho Levels of Cognitive Functioning VI and VII.

Based on ANCOVA and the percentage of the total variance uniquely explained by the measure, the Partial (Subtests 3 and 4) score provided the strongest measure for differentiation. Subtest 4 provided the second and the Composite (Subtests 1 to 4) the third best measures.

In combination, these findings are in agreement with the global disorganization theory (Hagen, 1984). They support the view that language processing and formulation abilities in patients after traumatic head injury are either heavily influenced or created by cognitive dysfunction. The finding that metaphoric interpretation and matching ability differentiated groups rated at Rancho Levels VI and VII agrees with previous observations of reductions in abstract thought after traumatic head injury (Thomsen, 1975). It suggests, however, that the degree of impairment of abstract thought will depend upon the level of recovery of cognitive functions.

Patients rated at Rancho Levels of Cognitive Functioning VI and VII were also differentiated by a combination of scores for interpreting and matching metaphors and recreating intents in complex sentences in response to illustrated contexts, the Partial score. This suggests that planning for language production, a task that requires conceptual integration and synthesis of semantic, syntactic, and pragmatic variables (Bock, 1982), was also influenced by the level of recovery of cognitive functioning.

A third measure, combining the scores on the four major subtests of the Test of Language Competence, the Composite, also differentiated patients rated at Rancho Levels of Cognitive Functioning VI and VII. The Composite incorporates measures of ability to give alternative interpretations of ambiguities in sentences and to make two plausible inferences about intervening event chains in a given situation. This finding suggests that cognitive linguistic flexibility (i.e., divergent production) was influenced by the relative level of recovery of cognitive functioning. This observation agrees with the perception that the language disorganization observed after traumatic head injury results from a breakdown of ability to deal differentially with stimuli and to shift cognitive set (Hagen, 1984).

Comparisons of Partial and Composite standard scores with the Test of Language Competence norms for 18-year-olds indicated that the measures of recovered linguistic competence by patients rated at Rancho Levels of Cognitive Functioning VII and VIII clustered around the average normal. Individual variations fell within the normal range. In contrast, the measures of recovered linguistic competence of patients rated at Rancho Level of Cognitive Functioning VI clustered at the lower limits of the normal range. Individual variations were large and covered the average and the below-average normal ranges. In combination, the findings contradict previous observations that patients with traumatic head injury perform within normal limits on tests of aphasia (Milton et al., 1984). The difference can be reconciled by the fact that Milton et al. (1984) did not rate their patients for relative level of cognitive functioning.

The standard scores for Subtest 4 (Interpreting Metaphoric Expressions) showed that the measures of metaphoric ability of patients rated at Rancho Levels of Cognitive Functioning VII and VIII clustered above average normal and within the normal range. In contrast, the measures of metaphoric ability of patients rated at Rancho Level of Cognitive Functioning VI clustered below average normal with considerable individual variation.

This study did not find that patients rated at Rancho Levels of Cognitive Functioning VI, VII, and VIII differed on the paired associate word recall task. Nor did patients with relatively short (0 to 2 weeks) or long (4 to 14 weeks) durations of coma and amnesia obtain different measures of linguistic competence or paired associate word recall. These findings do not contradict observations of significant negative relationships between duration of coma and amnesia and recovery of memory span for digits (Brooks, 1983; Levin, Benton, & Grossman, 1982). There were substantive, but nonsignificant, differences between the means for remembering word pairs in the two groups formed on the basis of relative duration of coma and amnesia. This suggests that relatively longer durations of coma and amnesia may have resulted in difficulties with a deeper level of processing (Type II memory) in some of the patients in this study.

Several patients commented on the adolescent slant of the items of the Test of Language Competence. Minor modifications of items on Subtests 2 and 4, which should not interfere with the use of the norms, should minimize this bias. The findings of this study supported a need for an adult bias in a test of linguistic competence. The Test of Language Competence for Adults (Wiig & Secord, in press), an upwards and more complex extension of the Test of Language Competence, was designed in response to this perceived need.

The present findings and conclusions should be interpreted within the limitations of the study. The number of desirable subjects was severely limited. This was due to the relatively small population of patients with traumatic head injury and to the stringent selection criteria outlined for the study.

Acknowledgments. The authors thank Adele Gagne and Joe Piette for their contributions to data collection. Appreciation is also extended to Phyllis Meyer for her valuable input and to Bill Insko, William Hoffey, and Chris Ingalls for their suggestions for design and data analysis. This study was made possible through the cooperation of the Head Injury Center at Lewis Bay, a part of the New Medico Head Injury System.

References

Allen, R.R., & Brown, K.L. (1977). *Developing communication competence in children.* Skokie, IL: National Textbook.

Alvy, K.T. (1973). The development of listener-adapted communications in grade-school children from different social-class backgrounds. *Genetic Psychology Monographs, 87,* 33–104.

Anglin, T. (1977). *Word, object, and conceptual development.* New York: W.W. Norton.

Austin, T.T. (1962). *How to do things with words.* Cambridge, MA: Harvard University Press.

Baddeley, A.D. (1970). Estimating the short-term component in free recall. *British Journal of Psychology, 61,* 13–15.

Baker, L. (1982). An evaluation of the role of metacognitive deficits in learning disabilities. *Topics in Learning and Learning Disabilities, 2,* 27–36.

Bernstein-Ellis, E., Wertz, R.T., Dronkers, N.F., & Milton, S.B. (1985). PICA performance by traumatically brain injured and left hemisphere CVA patients. In R.H. Brookshire (Ed.), *Clinical aphasiology: Conference proceedings, 1985, (pp. 97–*106). Minneapolis: BRK Publishers.

Bever, T.G., Garrett, M.F., & Hurtig, R. (1973). The interaction of perceptual processes and ambiguous sentences. *Memory and Cognition, 1,* 277–286.

Bock, T.K. (1982). Toward a cognitive psychology of syntax: Information processing contributions to sentence formulation. *Psychological Review, 89,* 1–47.

Brooks, D.N. (1976). Wechsler Memory Scale performance and its relationship to brain damage after severe closed head injury. *Journal of Neurology, Neurosurgery, and Psychiatry, 39,* 593.

Brooks, D.N. (1980). Cognitive sequelae in relationship to early indices of severity of brain damage after severe blunt head injury. *Journal of Neurology, Neurosurgery, and Psychiatry, 43,* 529.

Brooks, D.N. (1983). Disorders of memory. In M. Rosenthal (Ed.), *Rehabilitation of the head injured adult.* Philadelphia: F.A. Davis.

Carey, P., Mehler, F., & Bever, T. (1970). Judging the veracity of ambiguous sentences. *Journal of Verbal Learning and Verbal Behavior, 9,* 243–254.

Chafe, W. (1976). Givenness, contrastiveness, definiteness, subjects, topics, and point of view. In C. Li (Ed.), *Subject and topic* (pp. 25–55). New York: Academic Press.

Crowder, R.G. (1976). *Principles of learning and memory.* Hillsdale, NJ: Erlbaum.

Delia, J., & Clark, R.A. (1977). Cognitive complexity, social perception, and the development of listener-adapted communication in six-, eight-, ten-, and twelve-year-old boys. *Communication Monographs, 4,* 326–345.

Dunn, L.M., & Dunn, L.M. (1981). *Peabody Picture Vocabulary Test-Revised.* Circle Pines, MN: American Guidance Service.

Fillmore, C. (1968). The case for case. In E. Bach & R. Harms (Eds.), *Universals in linguistic theory.* New York: Holt, Rinehart & Winston.

Fodor, J.A., & Garrett, M.F. (1967). Some syntactic determinants of sentential complexity. *Perception and Psychophysics, 2,* 289–296.

Garoutte, B., & Aird, R.B. (1984). Behavioral effects of head injury. *Psychiatric Annals, 14,* 507–514.

Goodglass, H., & Kaplan, E. (1983). *The assessment of aphasia and related disorders* (2nd ed.). Philadelphia: Lea & Febiger.

Guilford, J.P. (1967). *The nature of human intelligence.* New York: McGraw-Hill.

Hagen, C. (1982). Language-cognitive disorganization following closed head injury: A conceptualization. In L.E. Trexler (ed.), *Cognitive rehabilitation: Conceptualization and intervention.* New York: Plenum Press.

Hagen, C. (1984). Language disorders in head trauma. In A. Holland (Ed.), *Language disorders in adults.* San Diego: College-Hill.

Hagen, C., Malkmus, D., Durham, P., & Bowman, K. (1979). Levels of cognitive functioning. In *Rehabilitation of the head injured adult: Comprehensive physical manage-*

ment (pp. 87–89). Downey, CA: Professional Staff Association of Rancho Los Amigos Hospital.
Heilman, K.M., Safron, A., & Geschwind, N. (1971). Closed head trauma and aphasia. *Journal of Neurology, Neurosurgery, and Psychiatry, 34,* 265–269.
Holland, A.L. (1980). *Communicative abilities in daily living: A test of functional communication in aphasic adults.* Baltimore: University Park Press.
Holland, A.L. (1982). When is aphasia aphasia?: The problem of closed head injury. In R.H. Brookshire (Ed.), *Clinical aphasiology: Conference proceedings, 1982* (pp. 345–349). Minneapolis: BRK Publishers.
Kaplan, E., Goodglass, H., & Weintraub, S. (1976). *Boston Naming Test.* Boston: VA Hospital.
Kertesz, A. (1981). *Western Aphasia Battery.* New York: Grune & Stratton.
Lakoff, G., & Johnson, M. (1980). *Metaphors we live by.* Chicago: Chicago University Press.
Levin, H.S., Benton, A.L., & Grossman, R.G. (1982). *Neurobehavioral consequences of closed head injury.* New York: Oxford University Press.
Levin, H.S., Grossman, R.G., & Kelly, P.J. (1976). Aphasic disorder in patients with closed head injury. *Journal of Neurology, Neurosurgery, and Psychiatry, 39,* 1062–1070.
Malkmus, D. (1979). Factors influencing management and outcome: Cognitive considerations. In *Rehabilitation of the head injured adult: Comprehensive physical management* (pp. 21–23). Downey, CA: Professional Staff Association of Rancho Los Amigos Hospital.
Malkmus, D. (1983). Integrating cognitive strategies into the physical therapy setting. *Physical Therapy, 63,* 1952–1959.
Malkmus, D., Booth, B.J., & Doyle, M. (1980). Meeting the challenge of the agitated patient. In *Rehabilitation of the head injured adult: Comprehensive management* (pp. 43–46). Downey, CA: Professional Staff Association of Rancho Los Amigos Hospital.
MacKay, D.G., & Bever, T.G. (1967). In search of ambiguity. *Perception and Psychophysics, 2,* 193–200.
Meichenbaum, D. (1977). *Cognitive behavior modification: An integrative approach.* New York: Plenum Press.
Milton, S.B., Prutting, C.A., & Binder, G.M. (1984). Appraisal of communicative competence in head injured adults. In R.H. Brookshire (Ed.), *Clinical aphasiology: Conference proceedings, 1984* (pp. 114–123). Minneapolis: BRK Publishers.
Milton, S.B., Turnstall, C.M., & Wertz, R.T. (1983). Dysnomia: A rose by any other name may require elaborate description. In R.H. Brookshire (Ed.), *Clinical aphasiology: Conference proceedings, 1983* (pp. 137–149). Minneapolis: BRK Publishers.
Porch, B.E. (1981). *The Porch Index of Communicative Ability: Administration, scoring, and interpretation* (Vol. 2). Palo Alto: Consulting Psychologists Press.
Reid, K., & Hresko, W.P. (1981). *A cognitive approach to learning disabilities.* New York: McGraw-Hill.
Sarno, M. (1980). The nature of verbal impairment of closed head injury. *Journal of Nervous and Mental Disease, 168,* 685–692.
Sarno, M. (1984). Verbal impairment after closed head injury: Report of a replication study. *Journal of Nervous and Mental Disease, 172,* 475–479.
Schank, R.C. (1982). *Reading and understanding: Teaching from the perspective of artificial intelligence.* Hillsdale, NJ: Erlbaum.
Schank, R.C., & Abelson, R. (1977). *Scripts, goals, plans, and understanding.* Hillsdale, NJ: Erlbaum.

Searle, T.R. (1969). *Speech acts: An essay on the philosophy of language.* Cambridge, England: Cambridge University Press.
Strub, R.L., & Black, F.W. (1985). *The mental status examination in neurology,* (2nd ed.). Philadelphia: F.A. Davis.
Thomsen, I.V. (1975). Evaluation and outcome of aphasia in patients with severe closed head trauma. *Journal of Neurology, Neurosurgery, and Psychiatry, 38,* 713–718.
Thomsen, I.V. (1976). Evaluation and outcome of traumatic aphasia in patients with severe verified focal lesions. *Folia Phoniatrica, 28,* 362–377.
Torgesen, J.K. (1977). Memorization processes in reading-disabled children. *Journal of Educational Psychology, 69,* 571–578.
Waterhouse, L., & Fein, D. (1982). Language skills in developmentally disabled children. *Brain and Language, 15,* 307–333.
Wiig, E.H. (1984). Language disabilities in adolescents: A question of cognitive strategies. *Topics in Language Disorders, 4,* 41–58.
Wiig, E.H., & Becker-Caplan, L. (1984). Linguistic retrieval strategies and word-finding difficulties among children with language disabilities. *Topics in Language Disorders, 4,* 1–18.
Wiig, E.H., & Secord, W. (1985). *Test of Language Competence.* San Antonio: Psychological Corp.
Wiig, E.H., & Secord, W. (in press). *Test of language competence for adults.* San Antonio: Psychological Corp.
Winner, E., Rosenstiel, A.K., & Gardner, H. (1976). The development of metaphoric understanding. *Developmental Psychology, 12,* 289–297.

Appendix 7. A Test of Language Competence: Description

Subtest 1, Understanding Ambiguous Sentences, contains six lexical and seven structural ambiguities. Illustrative items are: 1) "The roar of the fans disturbed the team" (lexical ambiguity), 2) "Bob did not blame the girl as much as her mother" (surface structure ambiguity), and 3) "I don't know about you, but visiting relatives can be a nuisance" (deep structure ambiguity). Subjects are asked to give two spoken interpretations of each item. Responses are given 3 points for two accurate, 1 for a single accurate, and 0 for an inaccurate or no response. The subtest has its basis in models of the resolution of ambiguities and evidence that ability to give alternative interpretations for decontextualized ambiguous sentences relates to linguistic competence (Bever, Garrett, & Hurtig, 1973; Carey, Mehler, & Bever, 1970; Fodor & Garrett, 1967; MacKay & Bever, 1967).

Subtest 2, Making Inferences, contains 12 items. Each item features two propositions, one that begins a situational script and one that ends it. Item 10 illustrates the format.

Item 10. Rick worked harder than anyone else on his project. He met with his teacher after school to talk about his bad grade.
Rick met with the teacher because:
(a) The teacher never graded Rick's project.
(b) Rick did not feel he had done a sloppy job.

(c) He realized he might have misunderstood the assignment.
(d) His work was better than anyone else's.

Subjects are asked to identify two plausible intervening events from among four spoken and printed choices. The propositions featured in the items refer to common causal event chains in situational and instrumental scripts. Responses are given 3 points for identifying two plausible inferences, 1 for one plausible inference, and 0 for inaccurate or no responses. The subtest has its basis in scriptal models (Schank, 1982; Schank & Abelson, 1977).

Subtest 3, Recreating Sentences, contains 13 items, each featuring an illustration of a common situation with two or more potential speakers. Each item gives three lexical units, one a conjunction, conjunctive, or correlative, which must be incorporated in the response. The remaining words are from the verb, noun, adverbial, and/or modifier cases. As an example, Item 10 features an illustration of the fruit and vegetable shelves in a supermarket. The stimulus words are: *neither week were.* Subjects are asked to reconstruct what someone could have said in the situation with the constraints that (a) the response must be one sentence and (b) all words must be contained in it. Responses are first scored holistically for semantic, syntactic, and pragmatic intactness. Intact propositions are scored 3, responses with deviations 1, and bizarre or no responses 0. A word score is given next. Sentences with all stimulus words are scored 3, with two 1, and with one or none 0. The holistic and word scores are added to obtain an item score. The task has its base in speech act theory, case grammar, and information-processing models (Austin, 1962; Bock, 1982; Chafe, 1976; Fillmore, 1968; Searle, 1969).

Subtest 4, Understanding Metaphoric Expressions, contains 12 items. Each gives a reference to a situation and a metaphoric expression. Subjects first interpret the expression. Next, four choices (a matching, an opposite, a nonrelated metaphoric, and a literal expression) are presented for identifying the figurative expression with the same meaning as the sample. As an example, Item 2 describes the situation as involving two students who are moving to a new town. The metaphoric expression is "There is rough sailing ahead for us." The four choices are: (a) The waves are going to make it hard to sail (literal), (b) The rough times are behind us now (opposite), (c) It took the wind out of our sails (nonrelated metaphor), and (d) We will be facing a hard road (matching metaphor). Responses are scored 3 for an accurate interpretation and match, 1 for an accurate interpretation or match, and 0 for inaccurate or no responses. The task has its basis in the metaphoric concept model (Lakoff & Johnson, 1980).

The Supplemental Task, Remembering Word Pairs, features 16 word pairs, selected to be familiar (acquired by Grade 5), mono- or disyllabic, and to represent four associatively mediated word categories (paradigmatic, spatial, temporal, unrelated). Four word lists in different degrees of randomization were designed, two for presentation and two for recall. The task has its bases in levels of processing models of verbal memory (Baddeley, 1970; Crowder, 1976). Relative to the models, the repeated paired associate paradigm should result in improved recall after a second presentation, if the repetition led to a deeper level of processing (Type II). Conversely, repeated processing at the same level (Type I) for both presentations should result in no significant increase in recall. The task is scored by adding the number of word pairs recalled on Elicitation Lists A and B.

8
A Paradigm Shift in Memory Rehabilitation

CATHERINE A. MATEER and MCKAY MOORE SOHLBERG

Reduced memory capacity is the complaint most frequently voiced by individuals who have suffered a closed head injury. Recent literature indicates that 70% of persons with traumatic brain injury continue to experience significant memory difficulties at 1 year postinjury (Brooks, 1983). Since memory is a primary cognitive process critical for successful functioning in even the most basic functions of everyday living, memory impairment is often one of the most debilitating deficits following traumatic injury. Decreased performance in memory can affect all aspects of the rehabilitation process and can have devastating effects on a person's educational or vocational goals as well as on independent living status. In this chapter, we briefly review traditional approaches to memory "retraining," provide rationale for a more ecologically valid approach to the study of memory disorders, and describe a three-pronged approach to memory rehabilitation.

Although the degree and nature of memory deficits differ among individuals, several patterns of impairment are commonly seen in the traumatically brain-injured population. Immediately following brain injury or with gradual recovery from coma, patients may not be able to retain any information from one moment to the next. This early, severe disruption of memory is termed *posttraumatic amnesia*. Its persistence is often indicative of a more profound brain injury. Patients who are in this state may exhibit such behaviors as repetitious question asking where the same questions are posed over and over. Often this state is associated with confusion and disorientation to place, time, and circumstances. In almost all cases, patients with traumatic brain injury recover consistent orientation. Many are left, however, with residual impairments in learning and retaining new information.

Traditional Approaches to Memory Rehabilitation

Although there is some literature, often of a popular nature, on enhancing memory skills in normal individuals, limited research is available on remediation of memory disorders. Two broad approaches have been utilized. The first involves use of exercises, repetitive practice, or drills that have *restoration* of memory as their goal. Commonly included in this approach are word- or list-learning tasks or paragraph-recall tasks. Despite the face value of such activities, published studies utilizing these approaches have repeatedly documented their failures in either enhancing scores on untrained memory tasks or, of greater importance, in impacting functional memory outside the clinic (Godfrey & Knight, 1985; Prigatano et al., 1984; Schacter, Rich & Stampp, 1985). Despite the lack of evidence that this muscle-building approach has any generalizable effects on memory enhancement, repetitive drilling is the approach taken in almost all of the published computer programs for so-called "memory retraining." Currently available programs rarely, if ever, have been evaluated for effectiveness, and in our own clinic, no memory-oriented computer program has been found useful in impacting memory.

The second approach commonly used in memory rehabilitation involves training of strategies or techniques for memory compensation. Such strategies variously focus on enhancing organization of information to be recalled, rehearsing of information to be remembered, or training of specific mnemonic devices such as peg words or visual imagery. Some studies have suggested that recall performance in memory-disordered patients can be improved through training use of such internal mnemonic learning schemes (Cermak, 1975; Crovitz, 1979; Gasparrini & Satz, 1979; Gianutsos & Gianutsos, 1979; Wilson, 1981, 1982). None of these studies, however, has provided support that use of these strategies generalizes to naturalistic settings.

On the face of it, the utility of such approaches should be suspect. These techniques place heavy demands on patients' already deficient cognitive systems, rendering them ineffectual for many persons with significantly compromised intellectual functions (Baddeley, 1982; Butters & Cermak, 1980; Schacter et al., 1985). They also presume to impose an approach to analyzing information or developing associations that cannot be explicitly observed or measured. Finally, it is very hard to imagine ways in which internally generated strategies, such as imagery techniques or verbal associations, could be utilized to begin to remember the myriad of facts, events, people, activities, or future intended actions to be remembered in daily life. In our own experience, attempts to utilize such procedures have been useful only for acquisition of very specific, small bodies of information (e.g., a medication schedule).

Toward an Ecological Approach to Memory Rehabilitation

A review of the memory rehabilitation literature suggests minimal gains in memory as measured by neuropsychological testing and no gains in memory function as measured by extra-laboratory assessments following traditional treatment (Godfrey & Knight, 1985; Prigatano et al., 1984; Schacter et al., 1985). One reason for these failures may be that current treatment techniques simply lack sufficient ecological validity to impact and enhance memory functioning in our patients' everyday world.

In recent years, there has been increasing interest in the study of human cognition in naturalistic contexts (Bronfenbrenner, 1979; Cole, Hood, & McDermott, 1978; Rogoff & Lobe, 1984). The shift in emphasis from descriptions of cognition generated from laboratory experiments to consideration of environmental and contextual variables has generally been limited to the realm of normal cognition (Baddeley & Wilkins, 1984; Bronfenbrenner, 1979; Levy & Loftus, 1984; Neisser, 1982). Much is known about cognitive and experimental variables related to memory that operate within controlled experimental designs. Results from such studies, however, lack the scope and functional context necessary to apply experimentally derived principles to the evaluation or rehabilitation of memory in persons with acquired neurological damage. Theories of memory are often so closely bound to particular laboratory paradigms that they limit practical application.

Current memory assessment and treatment techniques used with the brain-injured population rarely, if ever, reflect information derived from studies of everyday memory. For instance, studies investigating memory mechanisms as they operate in naturalistic contexts have identified prospective memory or the ability to remember to perform future actions as a valid class of memory behavior requisite for successful functioning in the everyday world (Harris & Wilkins, 1984; Kreutzer, Leonard, & Falvell, 1975; Meacham & Dumitru, 1976; Meacham & Leiman, 1982; Wilkins & Baddeley, 1978). Prospective memory includes such behaviors as remembering to keep an appointment, return a phone call, or take medications. Although this component of memory appears to have essential applications to naturalistic uses of memory, it is currently not addressed in the clinical management of patients exhibiting memory impairments. The majority of clinicians typically employ only retrospective memory assessment and treatment techniques, using laboratory-based tasks that are concerned with the recall of new information (Sunderland, Harris, & Baddeley, 1984). Treatment activities such as paragraph recall, picture recognition, training of mnemonic strategies, list learning, and associative pairing are restricted to recall activities. In very few respects do any of these treatment approaches approximate naturalistic uses of memory.

Results of a Survey of Forgetting Experiences

A better understanding of the memory factors operating in naturalistic contexts is essential before assessment and treatment tools that have relevance to real-world functioning can be developed. One technique that has proven fruitful in gathering information about everyday functional memory is the use of memory questionnaires (Herrmann, 1984). This method involves information gathering via questionnaires or surveys that elicit information concerning how people perceive various aspects of their memory function. Such a method of investigation is useful because it provides access to information about everyday memory functioning otherwise unavailable in laboratory research (Herrmann, 1984;

Sunderland et al., 1984). Questionnaire results describing how persons with both normal and disordered memory systems perceive their individual memory behavior have been reported (Broadbent, Cooper, Fitzgerald, & Parkes, 1982; Herrmann & Neisser, 1978; Martin, 1983; Sunderland, Harris, & Baddeley, 1983). Currently, however, little information is available regarding how head-injured persons perceive their memory functioning.

We developed and administered a memory questionnaire describing various types of memory failure or forgetting experiences to a large number of brain-injured individuals and normal controls (Mateer, Sohlberg, & Crineon, 1987). The goal was to ascertain the type of forgetting experiences perceived by both brain-injured and non-brain-injured individuals as most prominent or problematic. To date, there has been no attempt to measure the type and frequency of memory failures as perceived by head-injured patients. Such information is crucial for guiding the assessment and treatment of memory impairments suffered by this population. It is also potentially useful in gaining a tool for better understanding of potential discrepancies between measured and perceived memory capabilities.

Based on a review of the current memory literature, we hypothesized six distinct classes of memory, potentially useful in describing the type and frequency of memory failure experienced in brain-injured patients. They included anterograde episodic and semantic memory, retrograde episodic and semantic memory, working memory, and prospective memory. These six memory categories formed the basis for the theoretical construct used in the questionnaire. Samples of forgetting experiences related to each of these types of memory were generated. Brain-injured and control respondents read each item and then ranked them on a frequency-of-occurrence scale.

A rationally derived set of 30 statements relating to these six recognized classes of memory was developed. Instructions indicated that a 5-point rating scale referenced to frequency be completed for each statement. Three copies of the questionnaire and a cover letter were sent to 300 randomly selected personal residences on the Washington State Head Injury Foundation mailing list (900 total questionnaires). A cover letter sent with the questionnaires described the reason for the study and asked that one be completed by an individual in the family who had sustained a brain injury, and one or two more by non-brain-injured family members. Three hundred thirty-seven completed questionnaires were returned in an 8-week period. In addition to completing the rating scales for each of the statements, self-report information was completed regarding head injury (yes/no), coma (yes/no), length of coma, time postonset, sex, age, and current employment (yes/no).

Analysis of responses to the survey questionnaire was completed for a sample of 178 brain-injured and 157 control subjects; 121 of the brain-injured cases reported associated coma of greater than 24 hours, 57 did not. Analysis of survey responses yielded four separate Memory Factors, which were labeled Attention/Prospective Memory, Retrograde Memory, Anterograde Memory, and Historical/Overlearned Memory. Mean reports of frequency of memory failure are plotted for the four Memory Factors and three subject groups (head injury with coma, head injury without coma, and controls) in Figure 8.1.

Almost half of the total variance (47%) in responses to the questionnaire was accounted for by frequency ratings on items that loaded on the Attention/Prospective Memory Factor. Interestingly, questions related to Prospective Memory and to Attention loaded on the same factor rather than on separate factors. This suggests that the ability to carry out future intended actions depends heavily on attention, perhaps in the form of vigilance relative to time and situational cues. In addition to the common factor loading, forgetting experiences related to Prospective Memory and Attention were perceived as occurring most frequently. In every subject group, the mean frequency rating for forgetting related to these two areas was higher than that for any of the other three factors. While this study suggests that both brain-injured and non-brain-injured individuals ranked failures of prospective memory as occurring most often, this critical component of everyday memory has yet to be critically examined in either population. To date, there are no established assessment or treatment tools available for remediating prospective memory. Development of such procedures is clearly warranted.

A second major finding of the memory survey relates to outcome of the factor analysis of questions regarding perceived frequency of various kinds of forgetting experiences. Rather than confirming the six originally hypothesized categories of memory, the factor analysis yielded a four-factor structure. The episodic and semantic dissociations hypothesized for anterograde and retrograde memory were not upheld in the analysis of perceived memory difficulty. We are not suggesting that these distinctions are not valid clinically, as we have found them useful and important. It may be that questions on the survey simply did not adequately capture salient differences critical to episodic/semantic distinctions or dissociations. We believe our failure to find such distinctions in the analysis further points up, at least in part, the degree to which these distinctions have not yet been adequately described or conceptualized in reference to everyday experience.

The third result to be discussed relates to the pattern of reported frequency of memory failure across and within the three reporting groups. The general pattern of perceived memory dysfunction relative to the four-factor scales was relatively common across the four groups. Just as all groups perceived Attention and Prospective Memory as being most problematic, all groups perceived aspects of Historical or Overlearned Memory to be least interfering. While Anterograde and Retrograde Memory were reported to be of essentially equal and intermediate difficulty for controls and individuals who sustained brain injury without coma, individuals who had sustained coma perceived memory for new experiences and information (Anterograde Memory) as being more problematic than recall of events or information experienced or acquired prior to injury. Given the literature on the effects of brain injury, it is this latter group for whom significant anterograde relative to retrograde memory loss would be predicted. This finding lends a degree of face validity to the study in that self-report results appears to be reflecting predictable outcomes.

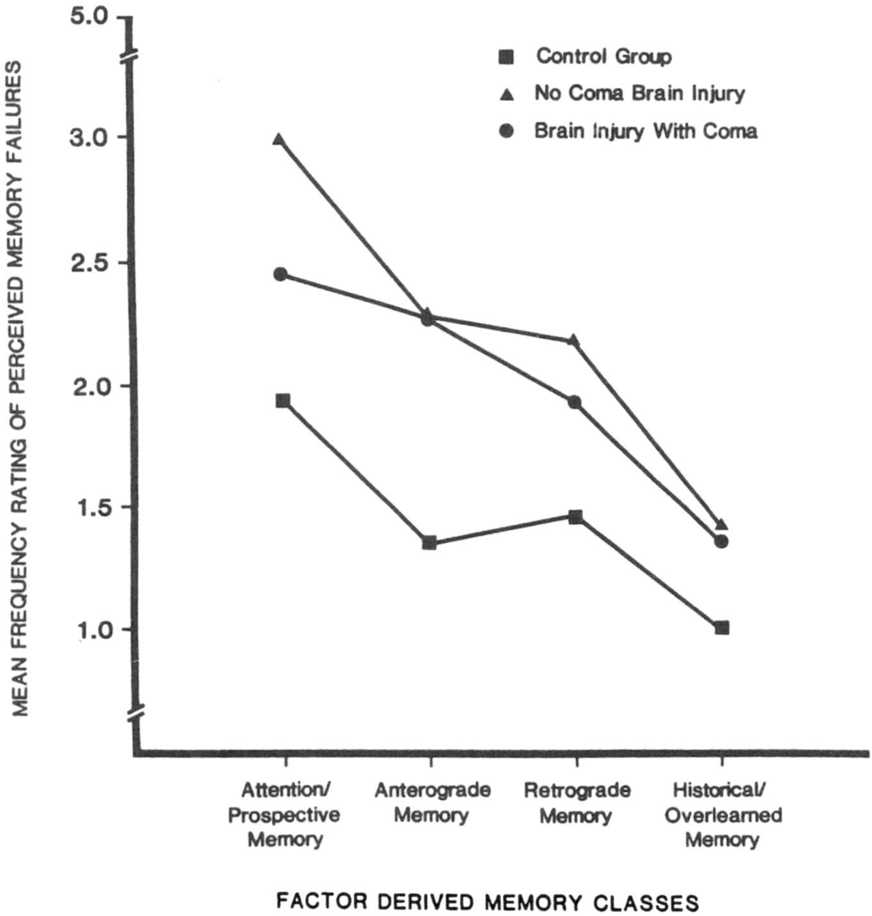

FIGURE 8.1. Results of a questionnaire regarding perceived frequency of memory failure. Mean frequency ratings for the four factor-derived categories of memory loss for three subject groups: control, brain injury with coma (>24 hours), brain injury without coma. All groups perceive memory failures related to attention deficits and future intended actions as most frequent and problematic. (From Mateer, Sohlberg, and Crineon, 1987.)

The questionnaire survey revealed that memory failures relating to prospective memory and attention are perceived as occurring the most often for both groups. This suggests that most individuals are more concerned with their ability to remember to perform future actions (Prospective Memory) and with attention-based forgetting experiences (e.g., holding numbers in their head, remembering what they went into another room for) than they are with other types of memory such as the recall of semantic information. Those results prompted us to further investigate the prospective memory functioning of the brain-injured persons with whom we worked. We felt this was necessary in order that our treatments would be effective in addressing memory impairments in naturalistic contexts. A paradigm shift in the clinical management of memory impairments is on the horizon with movement toward the use of assessment and treatment tools that have ecological validity. Treatment of memory breakdowns in functional components of memory, such as prospective memory, is critical if rehabilitation is to successfully impact the lives of patients with memory disorders.

A Three-Pronged Approach to Memory Rehabilitation

As reviewed earlier in this chapter, there is limited research available examining the remediation of memory disorders. For the most part, the research that is available does not shed favorable light on the rehabilitation potential of memory (Butters & Cermak, 1980; Godfrey & Knight, 1985; Schacter et al., 1985). Recent evidence suggests, however, that in the past, researchers and clinicians have been entirely too narrow and restricted in their view of memory (Mateer, et al., 1987). Results from our own studies at Good Samaritan Hospital Center for Cognitive Rehabilitation suggest that memory problems are amenable to treatment, given careful matching between the type of treatment and the presenting symptoms (Mateer & Sohlberg, 1986).

Memory impairment does not reflect a unitary functional deficit. We know that profound disruption of memory, amnesia, varies with the site of cerebral lesion. Amnesia that results from a lesion of the dorsomedial thalamus (diencephalic amnesia) has a different presentation than that resulting from damage to the mesial temporal regions (bitemporal amnesia). For example, amnesics with mesial temporal damage forget at a much faster rate on recognition tasks than patients with diencephalic damage (Patient NA and Korsakoff patients) who exhibit a normal rate of forgetting once they have learned the material (Squire & Cohen, 1982; Hupper & Piercy, 1979; Weingartner & Parker, 1984).

Although most traumatically brain-injured patients do not have focal or easily identifiable lesions, the notion that there are different types of memory problems requiring different treatment approaches still holds true. It is important to match a memory rehabilitation program with the specific constellation of memory sequelae.

The first step in arriving at an appropriate marriage between disorder and treatment is to perform a comprehensive memory assessment. A thorough evaluation of memory is crucial in order to adequately understand the nature of the memory problem. Current diagnostic tests, however, tend to have a very limited scope, addressing only retrospective memory, recall, or recognition ability. The most widely used assessment procedures include the Wechsler Memory Scale (Wechsler, 1945), the Auditory Verbal Learning Test (Rey, 1964), the Selective Reminding Test (Buschke & Fuld, 1974), and the Randt Memory Test (Randt, Brown, & Osborne, 1980). The major focus of each of these evaluation tools is recall ability. Evaluation of prospective memory ability and attentional processing, as well as recall ability, is essential for understanding the nature of a memory impairment. It is also critical to analyze *why* an individual fails on a particular memory test and to examine underlying factors potentially responsible for a memory failure. For example, failure on a semantic recall test may reflect a primary attention deficit rather than a primary memory impairment. Examination of results on other diagnostic tests sensitive to attention would be crucial for sorting out the nature of the impairment.

To address the different constellations of memory problems, we have developed a three-pronged approach to memory rehabilitation that has proven very effective in enhancing memory function in persons who have sustained traumatic brain injury. The memory model consists of three distinct treatment programs including: 1) Attention Process Training (APT) (Sohlberg & Mateer, 1986a), 2) Prospective Memory Process Training (PROMPT) (Sohlberg & Mateer, 1986b), and 3) Memory Notebook Training (Sohlberg & Mateer, 1987). Each of the three treatment programs are described with accompanying supportive experimental and clinical data.

Attention Process Training

Deficits in attention and concentration often go unrecognized or are misdiagnosed in the assessment of cognitive functions following diffuse brain injury. Disruption of the physiological systems critical to the regulation of attention may occur as the result of seemingly minor, as well as severe, neurological damage. Deficits that initially present as memory impairments are often found to reflect underlying impairments in attention. For many individuals, the primary deficit is an attention problem rather than a true memory disorder. Although the severity of an attention deficit nearly always lessens over the course of recovery, significant deficits in attention and concentration are often present many months or even years postinjury (Sohlberg & Mateer, 1987).

In the past, clinical models of attention have been largely restricted to the domain of asymmetries in spatial responsiveness or neglect. The experimental literature views attention in a much broader framework, but this has not been tied to clinical phenomena. A broadly based view of attention served as the basis for the development of Attention Process Training (APT) (Sohlberg & Mateer, 1986a). Briefly, attention was conceptualized as the capacity to focus on particular stimuli over time and to manipulate flexibly the information. Examples of cognitive tasks that are likely to reflect attentional deficits based on the APT model include: backward digit span, serial number sets, Trails B, and backwards spelling.

There is far from universal agreement in the information-processing literature regarding the mechanism of attention. Most models of attention are based on the human information-processing approach first introduced by Broadbent (1958). According to these models, attention is usually viewed as a selectivity phenomenon by means of which target stimuli receive priority processing over concurrent nontarget stimuli. That is, attention is considered to be the process by which one selectively responds to the specific event and is able to inhibit responding to a simultaneous event (Johnston & Wilson, 1980).

A shortcoming of the selectivity models is that they often stop at the level of signal detection or target selection. Additional processing of information tends not to be addressed in these theories. A more comprehensive view of attention is necessary to adequately describe the attention deficits observed in brain-injured populations that often manifest as decreased memory ability.

The theoretical construct of working memory as described by Baddeley & Hitch (1974) and Baddeley (1981) does begin to address the comprehensive nature of attention. The Central Executive, one component of Baddeley's model, is hypothesized to provide for temporary storage of information. The capacity for such temporary storage allows for the division of attention during information processing. Modeled as a controller of memory, the Central Executive allows information to be held in short-term storage while attention is temporarily shifted to other stimuli. This model thus incorporates additional levels of information processing. The problem with all the current models of attention, however, is that none adequately address the *clinical* phenomenon of attention deficits or their remediation. The few treatment programs for attention that do exist tend to be task oriented without a strong theoretical basis. At best, treatment programs address restrictive components of attentional requirements.

In response to the need for an adequate model on which to base treatment of attention disorders, we (Sohlberg & Mateer, 1986a, 1987) developed a clinical treatment program that considered attention to be a comprehensive and multilevel functional process. This treatment program is called Attention Process Training (APT). It considered attention as a multidimensional cognitive capacity including the following five levels of attention: Focused Attention, Sustained Attention, Selective Attention, Alternating Attention, and Divided Attention. Descriptions of each level of the model are as follows:

Focused Attention: The ability to respond discretely to specific visual, auditory, or tactile stimuli

Sustained Attention: The ability to maintain a consistent behavioral response during continuous or repetitive activity

Selective Attention: The ability to maintain a cognitive set that requires activation and inhibition of responses dependent upon discrimination of stimuli

Alternating Attention: The capacity for mental flexibility that allows for moving between tasks having different cognitive requirements

Divided Attention: The ability to simultaneously respond to multiple tasks

Hierarchies of treatment tasks were developed for each of the five levels of the attention model. Therapy was conducted using tasks and treatment materials as outlined in Attention Process Training (Sohlberg & Mateer, 1986a). A multiple baseline across cognitive areas (Hersen & Barlow, 1976) was used to assess the effectiveness of the APT program in four brain-injured subjects (Sohlberg, 1985; Sohlberg & Mateer, 1987). Previous research (Gianutsos, 1981; Gianutsos & Gianutsos, 1979) has established the practicality of using the single-case design to study the retraining of cognitive processes in individuals.

The subjects were participants at the Good Samaritan Hospital Center for Cognitive Rehabilitation, a postmedical day treatment brain injury program. They were randomly selected from a consecutive series of admissions to the program. Subjects varied widely in both nature of injury and time postonset. The study examined the relationship between the implementation of APT and changes in attentional skills as measured by the Paced Auditory Serial Addition Task (PASAT) (Gronwall, 1977), a neuropsychological test sensitive to attention deficits. To establish a functional relationship it was necessary to observe changes in attention and plot improvement over time. A multiple baseline design was utilized, which measured simultaneous changes in a second cognitive process area, visual processing. The measure used to assess visual processing abilities was the Spatial Relations Subtest (SR) from the Woodcock-Johnson Psychoeducational Battery (Woodcock & Johnson, 1977). This is a test of spatial perception and judgment that requires the subject to identify discrete spatial components that would fit together to form the whole target figure.

Scores on both the PASAT and SR were obtained at regular intervals over the course of 30 weeks. Once subjects met individually determined criterion levels for the specific treatment tasks in each of the five levels of the attention training model (APT), remediation of visual processing skills was initiated. To control treatment order effects, the above sequence was reversed for one subject (04) who received training in visual processing prior to attention training.

Research findings for each of the four subjects are displayed using a multiple baseline across cognitive areas. Data for each subject are represented in a pair of vertically oriented graphs (see Figures 8.2 through 8.5). The ordinant on the top graph represents PASAT scores used to measure changes in attention ability. The ordinant on the bottom graph represents raw scores on the SR used to measure changes in visual processing. The abscissa on both graphs corresponds to both weeks of treatment (lower scale) and the treatment phase (upper scale). Scores to the left of the heavy striped line represent the pretreatment baseline measures.

Results indicate that in the subjects who presented with mild to moderate attention deficits (02 and 03) indicated by PASAT scores within 2 standard deviations of the mean, attention skills increased to within normal limits. The subjects with severe attention impairment (01 and 04), whose PASAT scores were greater than 3 standard deviations below the mean, achieved scores within the mildly impaired range following attention training. Improvements in attention in all cases remained above baseline levels following cessation of specific attention training for periods of as long as 8 months, which was the longest period of measurement. These results demonstrate the potential for improvement of attention deficits in brain-injured persons given specific attention training. They also support the general effectiveness of the APT training model.

Results in this study further support the use of a process-specific approach to cognitive rehabilitation. The data suggest that although there may be some impact on attention skills following any focused cognitive treatment (i.e., visual processing), more significant improvement is made following specific attention

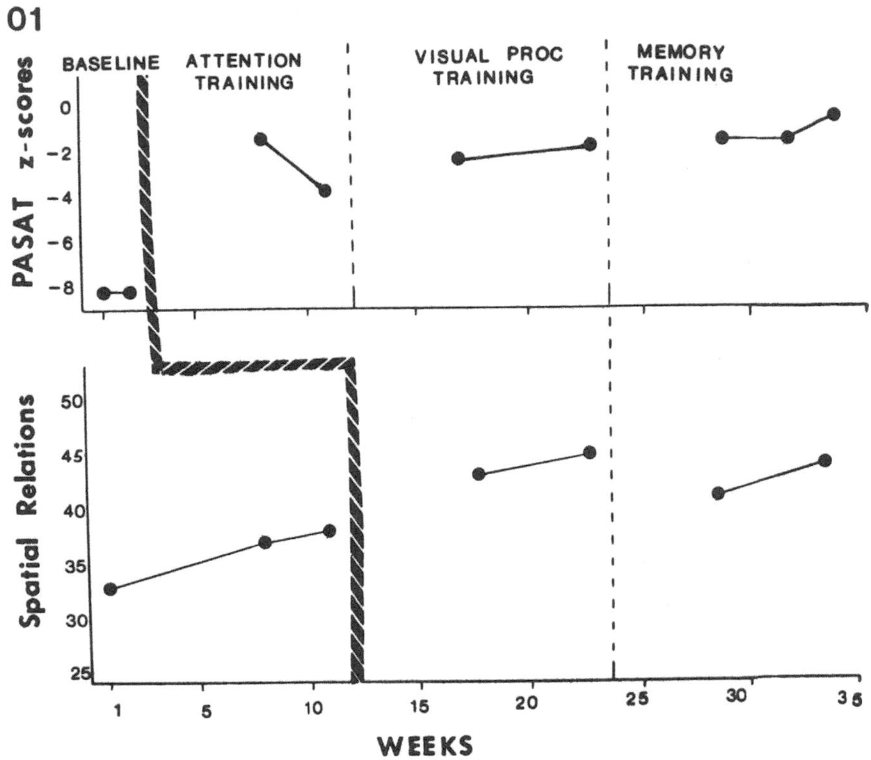

FIGURE 8.2. Results of attention training in Subject 01 using a multiple baseline across cognitive areas (attention, visual processing, and memory).

training. In Subject 04, gains in attention are evidenced during the baseline condition during which there was visual processing training but no specific remediation of attention. However, these gains appear to level off and more dramatic increases are seen following specific attention training. In Subjects 02 and 03, analogous results were found relative to visual processing ability. Visual processing-based SR scores remained stable during the period of attention training, despite improved PASAT scores, and increased only after the initiation of visual process training. This double dissociation provides powerful support for independent improvements in specific cognitive areas with process-specified training. The clinical implication is that therapy directed toward the remediation of underlying deficit processes should be encouraged.

The importance of addressing attention as a potential factor underlying memory problems has been sorely ignored. The preliminary data gathered on individuals who have completed APT strongly support the notion that increased attention ability for select patients results in improved memory. Table 8.1 provides data for five subjects who completed Attention Process Training and subsequently demonstrated significant improvement in memory ability as measured

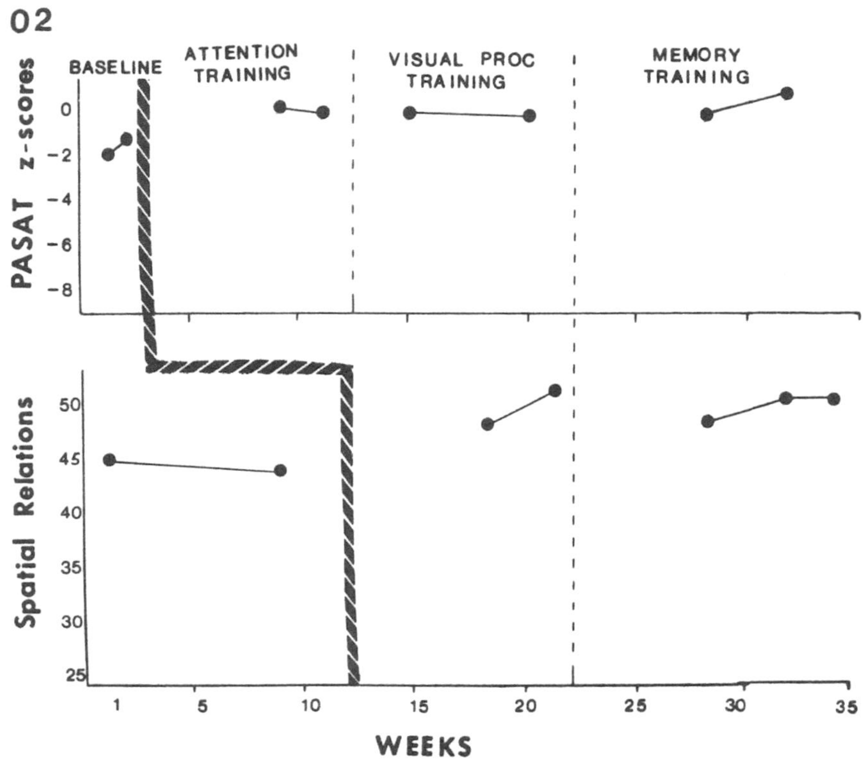

FIGURE 8.3. Results of attention training in Subject 02 using a multiple baseline across cognitive areas (attention, visual processing, and memory).

by the Five Items Subtest (Acquisition and Delayed Recall scores) from the Randt Memory Test. Each subject improved at least 1 standard deviation on both recall measurements even though they had received no formal memory training (with the exception of memory notebook training). Attention skills, as measured by Trial 1 of the PASAT, also improved at least 1 standard deviation. Each of these subjects initially presented with severe attentional deficits as indicated by results on the PASAT.

These results have important implications for the treatment of memory disorders. If some individuals exhibit memory disorders that are more fundamentally related to attention disorders, then, given that attention is amenable to treatment (supported by the aforementioned study), memory problems may be treatable. Current clinical literature has suggested that memory rehabilitation is not a viable option; however, it may be that we have not been utilizing the appropriate treatment methodology. It appears that there are some individuals who have attentionally based memory problems that may be identified through the use of neuropsychological measures sensitive to attention in conjunction with behavioral observations and interview. This may be followed by a cognitive

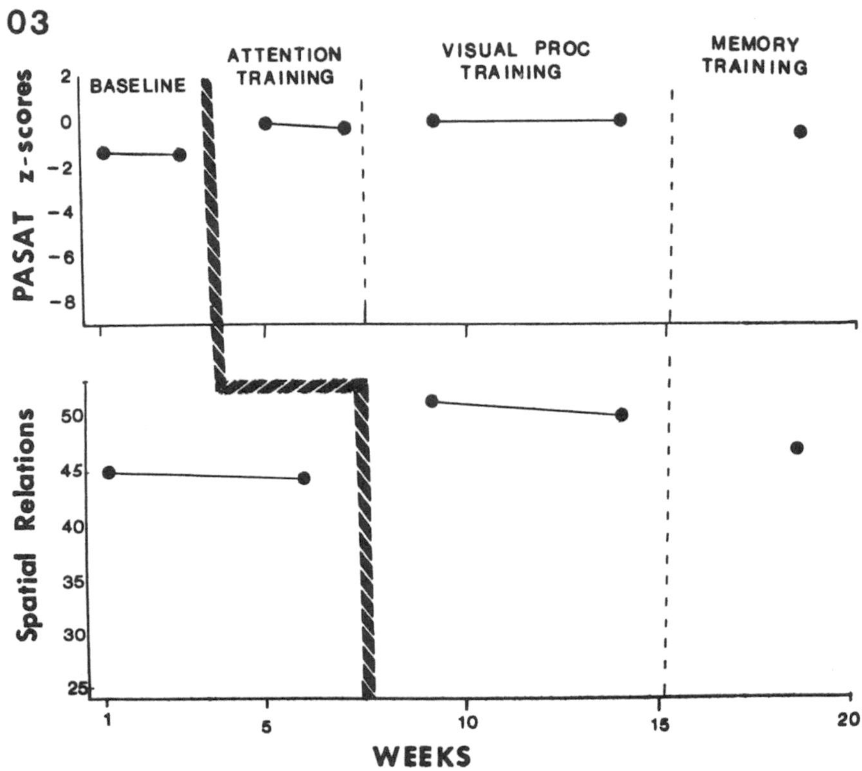

FIGURE 8.4. Results of attention training in Subject 03 using a multiple baseline across cognitive areas (attention, visual processing, and memory).

rehabilitation program specifically targeted toward remediation of attention deficits such as APT.

Prospective Memory Process Training

In the past, clinical models of memory have often been tied to the classical structural model that viewed memory as a dual time-based system (Squire, 1975; Walker, 1976). There was a tendency to look at memory solely as a dichotomous storage system of long- versus short-term memory. Again, the clinical emphasis was heavily weighted on retrospective memory with the length of delay on recall tasks operating as the variable parameter used to assess and treat memory. Subsequently, new hypotheses were formed and memory was conceptualized according to levels of processing rather than according to a store-based mechanism (Butters & Cermak, 1980; Cermak, 1982; Craik & Lockhart, 1972). The most commonly discussed processes or components of memory include: attention, encoding, storage, consolidation, and retrieval (Huppert & Piercy, 1982; McDowall, 1984; Posner, 1984; Squire & Butters, 1984). We know that to suc-

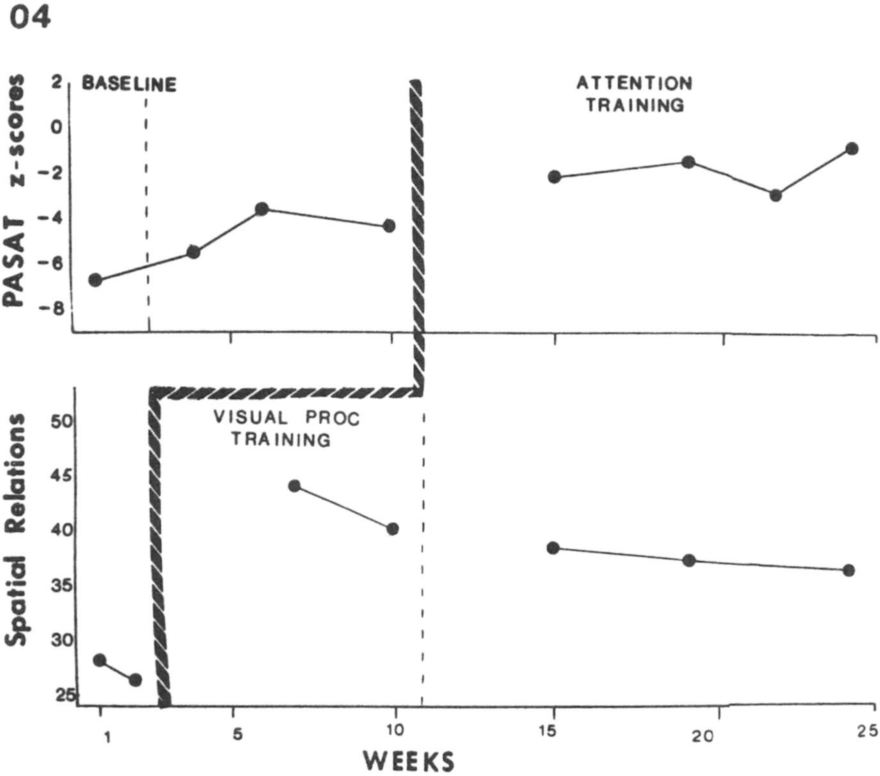

FIGURE 8.5. Results of attention training in Subject 04 using a multiple baseline (reversal) across cognitive areas (attention and visual processing).

cessfully remember an item there must be a mechanism or series of steps for adequately getting the information into the brain as well as for recalling it.

Unfortunately, treatment models have not yet begun to reflect our knowledge of levels of processing. Again, most diagnostic and treatment tools focused on the end process of retrieval. A new evaluation and treatment paradigm that does appear to address the different levels of processing is Prospective Memory Process Training (PROMPT) (Sohlberg, 1986; Sohlberg & Mateer, 1986b). For those patients who present with a primary memory deficit (as opposed to an attentionally based problem) and exhibit difficulty with the encoding and/or recall of information, PROMPT offers an effective means of management.

The overall goal of PROMPT is to systematically extend the amount of time an individual is able to remember to carry out specified tasks. The subject is provided with a target task and a target time for initiating the task. The act of continually updating memory traces, as the target time approaches, exercises the encoding mechanism as well as the retrieval mechanism (Sohlberg, 1986).

Treatment may be carried out in either a single- or dual-treatment paradigm depending upon whether or not the patient is performing a simultaneous distrac-

TABLE 8.1. Memory improvement following Attention Process Training.

Subject	Length of time postinjury at initiation of treatment (months)	PASAT z-score Trial 1		Randt Memory Test (Five items subtest-scaled score)			
				Acquisition		Delayed recall	
		Pre	Post	Pre	Post	Pre	Post
01	24	−3.6	−1.6	7	10	7	11
02	52	−2.5	.4	4	8	4	9
03	28	−3.3	−1.4	7	10	6	10
04	30	−5.0	−1.0	5	8	7	10
05	33	−1.0	.4	8	10	7	11

tor task during the waiting period. In the dual-task format, there is a heavier load on memory since the patient must hold on to the prospective memory task as well as engage in simultaneous cognitive tasks. Time is usually extended by 2-minute intervals following five consecutively correct responses.

Initial results from PROMPT are very encouraging. Three severely impaired closed head injury subjects underwent training using PROMPT (see Table 8.2). Following training, all three were able to complete prospective memory tasks 15 minutes from task presentation using the single-task paradigm (the limit of time to which treatment was extended). Simultaneous improvements were noted on the standard score (memory index) of the Randt Memory Test. Length of training for PROMPT varied from 4 to 12 weeks. Individuals were given prospective memory tasks at least 3 times a day, 4 days each week. These are very exciting results given the current literature reports of low potential for memory improvement in brain-injured subjects with postacute cognitive rehabilitation (Butters & Cermak, 1980; Godfrey & Knight, 1985; Schacter et al., 1985). Prospective memory tasks also more closely approximate naturalistic or real-life demands on memory. A more ecologically valid approach to memory rehabilitation is essential if clinicians are to impact vocational and independent living status. Initial results in this area suggest that prospective memory training could offer a new frontier in memory rehabilitation research.

Memory Notebook Training

It is important to recognize that for patients with more severe memory impairment, memory may improve given Prospective Memory Process Training, but the residual disability is often too great to allow for successful, independent functioning in the everyday world. There is a need for compensatory techniques that can minimize the barriers to independent living and vocational success that are so common with severe memory impairment.

In the past, clinicians have responded to this need for compensatory techniques in two ways. First, they have provided training in the use of internal mnemonic learning schemes that focus on the organization of target information to be

TABLE 8.2. Memory improvement following Prospective Memory Process Training (PROMPT).

Subject	Number of months postonset	Initial length of prospective memory ability (minutes)	Length of prospective memory ability following PROMPT (minutes) (15=max)	Randt Memory Test Memory Index	
				Pre-PROMPT	Post-PROMPT
01	15	.5	15	33	65
02	36	3.0	15	79	86
03	17	.5	15	40	73

recalled. Examples of such strategies include peg words, visual imagery, and associative pairing. As discussed earlier, none of the research studies examining these procedures has provided evidence that the use of these strategies generalizes to naturalistic settings (Cermak, 1975; Crovitz, 1979; Gasparrini & Satz, 1979; Gianutsos & Gianutsos, 1979).

The second compensatory technique that clinicians have utilized is written external memory aids such as memory notebooks. Often, however, these aids are given with minimal instruction or training in their use and are unsystematic in their design. A commonly reported experience of clinicians is that memory notebooks are rejected by patients or short-lived in their use outside the clinical setting. There is currently a dearth in research on the effectiveness of memory notebooks and other external compensatory aids and on appropriate methods for training their use.

In consideration of clinicians' widespread and often unsuccessful use of memory notebooks as external memory aids, as well as the need to provide more severely disordered patients with the means to compensate for residual memory difficulties, we developed theoretically based, systematic, formal training procedures to teach the use of a memory notebook (Sohlberg & Mateer, 1987). Previously, no established training protocols have been available. The theoretical foundations for these procedures come from the learning theory literature as well as from studies of preserved learning in amnesics.

Initially, memory notebooks must be designed that meet the specific needs of a patient. A first step in this process requires that the clinician perform a needs assessment to determine what an individual will require in his or her particular living and/or work setting. Based on the information gleaned from a needs assessment, different sections in the notebook are devoted to meeting different needs (see Table 8.3). For example, some patients may require an orientation section with pertinent autobiographical information, while others may not have difficulty with this type of information. Almost every notebook will contain a Calendar Section to allow recording of future dates and appointments, an Events Diary Section to log hourly events that are occurring, and a Things-To-Do Section to provide a place to record future intended actions.

Successful compliance for spontaneous and functional use of a memory notebook is predicated upon the implementation of appropriate, systematic training

TABLE 8.3. List of possible notebook sections.

Orientation:	Narrative autobiographical information concerning personal data and/or information surrounding the brain injury
Memory Log:	Contains forms for charting hourly information about what patient has done; diary of daily information
Calendar:	Calendars with dates and times that would allow a patient to schedule appointments and dates
Things to Do:	Contains forms for recording errands and intended future actions; includes place to mark due date and completion date
Transportation:	Contains maps and/or bus information to frequented places such as work, schools, store, bank, etc.
Feelings Log:	Contains forms to chart feelings relative to specific incidences or times
Names:	Contains forms to record names and identifying information of new people
Today at Work:	Various forms have been adapted for specific vocation and settings that allow individuals to record the necessary information to perform their job duties

procedures. Researchers in learning theory (Liberty, Haring, & White, 1980; White, 1984; White and Haring, 1980) identify three phases of learning critical for mastering new skills that may be applied to memory notebook training. These phases include Acquisition, Application, and Adaptation. Efficiency Building is an essential learning parameter that must also be incorporated within each of these learning phases. The authors note that each phase imposes somewhat different demands upon a learner and requires adjustment in instructional strategies if continued progress toward mastery is to be realized. Examination of learning phases and the corresponding instructional methodologies necessary for complete mastery of the new skill yields exciting possibilities relative to training of brain-injured adults to successfully manage a memory notebook. Teaching a new skill to an individual with compromised new learning ability requires careful planning of instruction. The outcome of instruction needs to be skill acquisition with enough fluency or efficiency to allow appropriate skill application in different environments (i.e., spontaneous independent use of the memory notebook across settings). Breaking up instruction into the learning phases of Acquisition, Application and Adapatation has proven successful in training memory-disordered adults to utilize memory notebook systems.

Acquisition refers to that stage of learning whereby the clinician is trying to build a behavior, the patient is learning *how* to perform a certain skill. In the case of memory notebook use, the patient needs to become familiar with the purpose and use of each different section in the notebook. Acquisition is the initial didactic learning stage in which the patient acquires basic competence with notebook use. This familiarization training is achieved through repetitive administration of questions regarding notebook contents and use specific to that patient's individual notebook.

The second stage of learning, Application, refers to learning *when* and *where* to utilize a new skill. It is not enough to simply know *how* to perform a task; in order to be successful, a person must be able to apply that skill to the appropriate situation. The use of role play provides an excellent training format to facilitate application of appropriate notebook use. The clinician can administer role play events either in person or simulate phone situations by telephoning the patient from a nearby telephone. The patient is given feedback regarding performance, and these variables are then scored on a data collection chart.

The third phase of learning is termed Adaptation. Adaptation corresponds to that learning stage wherein an individual demonstrates the ability to adapt and modify skill use to accommodate novel situations. Because it is not possible to role play every situation in which a patient might encounter a need to utilize the memory notebook system, it is important that the Adaptation phase of learning be adequately addressed. This is best accomplished via training in naturalistic settings. The clinician accompanies the patient out in the community or in naturalistic settings within the medical facility (e.g., gift shop or cafeteria) and scores performance on notebook use.

The above three training phases constitute a sequence of instruction that would establish basic skills for memory notebook use. Each level of instruction must also incorporate Efficiency Building. Efficiency Building is the instructional process that ensures that a patient will actually use this skill.

The establishment of efficiency aims or performance criteria that will allow a patient to maintain and use this skill must be established for each instructional phase in order for the clinician to determine when the patient can move on to the next level (see Table 8.4). For the purposes of memory notebook use, efficiency aims consist of accuracy and consistency measures that result in skill maintenance and use. The values were determined by examination of the data from 12 individuals who successfully learned to learn the memory notebook system.

The adaptation of a theoretical learning model provides a conceptual basis for the formalized instructional procedures used to train memory notebook use. Examination of preserved learning in amnesics further provides a methodology for how individuals with severe impairments can best learn. Areas of preserved learning and memory in severely amnesic patients may include perceptual motor skills (Cohen, 1984; Craik & Lockhart, 1972), memory for overlearned information (Cohen, 1984), and responsivity to repetition priming effects (Cohen, 1984; Warrington, 1982). A type of preserved learning that has been much discussed is procedural memory (Cohen & Squire, 1980; Fisk & Schrieder, 1984). Procedural memory refers to the type of "noncognitive learning" wherein an individual can learn an automatic behavioral sequence. This ability to learn procedures or motor sequences, even in the absence of conscious awareness of learning, is frequently spared in even severely amnestic patients. The training procedures outlined in this section depend heavily upon intact procedural memory. Establishment of instructional sequences including the repetitive administration of questions and answers regarding notebook use and contents (Acquisition phase), a repetitive role play giving practice with the mechanics of notebook use (Application), and community training allowing further notebook practice (Adaptation) all utilized the spared procedural memory that has been documented in this population.

TABLE 8.4. Stages of training-memory book use.

Training phase	Description
Acquisition	Learn names, purpose, and use of each notebook section via question/answer format
Efficiency goal	100% accuracy on questions for 5 consecutive days
Application	Learn appropriate methods of recording in notebook via role-play situations
Efficiency goal	100% accuracy of response to three role-play situations with no cueing on 2 consecutive days
Adaptation	Demonstrate appropriate notebook use in naturalistic settings via community training
Efficiency goal	Receive a score of 4 for two situations on 2 consecutive days

We have used these techniques to teach a compensatory memory system to three globally amnestic patients and many other patients with severely impaired memory function. All three amnestic patients, following a 6- to 8-month daily outpatient program, are using the compensatory systems to support independent living and all are gainfully employed; yet none of the three improved substantially on formal measures of recall performance. There have been other reported attempts to utilize aspects of preserved memory to teach specific knowledge or skills used in everyday life. Glisky & Schacter (1986) have reported success in using a visual priming task (method of vanishing cues) to teach a body of specific knowledge about computer use to severely amnesic patients, and Schacter (1986) has presented a single case for whom these skills were extended to a specific employment situation.

An important feature of the memory notebook system herein described is that a heavy emphasis is placed on the ability to record and follow up on intended future actions. As discussed, the ability to remember to carry out actions in the future, to remember to remember, has been termed *prospective memory.* In the aforementioned study involving a large survey of control and brain-injured individuals (Mateer et al., 1987), it was this kind of memory more than recall of information per se, that was most frequently experienced as problematic by both groups of subjects. Yet prospective memory is rarely ever addressed in traditional approaches to memory assessment or remediation. The ability to carry out needed or intended activity can make the crucial difference in allowing independent living or vocation.

Conclusions

In the past, researchers and clinicians have been too narrow in their view of memory. This has placed unfortunate limitations on the rehabilitation of memory disorders in patients with diffuse brain damage. This has necessitated a paradigm shift in memory rehabilitation away from a unitary focus on retrospective memory or recall toward a more comprehensive view of memory. Consideration of prospective memory, or the ability to remember future intentions, has allowed the development of memory training techniques as PROMPT, which result in enhanced memory functions in individuals with primary memory deficits. Recognition of prospective memory has further allowed clinicians to focus on functional aspects of memory. Devices such as memory notebooks, which provide a means for carrying out prospective tasks, can permit memory-disordered patients to live independently and pursue gainful employment. Similarly, the recognition of attention as an important aspect of memory has allowed for the development of training procedures (APT) that can restore memory functions in patients with attentionally based memory problems.

A comprehensive evaluation of memory, including examination of attentional processing and prospective memory ability, allows clinicians to match the appropriate treatment procedures with the existing disorder. This chapter argues for a more ecologically valid view of memory function and outlines a three-pronged approach to memory rehabilitation that includes Attention Process Training (APT), Prospective Memory Process Training (PROMPT), and Memory Notebook Training. In persons who exhibit memory impairment as a result of a primary deficit in attention, the first training program would be most appropriate. For persons with severe, more primary memory involvement, a combination of the latter two approaches would be advisable. There may be individuals who benefit from all three approaches. Fundamental consideration must be given to the type of memory disorders with which a patient presents. Today's diagnostic and treatment tools must continue to be expanded to meet this essential paradigm shift in memory rehabilitation, which offers optimistic, yet realistic, hope to persons experiencing memory impairment as the result of diffuse brain damage.

Acknowledgments. We wish to thank Good Samaritan Hospital for its support of clinical research within its brain injury rehabilitation programs and to express our appreciation to the memory-impaired patients from whom we have learned so much about the nature of memory disorders.

References

Baddeley, A.D. (1981). The concept of working memory: A view of its current state and probable future development. *Cognition, 10,* 17–23.

Baddeley, A.D. (1982). Amnesia: Minimal model and an interpretation. In L.S. Cermak (Ed.), *Human memory and amnesia* (pp. 305–330). Hillsdale, NJ: Erlbaum.

Baddeley, A.D., & Hitch, G.J. (1974). Working memory. In G. Bower (Ed.), *Recent Advances in Learning and Motivation* (Vol. 8, pp. 47–90). New York: Academic Press.

Baddeley, A.D., & Wilkins, A. (1984). Taking memory out of the laboratory. In J.S. Harris & P.E. Morris (Eds.), *Everyday memory actions and absent-mindedness.* New York: Academic Press.

Broadbent, D.E. (1958). *Perception and communication.* New York: Pergamon Press.
Broadbent, D.E., Cooper, P.F., Fitzgerald, P., & Parkes, K.R. (1982). The Cognitive Failure Questionnaire (C.F.Q.) and its correlates. *British Journal of Clinical Psychology, 2,* 1–16.
Bronfenbrenner, V. (1979). *The ecology of human development: Experiments by nature and design.* Cambridge, MA: Harvard University Press.
Brooks, N. (1983). Disorders of memory. In M. Rosenthal, E.R. Griffith, M.R. Bond & J.D. Miller (Eds.), *Rehabilitation of the head injured adult* (pp. 185–196). Philadelphia: F.A. Davis.
Buschke, H., & Fuld, P.A. (1974). Evaluations storage, retention, and retrieval in disordered memory and learning. *Neurology, 11,* 1019–1025.
Butters, N., & Cermak, L.S. (1980). *Alcoholic Korsakoff's Syndrome.* New York: Academic Press.
Cermak, L.S. (1975). Imagery as an aid to retrieval for Korsakoff patients. *Cortex, 11,* 163–169.
Cermak, L.S. (Ed.), (1982). *Human memory and amnesia.* Hillsdale, NJ: Erlbaum.
Cohen, N. (1984). Preserved learning capacity in amnesia: Evidence for multiple memory systems. In L. Squire & N. Butters (Eds.), *Neuropsychology of memory.* (pp. 83–103). New York: Guilford Press.
Cohen, N., & Squire, L. (1980). Preserved learning and retention of pattern-analyzing skills in amnesia: Dissociation of knowing how and of knowing that. *Science, 210,* 201–210.
Cole, M., Hood, L., & McDermott, R. (1978). *Ecological niche picking: Ecological invalidity as an axiom of experimental cognitive psychology.* New York University of California, San Diego, and The Rockefeller University.
Craik, F., & Lockhart, R. (1972). Levels of processing: A framework for memory research. *Journal of Verbal Learning and Verbal Behavior, 11,* 671–684.
Crovitz, H.F. (1979). Memory retraining in brain-damaged patients: The airplane list. *Cortex, 15,* 131–134.
Fisk, A., & Shreider, L. (1984). Memory as a function of attention level of processing and automatization. *Journal of Experimental Psychology: Learning, Memory and Cognition, 10,* 181–197.
Gasparrini, B., & Satz, P. (1979). A treatment for memory problems in left hemisphere CVA patients. *Journal of Clinical Neuropsychology, 91,* 66–73.
Gianutsos, R. (1981). Training the short- and long-term verbal recall of a postencephalitic amnesic. *Journal of Clinical Neuropsychology, 3,* 143–153.
Gianutsos, R., & Gianutsos, J. (1979). Rehabilitating the verbal recall of brain-injured patients by mnemonic training: An experimental demonstration using single-case methodology. *Journal of Clinical Neuropsychology, 2,* 117–135.
Glisky, E.L., & Schacter, D.L. (1986). Remediation of organic memory disorders: Current status and future prospects. *Journal of Head Trauma Rehabilitation, 1,* 54–63.
Godfrey, H., & Knight, R. (1985). Cognitive rehabilitation of memory functioning in amnesiac alcoholics. *Journal of Consulting and Clinical Psychology, 43,* 555–557.
Gronwall, D. (1977). Paced auditory serial addition task: A measure of recovery from concussion. *Perceptual and Motor Skills, 44,* 367–373.
Harris, J.E., & Wilkins, A.J. (1984). Remembering to do things: A forgotten topic. In J.E. Harris & P.E. Morris (Eds.), *Everyday memory actions and absent-mindedness.* New York: Academic Press.

Herrmann, D.J. (1984). Questionnaires about memory. In J.E. Harris & P.E. Morris (Eds.), *Everyday memory actions and absent-mindedness* (pp. 133–151). New York: Academic Press.

Herrmann, D.J., & Neisser, V. (1978). An inventory of everyday memory experiences. In M.M. Gruneberg, P.E. Morris, & R. Sykes (Eds.), *Practical aspects of memory.* New York: Academic Press.

Hersen, M., & Barlow, D. (1976). *Since case experimental designs: Strategies for studying behavior change.* New York: Pergamon Press.

Huppert, F., & Piercy, M. (1979). Normal and abnormal forgetting in organic amnesia: Effect of lows of lesion. *Cortex, 18,* 358–390.

Huppert, F., & Piercy M. (1982). In search of the functional lows of amnesic syndromes. In L. Cermak (Ed.), *Human memory and amnesia.* Hillsdale, NJ: Erlbaum.

Johnston, W., & Wilson, J. (1980). Perceptual processing of nontargets in an attention task. *Memory and Cognition, 8,* 372–377.

Kreutzer, M., Leonard, C., & Falvell, J. (1975). An interview study of children's knowledge about memory. *Monographs of the Society for Research in Child Development, 40* (1 Serial No. 159).

Levy, R., & Loftus, G. (1984). Compliance and memory. In J.E. Harris & P.E. Morris (Eds.), *Everyday memory actions and absent-mindedness.* New York: Academic Press.

Liberty, K., Haring, N., & White, O. (1980). Rules for data-based strategy decisions in instructional programs: Current research and instructional implications. In W. Sailor, B. Wilcox, & L. Brown (Eds.), *Methods of instruction for severely handicapped students.* Baltimore: Brookes.

Martin, M. (1983). Cognitive failure: Every day and laboratory performance. *Bulletin of the Psychonomic Society. 21,* 79–100.

Mateer, C., & Sohlberg, M.M. (1986). *Efficacy of attention and prospective memory training.* Unpublished paper presented at the University of Victoria Neuropsychology Workshop, Victoria, B.C.

Mateer, C., Sohlberg, M.M., & Crineon, J. (1987). Perceptions of memory function in individuals with closed head injury. *Journal of Head Trauma Rehabilitation, 2,* 74–84.

McDowall, J. (1984). Processing capacity and recall in amnesics and control subjects. In L. Squire & N. Butters (Eds.), *Neuropsychology of memory.* (pp. 63–66). New York: Guilford Press.

Meacham, J., & Dumitru, J. (1976). Prospective remembering and external retrieval cases. *J.S.A.S. Catalog of Selected Documents in Psychology, 5,* 65 (Ms No. 1284).

Meacham, J.A., & Leiman, B. (1982). Remembering to perform future actions. In V. Neisser (Ed.), *Memory observed, remembering in national contexts* (pp. 327–336). San Francisco: W.H. Freeman.

Neisser, V. (1982). Memory: What are the important questions? In V. Neisser (Ed.), *Memory observed* (pp. 3–19). San Francisco: W.H. Freeman.

Posner, M. (1984). Selective attention and storage of information. In J. Lynch, J. McGaugh, & N. Weinberger (Eds.), *Neurobiology of learning and memory* (pp. 89–104) New York: Guilford Press.

Prigatano, G., Fordyce, D., Zeiner, H., Roueche, J., Pepping, M., & Wood, B. (1984). Neuropsychological rehabilitation after closed head injury in young adults. *Journal of Neurology, Neurosurgery, and Neuropsychiatry, 47,* 505–513.

Randt, C.T., Brown, E.R., & Osborne, D.J., Jr. (1980). *A memory test for longitudinal measurement of mild to moderate deficits (Rev.).* Unpublished manuscript, Department of Neurology, New York University Medical Center.

Rey, A. (1964). *L'examen clinique en psychologie.* Paris: Presses Universitaires de France.
Rogoff, B., & Lobe, J. (1984). *Everyday cognition: Its development in social context.*
Schacter, D. (1986). *Preserved learning in memory disordered patients: Integrating theory and practice.* Presented at the National Head Injury Foundation Fifth Annual National Symposium, Chicago.
Schacter, D., Rich, S., & Stampp, A. (1985). Remediation of memory disorders: Experimental evaluation of the spaced-retrieval technique. *Journal of Clinical and Experimental Neuropsychology, 7,* 79–96.
Sohlberg, M.M. (1985). *Remediation of attention disorders.* Unpublished paper presented at Models and Techniques in Cognitive Rehabilitation Symposium, Indianapolis, IN.
Sohlberg, M.M. (1986). *Rehabilitation of memory disorders.* Unpublished paper presented at the Western Regional Conference of the American Speech Language and Hearing Association, Seattle, WA.
Sohlberg, M.M., & Mateer, C. (1986a). *Attention Process Training (APT).* Puyallup, WA: Association for Neuropsychological Research and Development.
Sohlberg, M.M., & Mateer, C. (1986b). *Prospective Memory Process Training (PROMPT).* Puyallup, WA: Association for Neuropsychological Research and Development.
Sohlberg, M.M., & Mateer, C. (1987). Effectiveness of an attention training program. *Journal of Clinical and Experimental Neuropsychology, 9,* 117–130.
Sohlberg, M.M., & Mateer, C. Effective training of memory notebook use in brain injured patients. Manuscript submitted for publication.
Squire, L. (1975). Short-term memory as a biological entity. In D. Deutch & J.A. Deutch (Eds.), *Short-term memory.* New York: Academic Press. pp. 1–40.
Squire, L., & Butters, N. (Ed.). (1984). *Neuropsychology of memory.* Hillsdale, NJ: Erlbaum.
Squire, L., & Cohen, N. (1982). Remote memory, retrograde amnesia, and the neuropsychology of memory. In L. Cermak (Ed.), *Human memory and amnesia.* Hillsdale, NJ: Erlbaum.
Sunderland, A., Harris, J.E., & Baddeley, A. (1983). Do laboratory tests predict everyday memory? A neuropsychological study. *Journal of Verbal Learning and Verbal Behaviors, 22,* 341–357.
Sunderland, A., Harris, J.E., & Baddeley, A.D. (1984). Assessing everyday memory after severe head injury. In J.E. Harris & P.E. Morris (Eds.), *Everyday memory actions and absent-mindedness.* New York: Academic Press.
Walker, K. (1976). Memory. In H. Kenneth Walker, W. Dallas Hall, J. Willis Hurst (Eds.) *Clinical methods: The history of the physical and laboratory examination* (pp 693–698). Boston: Butterworth.
Warrington, E. (1982). The double dissociation of short-and long-term memory deficits. In L. Cermak (Ed.), *Human memory and amnesia.* Hillsdale, NJ: Erlbaum.
Wechsler, D. (1945). A standardized memory scale for clinical use. *Journal of Psychology, 19,* 87–95.
Weingartner, H., & Parker, E. (1984). *Memory consolidation.* Hillsdale, NJ: Erlbaum.
White, O. (1984). Performance based decisions: When and what to change. In R. West & K. Young (Eds.), *Precision teaching: Instructional decision making, curriculum, and management and research.* Provo, UT: Utah State University, Department of Special Education.
White, O., & Haring, N. (1980). *Exceptional teaching* (2nd ed.). Columbus, OH: Merrill.

Wilkins, A., & Baddeley, A. (1978). Remembering to recall in everyday life: An approach to absent-mindedness. In M. Gruneberg, P. Morris, & R. Sykes (Eds.), *Practical aspects of memory.* New York: Academic Press.

Wilson, B. (1981). Teaching a patient to remember people's names after removal of a left temporal tumor. *Behavioral Psychotherapy, 9,* 338–344.

Wilson, B. (1982). Success and failure in memory training following a cerebral vascular accident. *Cortex,18,* 581–594.

Woodcock, R., & Johnson, B. (1977). *Woodcock-Johnson Psychioeducational Battery.* Boston: Teaching Resources Corp.

9
Closed Head Trauma: Somatic, Ophthalmic, and Cognitive Impairments in Nonhospitalized Patients

RICHARD E. CYTOWIC, DAVID A. STUMP, and DAVID C. LARNED

According to the National Head Injury Foundation (1986), 700,000 Americans sustain closed head injury annually from a variety of circumstances, including automobile accidents, work-related injuries, and athletic and domestic trauma. That 50,000 such persons are permanently impaired may not be widely appreciated, but even more interesting is the gray zone – a tremendously variable time during which patients suffer a range of neurobehavioral symptoms that keep them from work or usual activities and severely hamper interpersonal relationships and family life. The term usually applied is *postconcussion syndrome.*

Compared to penetrating missile wounds and open head injury, closed head trauma has excited little interest, except to fuel arguments about its validity as an organic brain disease, particularly when litigation is involved (Kelly, 1981; Kelly & Smith, 1981). This point of view may satisfy physicians whose wits are challenged by lack of gross abnormality on neurological examination and conventional tests. Few descriptive studies, and hardly any regarding treatment, exist for this troublesome population who are frequently told that nothing is wrong with them. Whatever its basis, the situation begs explanation and some treatment to hasten a return to functional status for so many unproductive, miserable patients.

Only recently has the focus shifted away from catastrophic head injury to objective assessment of sequelae of closed head trauma (Levin, Benton, & Grossman, 1982; Stuss et al., 1985). But even here, the study victims have some period of coma or have at least been hospitalized for up to 48 hours. *They are also referents to tertiary academic centers.* While validated statistics are lacking, the National Head Injury Foundation estimates that 80% of closed head trauma patients are initially seen by primary-care physicians; we suspect that many are never hospitalized but discharged from emergency facilities after observation or, since many are ambulatory, escape transport to the emergency room altogether and see a private physician at their own initiative. The combined morbidity and societal loss may assume an enormity hitherto unrecognized.

Capitol Neurology and Associated Specialties has a strong interest in head injuries that are not catastrophic. That is, our interest is in *shaking injuries of the brain.* Like many who treat head-injured patients, the physicians of Capitol

Neurology spend much time educating others—including physicians, families, attorneys, insurance companies, and juries—that these patients, who do not have glaring impairments, *do* have real brain injuries. Frequent is the disbelief of others who insist on abnormal x-rays and prolonged coma before accepting the fact that a brain injury has occurred. This disbelief is nearly axiomatic for patients who were not hospitalized immediately following their injury.

Fundamental facts are easily forgotten and one then loses the forest for a tree. Skull and brain tissues have different physical properties and are injured by quite different mechanical forces. No advanced training is required to notice fractures or focal hemorrhages, whereas the behavioral derangements that stem from diffuse axonal injury are beyond the recognition of most neurologists let alone the average practitioner. Once found, focal injuries tend to hold an interest out of all proportion to their significance. Those who treat head trauma need to separate injuries of the container from those of the contents, and focal lesions, which result from focal forces, from diffuse injury, which results from shearing forces applied to the inhomogenous nervous tissue. Acceleration—deceleration, whiplash, and commotio cerebrii are all types of shaking injuries of the brain. Unfortunately, the biomechanical factors that cause such injury are known to the majority of automotive engineers but to only a fraction of physicians.

We wish to underscore that the investigations at Capitol Neurology emphasize clinical decisions and finding answers to practical problems. Our waiting rooms are full of patients clamoring for help. Attorneys and insurers (who are assuming a larger role in the patient's true outcome) pose questions to which the answer is all too often unknown or uncertain. Many issues have just not received the attention of a proper study. We hope our work marks a little progress here. Underlying questions in this chapter are "Who do you need to work up among outpatients?" and "Who will have an unsatisfactory outcome?" This is an underserved population who have considerable morbidity and a rather large societal loss in economic terms. This is particularly true in the large managerial population of Washington, DC. We attempt here to construct a model that could be useful at initial patient encounters. To this end, a multivariate statistical analysis, including a maximum R-squared stepwise regression, is performed to detect the best model of variables discriminating between outcome groups. This multivariate analysis of regression technique supplements concepts of statistical significance with additional information concerning the efficiency of a particular model (namely, the amount of variance it can account for) in discriminating the groups. The task is to trim away useless predictor information—insignificant sources of variance—and arrive at the simplest representation of the data without reducing discriminatory accuracy. According to Ward and Jennings (1973), if a simple model and a less simple one can estimate sample means equally well, then the estimates of the simpler model will be closer to the parameter means than those produced by the less simple one.

For reasons mentioned above, the kind of patient described here is usually not seen at academic tertiary centers. Conversely, it is rare for the private sector to examine these patients in the detail that we do. Lastly, the kind of "clinical research" that comes out of tertiary centers may have little actual utility for the majority of clinicians in primary care. Practitioners in the field do not always have access to the kind of instrumentation or laboratory analysis on which the academic data are based. Emphasizing the practicality of clinical decision making, the variance separating out groups by outcome can be determined by clinical methods in conjunction with low-cost tests that are commonly available.

Method

The study group was 205 consecutive patients with closed head injuries. All patients were evaluated and treated by a single physician (REC) in an outpatient setting at Capitol Neurology according to current standards of practice. All tests and subsequent referrals were ordered by this physician.

Demographic data on age, sex, education, occupation, and handedness were obtained on every patient. Information regarding type of accident (e.g., work-related, automobile), loss of consciousness, and whether litigation was involved was also ascertained. Twenty-seven patients were lost to follow-up, leaving $N = 178$. Table 9.1 summarizes pertinent demographics of the whole study population.

Numerous symptoms were assessed in all 205 patients by both a self-administered checklist and structured interview by the physician. This checklist is reproduced in Appendix 9.A. (The version currently in use was revised to include a quantitative scale that rates target symptoms in severity from 1 to 10. Use of this self-rating sheet on subsequent visits permits objective evaluation of the patient's perception of improvement of target symptoms.) The frequency of these somatic, ophthalmic, and neurobehavioral symptoms for the study population as a whole is listed in Table 9.2. The frequency of abnormal results on further evaluation is shown in Table 9.3.

Explication of Symptoms and Clinical Evaluation

While the meaning of some symptoms, such as headache, may seem straightforward, we believe that an explication of symptom categories and target symptoms is in order to reduce ambiguity.

Headache

Our only attempt to differentiate headache types was to assign vascular headache to its own category. *Vascular headache* refers to an episodic, throbbing hemicrania, at times associated with nausea, visual symptoms, or Horner's syndrome. These migraine headaches have been described after mild head injury (Weiss, Stern, & Goldberg, 1984), but no convincing explanation for why trauma should induce migraine exists. These headaches respond well to conventional anti-migraine treatment. Unfortunately, careful history and examination of patients subsequently showed us that headaches are quite heterogenous in head injury patients. We now feel that the majority of posttraumatic headaches are due to

TABLE 9.1. Demographics of population by outcome groups.

Outcome	Age	Male/Female	Education	Black/White
Normal (n=91)	31.0 ± 9.3	31:60	12.4	62:29
Symptomatic (n=50)	35.1 ± 14.5	16:34	12.8	26:24
Impaired (n=37)	35.5 ± 11.9	18:19	12.8	19:18
Total	33.1 ± 11.7	65:113	12.6	107:71

Note. $N = 178$.

peripheral injuries, such as blunt trauma to the occipital nerves (left more common than right because of shoulder restraint design), cervical myodystonia involving the small muscles of the suboccipital triangle, and mechanical strain of the cervical spine including autonomic dysfunction. These conditions are discussed further below in the section on neck injury.

Memory Disturbance and Confusion

Not all subjective complaints that "I can't remember" are borne out by objective testing. Since patients lack the vocabulary for derivative aspects of cognition,

TABLE 9.2. Target symptoms.

Symptom	*N*	%
Headache	154	87
Vascular headache	13	7
Memory/confusion	104	58
Dizziness/vertigo/lightheadedness	89	50
Neck pain	80	45
Irritability/sonophobia	67	38
Sleep disturbance not due to pain	52	29
Depression/neurasthenia	49	28
Incoordination	37	21
Nausea/vomiting	36	21
Hearing/tinnitus	26	15
Personality change	14	8
Seizure	6	3
Blurry vision	73	41
Photophobia	47	26
Spots/flashes	38	21
Binocular fusion failure	31	17
Evidence of blunt trauma	51	27
Eye movement disorder	33	19
Smell abnormality	17	10

Note. $N = 178$.

TABLE 9.3. Frequency of abnormal results—whole group.

	No. abnormal/No. performed[a]	%
Neuropsychological assessment	48/64	75
Goldmann Visual Perimetry	76/104	73
Referred for ophthalmic exam	88/178	49
Laser surgery for retinal tears	13/88	15
Beck Depression Scale >20	18/119	15
EEG	8/43	6
CT scan	36/175	21
Posttraumatic stress syndrome	19	11

[a] Denominator indicates number of patients who had the test.

they may convey visuoconstructive and navigational difficulties, linguistic deficits, or complex perceptual abnormalities by simply saying that "I can't think" or "My memory is no good." Inclusion in this category is based on the *patient's perception* of impaired memory performance.

Dizziness

Dizziness includes true vertigo as well as lightheadedness or giddiness without a subjective sense of movement.

Neck Pain

The self-complaint of neck pain required the physical presence of myodystonia on examination (Ommaya, Hirsch, & Martinex, 1966; Travell, 1967, 1976; Travell & Simmons, 1983) to be included in this category. That is, a palpable increase in muscular tone in the posterior cervical muscles or suboccipital triangles. Palpation in these regions frequently discloses exquisitely painful trigger points. The most common locations are at Erb's point, mid trapezius, suboccipital triangles, transverse processes of C4, and the suprascapular region.

Sleep Disturbance

Sleep disturbance includes difficulty with sleep onset, fragmentation, and early morning awakening; we excluded all instances in which *pain* prevented onset or was the cause of nocturnal awakening.

We were impressed at how many of our patients complained of disturbed sleep *that was not due to pain.* Sleep onset appeared to be normal, but the sleep period became fragmented with frequent awakenings and lack of dreaming. This lack of dreaming resolved abruptly after many weeks, when the patient would report vivid dreams, in color, that were sometimes frightening. Residue from the actual trauma did not seem to be prominent in this rebound dreaming.

Ron, Algom, Hary, and Cohen (1980) demonstrated abnormal sleep patterns 6 months after concussion. Changes in REM sleep correlated with cognitive impairment. Prigatano, Stahl, Orr, and Zeiner (1982) described 10 patients, all comatose less than 24 hours, who complained of disturbed dreaming. All showed decreased Stage I sleep and an increased number of awakenings over controls. The percentage of REM was not correlated with complaints of decreased or absent dreaming or with memory impairment as measured by the Wechsler Memory Scale.

Depression/Neurasthenia

Depression/neurasthenia describes patients who are both anxious and depressed, complain of lassitude, and are disinclined to socialize with family or friends but are clearly not suffering from posttraumatic stress syndrome (American Psychiatric Association, 1980, p. 309), in whom rumination and flashbacks of the trauma are common, particularly when trying to fall asleep. Although they appear depressed clinically, they did not consistently have Beck Scale elevations above 20. This clinical impression of an agitated depression, congruent with their subjective complaints, was a major factor in prescribing Alprazolam, a drug that was marketed during this study. This use of this new drug in a subset of the study group is discussed in detail below.

Irritability/Sonophobia

These patients are most distinct. They prefer dark, quiet isolation as if overloaded by sensory stimuli. They startle at environmental sounds, such as the telephone, closing doors, clanking dishes, or shouting children, complain that the radio or television is too loud, frequently find more than one person talking at a time unpleasant and sometimes confusing, are astonished at the uncharacteristic ease and lability of their temper, and abhor sexual relations. Quite a few wore sunglasses. The sonophobia was unassuaged by most medications; relief was sometimes obtained with industrial earplugs (Cabot Corporation, Ear Division, 7911 Zionsville Road, Indianapolis, IN 46268).

Personality Change

Personality change or bizarre behavior was more often than not reported by others, and thus ascertainment may be incomplete.

Incoordination

Incoordination was historical. Patients volunteered that their sense of balance was impaired or else history was obtained that they stumbled, bumped into furniture or the walls, or had accidents reaching for or manipulating objects, usually in the kitchen or bathroom.

Seizure

Witnessed convulsions or history compatible with postictal symptoms were included. Some spells of sudden behavioral change or perceptual distortion were diagnosed as compatible with temporal lobe seizures and were included in this category if the EEG was abnormal. Such patients were placed on Carbamazepine.

Ophthalmic Symptoms

Vision is a psychophysical phenomenon that involves more than tracts from the retina and visual cortex, and patients with closed head trauma complain of a range of subjective visual symptoms, such as diplopia, blurring, "running together" of images when reading or working at video display screens, flashing photisms and obscurations of vision, distortion of parallax or apparent bending of straight lines, and photophobia. There are limitations to organic assessment, however, and a "standard" eye exam will disclose 20/20 acuity and normal motor activity in most patients with closed head trauma who perceive faulty vision. This paradox is explored further below.

The category of *spots/flashes* combines what is ordinarily considered floaters with symptoms of retinal traction, such as flashing lights, scintillating spots (central darkness, bright or colored), shadows or apparent bending of straight lines ("heat waves"). *Failure of binocular fusion* contains diplopia as well as "running together" of words or images while reading or watching television. Presumably, repetitive saccades, which require foveal fixation during these activities, strain the fusion mechanism more than other viewing activities. Visual fixation is foveal, fusion is cortical. The fusion mechanism is complex, sensorimotor, and believed to be derived from retinal-cortical point-to-point correspondence. Items in these categories are symptoms extracted during the history; objective eye movement abnormalities detected during the physical examination are described under "Eye Movement Disorders."

Floating spots and flashing lights ordinarily indicate disorders of the vitreous, usually with traction on the retina. These entopic photopsias (light flashes originating within the eye) are usually arch-shaped, achromatic, and not complex in form.

Evidence of Blunt Trauma

This includes obvious scars, hematomas, and abrasions. A specific entity here is traumatic neuritis of the supraorbital, infraorbital, and greater occipital nerves, diagnosed by exquisite sensitivity to palpation compared to the unaffected side. Normal subjects can withstand considerable manual pressure on these nerves where they emerge from the skull.

Eye Movement Disorders

While we did see a few gaze palsies (lateral rectus or superior oblique from an orbital blowout fracture), the most common finding was saccadic pursuit. That is, the replacement of the normal, smooth, low-velocity eye movements on following a target by a series of small amplitude jerky pursuit movements. Specific abnormalities on Goldmann perimetry are discussed in the section on ophthalmic impairments.

CT Scan Abnormalities

No patient had hemorrhage. Some had lucencies consistent with traumatic encephalomalacia and fluid collection. The most common CT finding was delayed symmetrical dilatation of the ventricles (ventriculomegaly) (Levin, Meyers, Grossman, & Sarwar, 1981).

Follow-Up Visits and Determination of End Point

Patients took one or more of the following tests: CT head scan, EEG, Goldmann visual perimetry, Beck Depression Scale, and neuropsychological assessment of higher cerebral function (HCF). The HCF battery is a modified Halstead-Reitan battery and consists of the Wechsler Adult Intelligence Scale–Revised, Wechsler Memory Scale, Aphasia Screening Test plus repetition and confrontation naming, Drawings on Command, Trail Making A and B, Reitan-Kløve sensory perceptual exam (single and simultaneous sensory discrimination in visual, auditory, and tactile modes; finger gnosis; stereognosis; fingertip graphesthesia); Form Board, Finger Tapping, Grip Dynamometry, and Minnesota Multiphasic Personality Inventory (MMPI).

Because confusion and memory difficulty is a common and troublesome issue in this patient population, compliance can be erratic. Our uniform procedure was to give every patient a 7-day medication box and instruct spouse or family in administration of medication or other aspects of their treatment. Written instructions on special pads labeled "patient instructions" were frequently given. An aggressive recall system was also used to ensure uniformity in keeping follow-up appointments at regular intervals.

We broke the 178 patients into three groups by outcome. Because all patients were uniformly treated by a single physician, our criterion for end point was the time of discharge from active care. This was largely a clinical judgment reached by the treating physician with the patient and his or her family. Prior to this, all patients were on continuous medication and monitored closely (every 1 to 4 weeks).

Patients in the *normal* category returned to their premorbid work or home environment free of medication and had no further follow-up appointments. Those in the *symptomatic* group continued to have symptoms that they felt were tolerable or acceptable and that were relieved by as-needed medication. None of the *impaired* group were judged to have a satisfactory outcome compared to their premorbid level: There was dissatisfaction by patient, physician, and family. *We acknowledge that the assessment of end point is fraught with difficulties in patients with head injury, but feel that a clinical judgment is practical.* The presence of an objective "abnormality" may not bother the individual patient and, conversely, lack of objective findings does not mean that the patient is carte blanche normal. In the absence of posttraumatic stress syndrome or other psychiatric diagnosis, the logical conclusion when testing fails to explain the patient's misery is that the testing instrument is insensitive to the pathophysiology, not that no pathology exists.

Examples that placed patients in the *impaired* group were persistence of symptoms such as headache, dizziness, visual symptoms that prevented them from performing work or home duties, monoparesis (usually from a lower motor neuron injury), gait disturbance, or a cognitive impairment that had plateaued and showed no further improvement by serial higher cerebral function testing. The assessment of higher cerebral function was probably the most meaningful objective measure.

Results

Multivariate Analysis by Outcome

We broke the patients into three groups by outcome. Table 9.4 shows these groups and the percentages of outcome variables. The criteria for inclusion in a particular group (normal, symptomatic, or impaired) is explained above. Selection is weighted toward clinical decision. A maximum *R*-square improvement stepwise regression was used to develop an *X*-variable model to separate the three groups. Based on an analysis of maximum *R*-squared improvement for dependent variable outcome, we eliminated those items that provided little explanation of the variance. These are: litigation, headache, vascular headache, nausea, hearing loss or tinnitus, abnormal eye movements, loss of smell, a Beck Scale >20, abnormal EEG, and whether or not the patient underwent laser surgery for a retinal tear.

Table 9.5 shows the best model using 10 of the predictor variables to explain the variance between the three outcome groups. Using all 10 variables, this model explains 22% of the variance. There is little added variance between a 7- and a 10-item model explanation. Note that 16% of the variance can be explained by simple clinical observations as opposed to the use of high technology testing. One needs to ask what each of these tests contributes to either treatment or prognosis of the individual patient.

The abnormalities found on CT scan are nonspecific, and add little information beyond that fact that some injury has occurred. The most common change is an increase in the ventricular size (ventriculomegaly) either based on the patient's age or by serial scanning over time. Ventriculomegaly presumably results from white matter loss due to diffuse axonal injury. While such findings may be interesting academically or serve as "proof" for litigation that a "real" injury has occurred, it does little to alter the clinical course. It may of course corroborate information obtained by HCF assessment or measurement of peripheral vision. These latter two assessments have much more practical significance.

How can the CT help in the clinical treatment? Initially, by ruling out a space-occupying lesion or cerebral edema. Pseudotumor cerebrii may also be suggested by CT by the usual criteria of slitlike ventricles and absence of cortical sulci over the convexity, for which case lumbar puncture and standard treatment may be warranted. Six such patients are present in our study group (four females, two males). Whereas cerebral edema is well known in comatose, hospitalized head

TABLE 9.4. Frequency of abnormality in three outcome groups.

Variable	% Normal ($N = 91$)	% Symptomatic ($N = 50$)	% Impaired ($N = 37$)
Loss of consciousness	40	46	51
Litigation[a]	80	80	81
Headache[a]	89	88	92
Vascular headache[a]	7	16	0
Memory/confusion	50	44	62
Dizziness	48	44	62
Neck pain	50	36	43
Irritability/sonophobia	41	28	51
Sleep disturbance	30	20	43
Depression/neurasthenia	34	16	32
Beck scale >20[a]	17 (11/65)	15 (4/27)	11 (3/27)
Incoordination	19	14	43
Nausea[a]	20	22	24
Hearing/tinnitus[a]	13	18	16
Personality change	13	2	27
Seizure	–	2	14
Blurry vision	53	32	73
Photophobia	24	28	35
Spots/flashing lights	25	10	43
Binocular fusion failure	21	22	27
Evidence of blunt trauma	24	24	38
Abnormal eye movements[a]	19	14	19
Anosmia[a]	9	6	11
Neuropsychological testing	50 (10/19)	63 (12/19)	100 (26/26)
EEG[a]	3 (2/73)	3 (1/37)	9 (3/32)
CT scan	11 (10/89)	20 (10/49)	43 (16/37)
Male:female	34:66	32:68	49:51
Black:white	68:32	52:48	51:49
Retinal laser surgery[a]	5/88	3/88	5/88
Visual perimetry abnormal	69 (40/57)	63 (12/19)	86 (24/28)
Duration of abnormal visual perimetry	72% normal at 4 mos; 14% abnormal at 2 yr	61% normal at 4 mos; 24% abnormal at 2 yr	29% normal at 4 mos; 43% abnormal at 2 yr

[a] Negligibly contributive to variance between groups.

TABLE 9.5. Best prediction for an X-Model variable.

											R-squared
1	Seizure										0.072
2	Seizure	Memory									0.111
3	Seizure	Memory	Age								0.140
4	Seizure	Memory	Age	Race							0.158
5	Seizure	Memory	Age	Race	CT						0.172
6	Seizure	Memory	Age	Race	CT	HCF					0.183
7	Seizure	Memory	Age	Race	CT	HCF	VF				0.194
8	Seizure	Memory	Age	HCF	BlnTr	Photo	VF	Depres			0.204
9	Seizure	Memory	Age	HCF	BlnTr	CT	Photo	Depres	VF		0.215
10	Seizure	Memory	Age	Race	CT	HCF	BlnTr	Depres	VF	Photo	0.222

Note. BlnTr = blunt trauma. VF = visual field; Photo = photophobia; Depres = depression.

trauma patients, there are few references on posttraumatic increased intracranial pressure pertinent to outpatients of this kind (Bennett & French, 1980). A speculative explanation suggests mild subarachnoid bleeding at the time of impact as the cause. In a study done soon after scanning became a clinical tool, Wiggins et al. (1978) elegantly demonstrated that the early EMI scanner could detect blood in the cerebrospinal fluid (CSF) only if it had a hematocrit value of 16%. Scott, New, & Davis (1974) and Patten (1968) also address the detection of CSF hemorrhage. While the ability of CT scanning to detect subarachnoid blood is much improved since the original EMI scan, that ability is not absolute. A mild elevation of CSF protein in these patients is supportive of a previous subarachnoid bleed and subsequent malabsorption of CSF. The patients in our group responded to acetazolamide; two required short-term use of prednisone.

Lastly, the CT can influence the long-term prognosis. For example, if ventriculomegaly or encephalomalacia is demonstrated, the physician may be more sanguine in suggesting a recovery to someone in college or to a professional who must have full command of his or her judgment and wits.

Compared to the influence of CT, practical recommendations can be made based on information obtained from HCF and perimetry. Patients may be advised not to drive or attempt a return to work in a hazardous environment until peripheral vision improves to satisfy Occupational Safety and Health Administration (OSHA) requirements. Objective abnormality on perimetry often satisfies patients whose subjective complaints interfere with reading or detailed visual work, particularly at computers and word processors. Patients perceive congruence between complaints and an abnormal visual plot that they can hold in their hands, but are only frustrated and bewildered if told "your eyes are all right."

Valuable information is also gained by HCF assessment, which both qualifies and quantifies the kinds of intellectual problems that the patient may face. Often concrete manipulations of their environment or biofeedback, external memory aids, and behavioral modification can aid to mitigate the difficulties that the cognitive impairments cause.

Ophthalmic Findings

That the majority of patients complain of subjective visual symptoms is obvious and confirmed by our data. Unfortunately, the standard of treatment in an outpatient setting is to measure acuity and intraocular pressure, perform a slit lamp exam and ophthalmoscopy, and advise the patient that "nothing is wrong with your eyes." One assumes that the neurologist or primary practitioner initiated ophthalmic referral in the first place. Only a *specific examination* for retinal tears and posterior vitreous detachments, and particular kinds of visual evaluations will detect organic abnormalities and also permit prediction of ultimate outcome.

All patients referred for ophthalmic evaluation during the course of this study were seen by a single ophthalmologist.* Undoubtedly, having an on-site ophthalmologist with expertise in retinal pathology was instrumental in being able to detect abnormalities in the first place. We refer to the fact that outpatients with mild head injury have not been examined in such detail previously. It is the *kind* of examination that is important, and not simply the fact of an ophthalmic referral itself.

Because of their peripheral location in the eye, retinal breaks, horseshoe tears, and posterior vitreous detachments require an active search for their detection. The posterior pole and fovea, which are usually the center of the clinician's attention, happen to be firmly adherent and therefore almost never injured. Thus, the hand-held ophthalmoscope does not reveal much in the early evaluation of these patients, who require a dilated fundus exam and indirect ophthalmoscopy.

A few patients had posttraumatic retinal edema, which resolved with time and without permanent visual loss. As a late sequela of injury, a few patients developed optic atrophy. Unfortunately, evoked potentials were not performed during this study period, although abnormalities with both auditory and visual evoked potentials have been noted in hospitalized patients (Benna, Bergamasco, Bianco, Gilli, Ferrero, & Pimessi, 1982; Rowe & Carlson, 1980).

After neutralization of refractive errors and elimination of intrinsic ocular disease, a visual field test assesses light and color discrimination. The peripheral retina is responsible for the outer limits of vision and measures on the average 60 degrees nasally and superiorly, 70 degrees inferiorly, and 90 degrees temporally. The physiological blind spot corresponding to the optic nerve is located 14 to 20 degrees temporal to fixation, approximately 2 degrees above and 5 degrees below the horizontal meridian. It is 7 to 8 degrees high and 5 to 6 degrees broad. A generalized, mild constriction of the visual field occurs with age, presumably due to peripheral retinal degeneration from relative anoxia of retinal tissue at the "end of the line" of the retinal circulation (Miller, 1982).

Figures 9.1 to 9.3 show characteristic visual field defects and support concussion to the optic nerves as a valid concept (Walsh, 1966). A common example

---

*David A. Newsom, M.D., is currently professor of opthamology and director of clinical research in retinal degenerations at Louisiana State University School of Medicine in New Orleans.

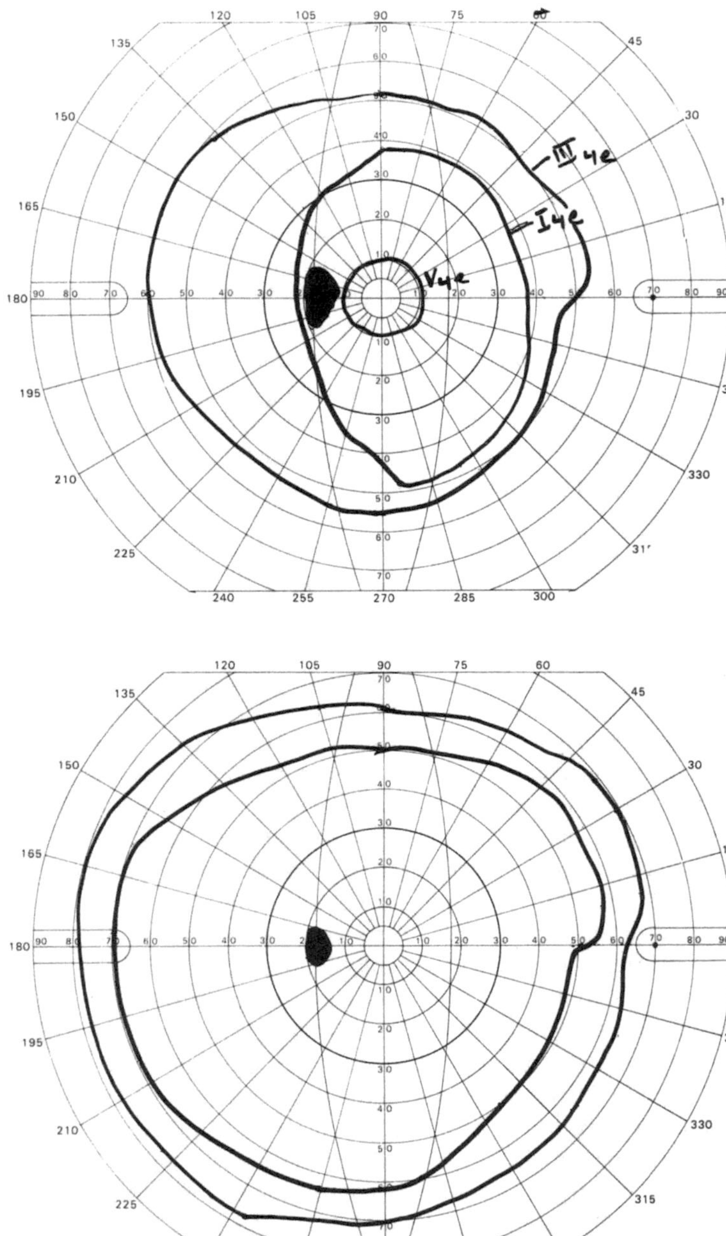

Left Eye

FIGURE 9.1. *Top:* visual field 5 days after injury. The right eye shows enlargement of the blind spot and a step defect at the horizontal meridian. The left eye shows generalized constriction. No central defects are found. *Bottom:* 3 weeks after injury. The left eye is normal and the right eye shows a mild nasal constriction.

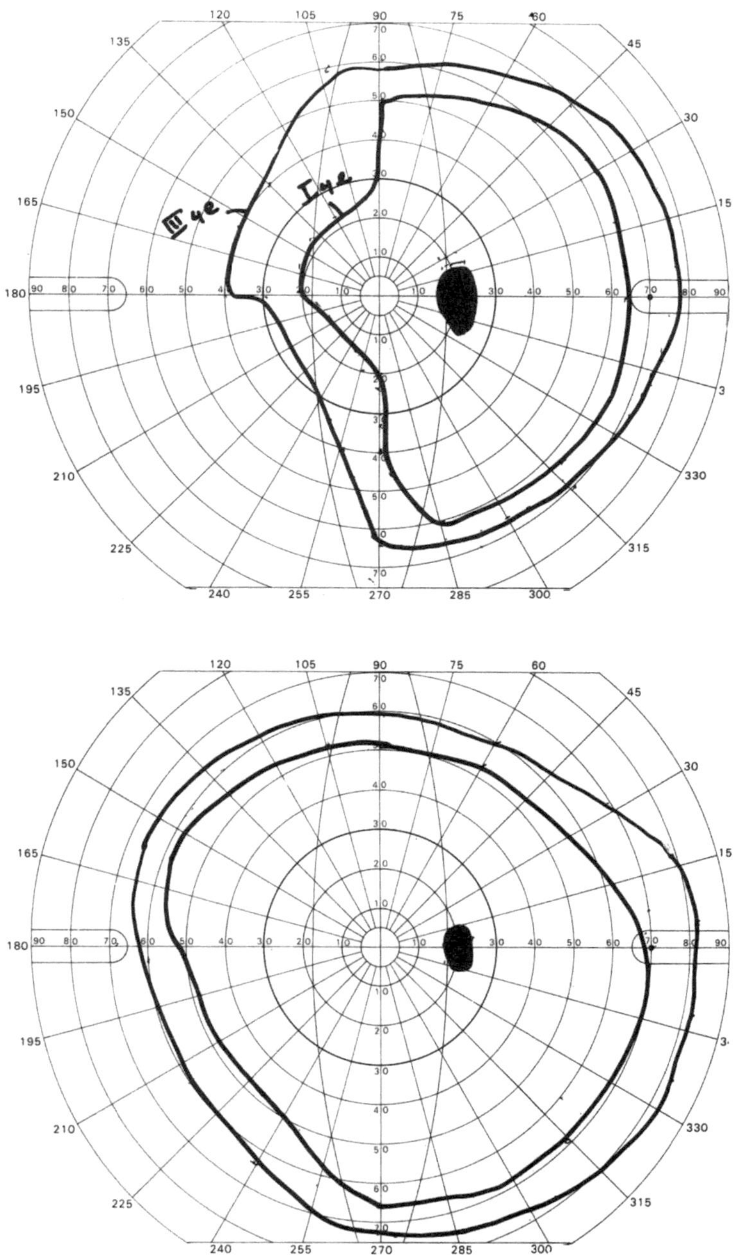

Right Eye

FIGURE 9.1. (*Continued*).

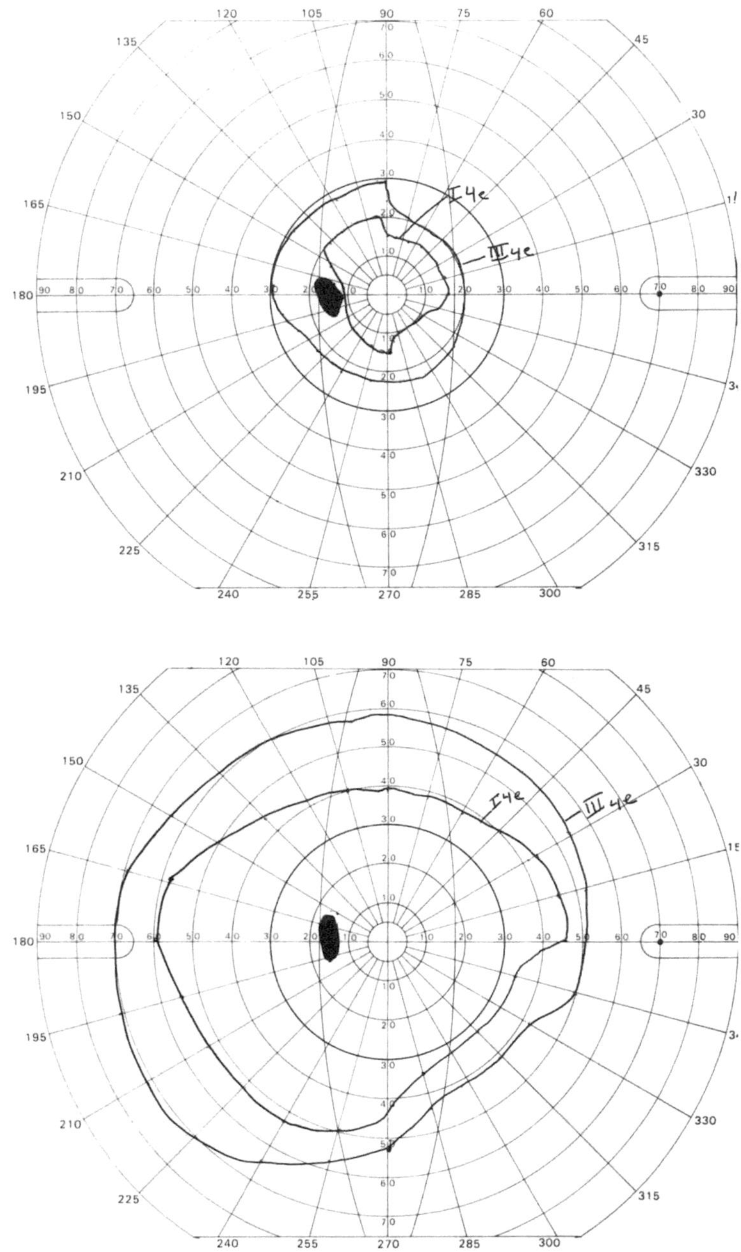

Left Eye

FIGURE 9.2. *Top:* 2 weeks after injury, both eyes show generalized constriction. *Bottom:* 4 months later eyes show improvement, with the right eye still showing constriction in the nasal and superior portions.

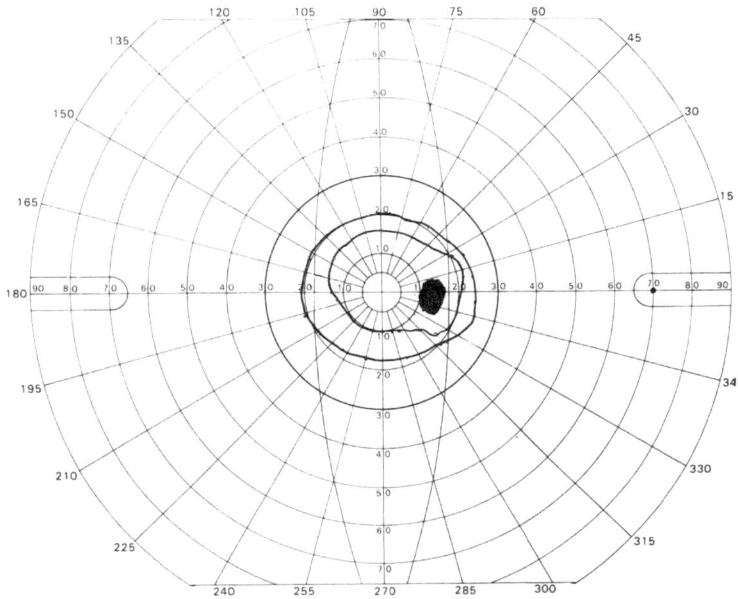

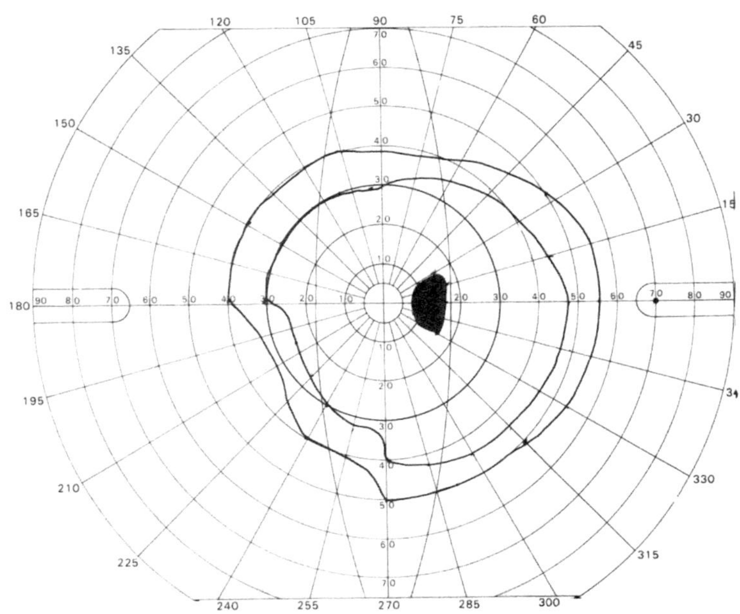

Right Eye

FIGURE 9.2. (*Continued*).

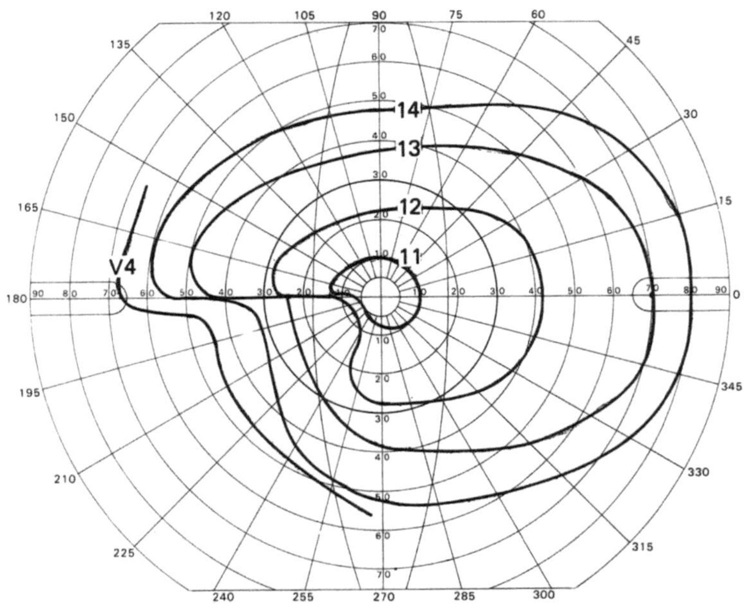

FIGURE 9.3. A typical infronasal step defect in the right eye.

of recovery of function without residual organic findings would be a blow to the back of the head producing momentary loss of vision without loss of consciousness.

The most common field defects are generalized constriction and enlargement of the blind spot, nasal (especially inferonasal) loss, and step defects along the nasal horizontal meridian. Rarely, an altitudinal defect is seen. These may be seen with either the peripheral or central isopters. In general neurology, nasal field defects are rare and indicate optic nerve lesions, often aneurysms of the anterior cerebral or anterior communicating arteries.

At the bottom of Table 9.4, one can find the percentage of patients who had abnormal visual fields in each of the three outcome groups, as well as the proportion of patients who had normalized at 4 months and those who remained abnormal at 2 years. Compared to 72% of patients in the *normal* outcome groups whose visual fields had returned to normal in 4 months, only 29% of those in the *impaired* group had resolution of their vision at 4 months.

The visual field defects resemble those seen in pseudotumor cerebrii (Wall & George, 1987). In this condition, the earliest field defects noted are nasal loss, especially inferonasal steps, and generalized constriction. In 40 eyes examined, Wall and George found constriction in 50% and inferonasal loss in 45%. They suggest that the frequency of defect detection is highly dependent on the visual field strategy used, and recommend the Armaly-Drance strategy (Armaly, 1969; Rock, Drance, & Morgan, 1973). This strategy of visual field testing is specifically sensitive to the central 30 degrees and the nasal horizontal meridian (Figure

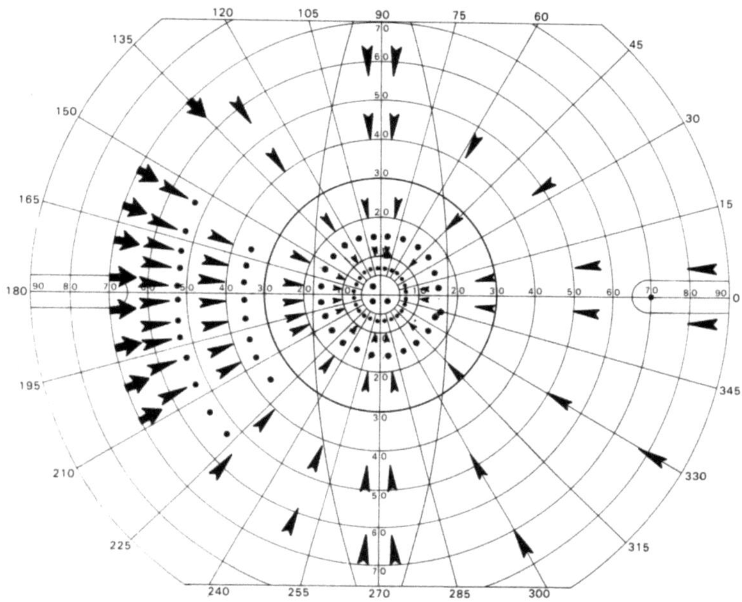

FIGURE 9.4. Modified Armaly-Drance visual field algorithm for the right eye for Goldmann perimetry, after Wall and George (1987). The *arrows* indicate test sites for kinetic perimetry and the *dots* indicate static sites. This strategy of visual field testing is biased to detect defects along the horizontal meridian.

9.4). Wall and George also feel that manual perimetry is superior to automated (octopus) threshold perimetry in defining step defects at the horizontal meridian.

An analysis of the perimetric fields suggests that these lesions are prechiasmal. The location of injury may be along the course of the optic nerve, where it is tethered at the optic foramen or where it pierces the globe. The optic nerve is relatively free to move within the orbit, is sheathed in dura, and is affected by intracranial pressure. The sudden rise of intrathoracic pressure from a steering wheel impact is transmitted to the intracranial and orbital compartments.

Table 9.6 shows an *X*-variable model that separates patients whose visual fields are abnormal for longer than 4 months regardless of their outcome. Again, over 20% of the variance can be accounted for by a model that uses clinical criteria.

EFFECT OF ALPRAZOLAM ON TIME TO END POINT

We were interested in finding out which treatment among the many options worked best for this outpatient population. The choice of modalities is broad and includes analgesics, narcotics, muscle relaxers, nonsteroidal anti-inflammatories, benzodiazepines, tricyclics, anticonvulsants, psychostimulants, and barbiturates. The wide range of choices indicates that no drug or class of drugs is uniformly successful in treating the various aspects of cerebral concussion and neck injury.

TABLE 9.6. X-Variable model separating patients whose visual fields are abnormal after 4 months regardless of outcome.

								R-squared
1 CT								0.044
2 Neck pain	CT							0.076
3 Neck pain	HCF	CT						0.111
4 Neck pain	HCF	Seizure	Age					0.146
5 Occupation	Neck	HCF	Seizure	Age				0.172
6 Occupation	Neck	HCF	Seizure	Fusion	Age			0.186
7 Occupation	Neck	HCF	Seizure	Fusion	Race	Age		0.220
8 Occupation	Neck	Irritab	HCF	Seizure	Fusion	Race	Age	0.223

Note. Irritab = irritability; Fusion = binocular fusion failure.

During the course of the series (1/82 to 10/84), Alprazolam was marketed as a new drug and therefore available among the options currently used to treat the population under study. Alprazolam was given to 54 patients as part of their medical treatment. We wished to eliminate effects of age and control for type and severity of injury. Of the 54, we selected 20 patients between 22 and 42 years who had at least 12 years of education and had had an automobile accident. Of the 205 subjects, 78 were eliminated from the study due to age, loss to follow-up, or because they had had accidents other than motor vehicle. Table 9.7 demonstrates the demographic equivalence of the groups. Table 9.8 details the similarity of the symptoms and treatment. Irritability/sonophobia was part of the clinical constellation that led to an impression of an agitated depression and that dictated the prescription of Alprazolam. Note that the Alprazolam group has a larger proportion of subjects who complained of irritability and sonophobia; otherwise the subjects were equivalent for severity and type of symptoms. All patients were either in the *normal* or *symptomatic* groups. No patient had posttraumatic stress syndrome.

TABLE 9.7. Demographic equivalence.

	Alprazolam	Controls
N	20	20
Sex	4 M, 16 F	4 M, 16 F
Age[a]	27.6 ± 4.9	27.8 ± 4.9
Education	13 ± 2.0	12.9 ± 1.89
Type of accident	Auto	Auto
Loss of consciousness	10/20	6/20
Outcome		
Normal	16/20	14/20
Symptomatic	4/20	6/20

[a] $t = 2.94$; $p =$ NS

TABLE 9.8. Frequency of symptoms and abnormal signs.

	Alprazolam	Controls	Total
Somatic-neurobehavioral			
Headache	18/20	17/20	35/40
Vascular headache	2/20	2/20	4/40
Memory/concentration	16/20	12/20	28/40
Dizziness/vertigo	15/20	13/20	28/40
Neck pain	10/20	11/20	21/40
Irritability/sonophobia	11/20	7/20	18/40
Sleep disorder not due to pain	8/20	5/20	13/40
Depression/neurasthenia	4/20	6/20	10/40
Incoordination	2/20	6/20	8/40
Nausea/vomiting	5/20	7/20	11/40
Hearing loss/tinnitus	2/20	5/20	7/40
Personality change	2/20	1/20	3/40
Menstrual irregularity	3/16 females	3/16	6/32
Ophthalmic			
Blurry vision	12/20	12/20	24/40
Photophobia	8/20	10/20	18/40
Spots/flashes	5/20	7/20	11/40
Binocular fusion failure	5/20	5/20	10/40
Neurological exam			
Evidence of blunt trauma	7/20	6/20	13/40
Eye movement disorders	5/20	3/20	8/40
Smell abnormality	4/20	1/20	5/40
Ancillary procedures			
Abnormal visual perimetry	13/15	12/15	25/30
Ophthalmology referral	12/20	14/20	26/40
Laser surgery	1/20	2/20	3/40
Abnormal CT	2/20	2/20	4/40

Twenty controls were chosen from the remaining group of patients. Controls were matched for age, sex, education, and severity of injury. Additionally, the Alprazolam patients were chosen such that they received either only Alprazolam or a combination of analgesics, muscle relaxers, or anti-motion sickness agents. The control patients were exposed to a similar range of drugs but did not receive other Benzodiazepines.

Patients who received Alprazolam had a more rapid recovery, as determined by the number of treatment days from the time of injury to end point, compared to subjects who received similar treatment but without Alproazolam (93 ± 60 versus 155 ± 110, $p < 0.05$). Injuries kept all patients from work.

We conclude that in nonhospitalized patients with moderate closed head trauma, Alprazolam improves the rate of recovery as determined by the number of days from injury to return to a status the patient equates as equivalent or acceptable relative to his or her premorbid status.

Correlation of Discrete Lesions Seen on Magnetic Resonance Imaging with Neuropsychological Assessment

A theme of this chapter is identification of abnormality in patients who have had a shaking injury or blunt trauma to the head. We have tried to show, too, that conventional tests and "standard" examinations fail to disclose the abnormality in patients with concussion. Conventional x-rays and even CT scans have been unrevealing in this patient group. In spite of this, clinicians continue to rely on "imaging" and other technical evaluations at the expense of an appropriate clinical examination or functional neuropsychological testing. Neuropsychologists need to make better inroads. A clinician is still much more likely to scan a patient who complains of memory impairment than to actually have his memory tested. This section shows that discrete structural lesions can be found in these patients, although the neuropsychological assessment still remains the investigation of choice.

Magnetic resonance imaging (MRI) technology became available in the Washington area in November 1984. At that time, Capitol Neurology entered into a collaboration with Magnetic Resonance Imaging Associates (MRIA) in the neighboring jurisdiction of Maryland. Although other magnets were regionally available, the device at MRIA was the first high-field/high-resolution scanner in our area. We knew of MRI's extraordinary sensitivity in detecting lesions not seen by CT. Patients with negative CTs but cognitive deficits demonstrable by higher cerebral function assessment seemed to be ideal patients for this new technology. At that point, active patients who already had abnormal higher cerebral function assessments were scanned with the hope of demonstrating anatomic lesions. These patients are not part of the previous group of 205 subjects.

Surprisingly, we did not see the gross lesions that we expected and that were subsequently described in the literature on hospitalized patients. Our scans were largely normal, but some initial patients had small lesions in white matter called *unidentified bright objects* (UBOs). These UBO's were located where the HCF said there was an abnormality.

The detection of abnormality and localization is done first by HCF, which is abnormal in all our patients. The hypothesis is that the MRI will either agree or not agree with the presence of an abnormality and its localization. HCF is the predictor and MRI is the confirmatory test. The data show that MRI is positive less than 50% of the time, but when it is, the congruence of lesion location is 80% (Table 9.9).

Table 9.9. Confirmatory accuracy of magnetic imaging.

	HCF	MRI	
Abnormality?	25/25	11/25	(44%)
Congruent localization		9/11	(82%)

TABLE 9.10. Correlation of lesions with HCF and MRI in concussion.

Age	Sex	Edu	Loc	Impact region	Lesion by HCF	Lesion by MRI	Date of accident	Days to HCF	Days to MRI
17	F	12	F	F	4,6	N	11/28/85	29	131
19	M	12	T	F	4,6	1,4	10/16/84	259	211
19	M	14	T	3,5	6	N	01/27/84	703	785
20	M	12	T	F	3	3	07/31/85	90	181
20	M	12	T	1,3	3	N	11/25/85	36	110
22	M	12	F	2	3,4,5,6	N	12/20/85	61	165
27	F	12	T	F,7	5,6	N	12/31/85	36	62
29	F	10	F	8	3,5	N	09/27/85	74	167
30	M	14	T	1,8	3,5,6	2,5,6	10/17/84	93	208
30	M	7	T	1,3	6	N	04/18/85	22	40
30	F	12	T	1	3,6	5	11/16/85	52	114
30	F	12	F	0	3,4,5,6	3,4,5,6	06/01/84	585	551
31	M	12	T	F,Z	1,3,5	3,4,5	10/01/84	116	207
32	F	12	F	0	5,6	N	11/02/85	24	121
33	M	12	T	3,Z,4	3,5	N	05/15/85	97	145
34	M	16	F	1,3	3,6	N	05/29/85	15	20
36	F	12	F	F,Z	3,5	3,6	04/01/85	39	364
38	F	12	T	3	3,5	3	03/22/85	42	297
39	M	12	F	1,2	3	1	11/20/85	48	101
40	F	13	F	3,8	3,5	N	03/09/85	55	88
44	F	14	F	F,0	6	N	05/01/83	851	950
45	F	18	F	2,8	F	N	01/24/86	33	105
51	M	18	T	1	3,6	N	10/29/85	49	129
52	M	18	F	F,0	3,5	5,6	01/24/86	33	101
55	F	19	T	0	5,6	6	12/13/83	679	693

Note. Edu = education; Loc = loss of consciousness.

In the 16 months between January 1985 and June 1986, 25 patients had both HCF and MRI done as part of their evaluation for closed head trauma. All were outpatients. None had gross deficits, but all were unable to function in their premorbid work or home environment.

Table 9.10 shows the population, localization of lesions by both tests, and the interval from the date of accident to the performance of the HCF and MRI. The mean age was 32.9 ± 10.7 and mean education was 13.2 ± 2.8 years.

Interpretation of the higher cerebral function assessment and localization of abnormality was done according to current standards of practice. Understandably, this involves judgment and experience on the neuropsychologist's part in deciding the *maximum site of impairment* in these patients who, by definition, have diffuse axonal injury. While some latitude of interpretation may be expected, we assume that independent analysis would be in agreement with the general nature and location of the abnormality. Figure 9.5 shows a sector system of four paired lateral locations plus rectilinear frontal, occipital, and vertex sites. These refer to site of impact and location of abnormality by HCF and MRI. Localization of the UBO is by visual inspection and assigning it to its appropriate sector.

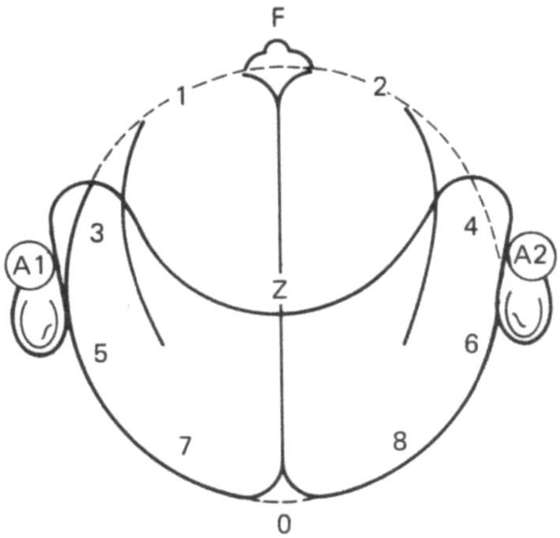

FIGURE 9.5. Sector system for localization of lesions by neuropsychological assessment and magnetic resonance imaging. There are four paired lateralized locations (frontal, temporal, parietal, and occipital) and three rectilinear locations frontal (F), occipital (O), and vertex (Z).

Technical Data and Images

Proton magnetic resonance imaging has soft tissue discrimination 500 times more sensitive than computerized x-ray tomography and is, consequently, more sensitive to abnormalities in the neuraxis. The basic principles of MRI, namely perturbation of hydrogen nuclei by specifically tuned radio frequency bombardment and computer reconstruction of the resultant signals, apply to all systems. The quality of the reconstructed images is dependent on signal-to-noise ratios (SNR), which are affected by several variables.

The available signal is roughly proportional to the strength of the ambient magnetic field, whereas the noise (which is mainly generated from the patient himself) is linear. Therefore, by simply increasing the field strength from 0.35 tesla to 1.5 tesla, one can achieve a fivefold increase in signal strength. This surplus of signal can be used to realize thin slices with a consequent increase in spatial resolution. Shorter imaging times are also possible, resulting in greater patient comfort and tolerance of the imaging procedure. The point is not so much that MRI systems can generate images of superior discrimination to CT scanning, but that high-field MRI systems have significant advantages over low- and mid-field systems.

The device used in our study was a SIGNA system (General Electric Medical Systems, Milwaukee, WI) operated at 1.5 tesla. Five-millimeter-thick localizing images are generated in the sagittal plane using a repetition time of 400 milliseconds (TR) and an echo delay of 20 milliseconds (TE). Two hundred fifty-six phase-encoded measurements are obtained by a single excitation over a 240-millimeter field of view. This yields a pixel size of 240/256 = 0.9 millimeter and a voxel size of 0.9 × 0.9 × 5 millimeters. Total imaging time is under 2 minutes. The images are reconstructed in a high-speed multitasking computer at approximately 2 seconds per image.

A cursor is placed at the foramen magnum and then at the vertex, and a prescription for a multislice acquisition in the axial plane is established. Fifteen to twenty 5-millimeter-thick locations are imaged using a 240-mm field of view, 256 × 256 matrix, a single excitation, TR of 2250 milliseconds and TEs of 20 and 80 milliseconds. This protocol yields two images per location, the 2250/20 or proton density image and a relatively T2-weighted study at 2250/80. Imaging time is approximately 11 minutes.

A third set of images is performed in patients with closed head trauma to evaluate the temporal lobes. These are also 5-millimeter slices in the coronal plane using the same protocol as for the axial plane. T1-weighted images (short TR, short TE) and inversion recovery sequences have not proved helpful in evaluating the temporal lobes. Some degradation of the temporal lobe areas by pulsation artifact from the carotid vessels is occasionally encountered, but can be corrected by swapping the frequency and phase encoding direction or, more recently, by gating the acquisition to the cardiac cycle. This latter scheme also results in an increase in SNR and a higher quality image. Figures 9.6 to 9.9 illustrate the UBOs in these patients with concussion. They are usually isolated white-matter signals best detected on T2-weighted images and are circumscribed. They appear singularly or multiply in white matter or at gray-white junction. When seen in the periventricular region, they are not subependymal but reside in the centrum

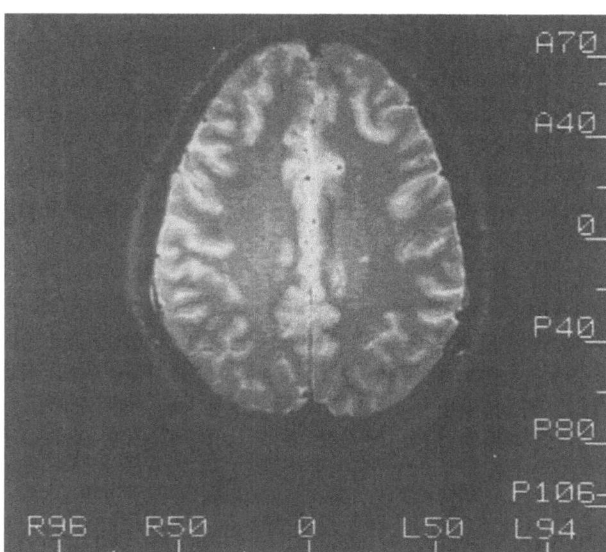

FIGURE 9.6. Single UBO in the left parietal white matter.

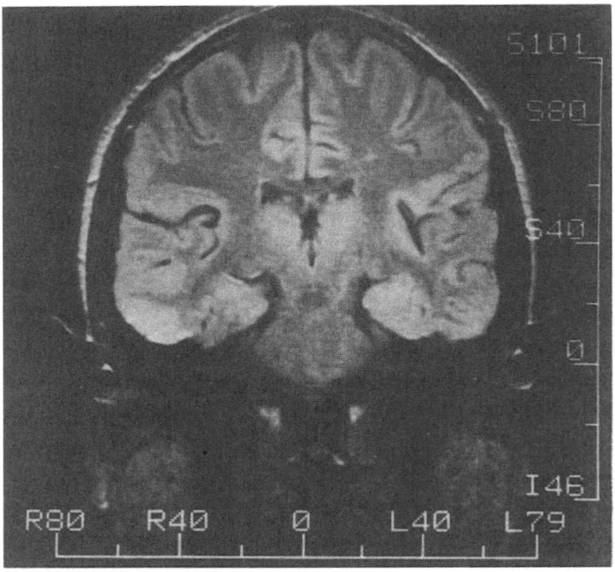

FIGURE 9.7. Coronal view showing single UBO in the corona radiata on the left. The post-traumatic UBOs do not hug the ventricles.

semiovale. Thus, there seems to be a predilection (which has not been tested by statistical evaluation) for the UBOs to be in white-matter tracts such as the locations of the short U fibers and association tracts.

Several important issues concerning these UBOs follow.

Controls

None of 25 age-sex match controls who had MRIs for reasons other than head trauma showed UBOs.

UBOs in Comparison to White-Matter Signals in Other Patient Populations

Trauma

Levin, Meyers, Grossman, & Sarwar (1985) described a patient with *severe* head injury: coma, increased intracranial pressure, hemiparesis, quadrantinopsia, language and memory difficulties by formal assessment. Five years after the injury, which left the patient grossly impaired, MRI demonstrated huge multifocal white-matter signals that were detected by a low-field low-resolution device.

Aging

UBOs are not seen in young adults. Nor are they necessarily related only to normal aging, since many octogenarians have no such lesions. In 151 patients

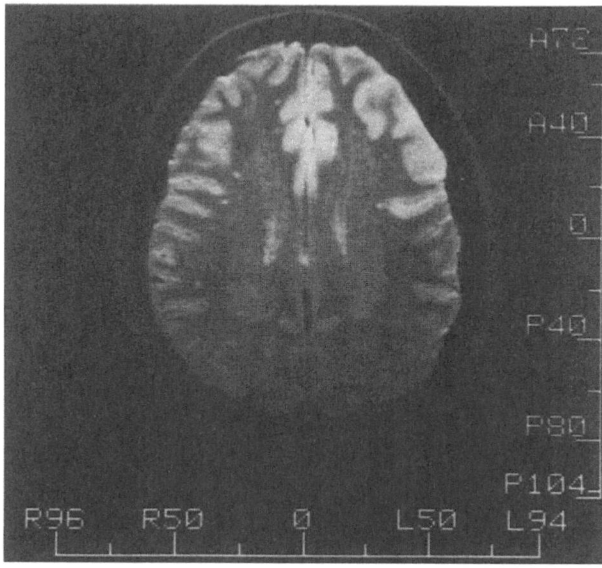

FIGURE 9.8. Multiple and bilateral UBOs. Note the asymmetry and location at gray-white junction.

over 50 years old, Gerard and Weisberg (1986) found periventricular lesions in 7.8% of those who had no cerebrovascular symptoms or risk factors. The figure jumped to 78.5% of those who did. Lesions in these patients are huge, symmetrical, and periventricular, with a predilection to cap the frontal and occipital horns. Some lesions in centrum semiovale and gray-white junction at the frontal poles are seen, but they are quite distinct from the UBOs that we demonstrate. Gerard detected these at a low magnetic field strength and with a low-resolution matrix.

Does the 7.8% of Gerard's patients who are over 50 and who have white-matter lesions represent the expected proportion of people in that age group who have had head trauma at some time in their lives? The question is moot, because his lesions are quite different from the UBOs we detect at a higher resolution.

Dementia and Stroke

Lesions more like UBOs are found – along with other gross lesions – in demented patients with stroke. Hershey, Modic, Greerough, and Jaffe (1987) studied 34 patients with a low-resolution magnet, and found a combination of lesions in old, sick patients. In some elderly patients, single subcortical lesions may be seen in conjunction with ventricular dilatation and cortical atrophy. Others show combination of periventricular white-matter signals that may coalesce and be seen with gray-matter signals.

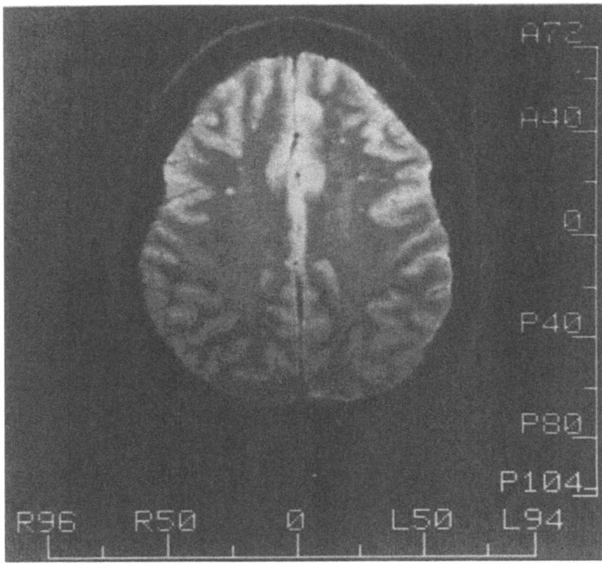

FIGURE 9.9. Multiple UBOs in frontal white matter (bilateral) and right parietal occipital region.

Table 9.11 summarizes the technical parameters of the various authors cited. In our outpatient population, we rarely see the large focal lesions that the low-field magnets detect. When we do, they are almost always in patients who have abnormal CT scans that show traumatic hemorrhage or cavitation and fluid collection following traumatic encephalomalacia.

What does the UBO represent? No one knows. UBOs are unlikely to represent a single etiology, but may be the final footprint of gliosis, stroke, demyelination, infection, inflammation, or whatever. These lesions appear different in size, location, and symmetry from those of multiple sclerosis. It would be of interest to see if boxers have such UBOs. In trauma, the UBO may represent rarefaction and axonal swelling similar to that seen by light microscopy in diffuse axonal injury (Adams, Graham, Murray, et al., 1982; Gennarelli, Thibault, Adams, et al., 1982; Holbourn, 1943; Ommaya, 1981; Oppenheimer, 1968; Strich, 1956, 1961, 1970). This is speculative, since anatomic correlations with the images have not been done. The best course at present may simply be to describe the signals and correlate them with the clinical and neuropsychological findings.

Time Factors

Early results indicated that a minimum time is necessary for the UBO lesions to appear. They may also resolve with time. Reference to Table 9.10 shows a large variation in the number of days from injury to performance of the MRI. This vari-

TABLE 9.11. Technical comparison of resolution.

Author	(0000)	Tesla	Matrix	Slice (mm)
Levin & Weisberg	(1985)	0.35	128×128	7
Gerard & Weisberg	(1986)	0.35	128×128	7
Weidmann et al.	(1987)	0.15	128×128	10
Hershey et al.	(1987)	1.0	256×256	10
Present study	(1987)	1.5	256×256	5

ation is due to the changing referral for obtaining MRI scans once the technology was available and once we began detecting the UBOs. In comparison, the variance in days from injury to performance of the HCF is accounted for by five outliers who were referred because of persistent cognitive deficits long after their injury.

In addressing the issue of when after injury the UBO appears and whether it resolves with time, examination of the data showed that patients with *normal* MRIs tended to be scanned either very early or very late after their injury.

Table 9.12 shows this time relationship with the outliers removed. These 18 patients were injured after March 1985. Separating into groups who had either a normal or abnormal MRI, there was no statistical difference from date of injury to the time of HCF (6 to 7 weeks postinjury).

However, by independent nondirectional t test ($p < .02$), patients who had an abnormal MRI were imaged significantly later than those patients who showed no MRI lesions (3.5 compared to almost 5 months).

Two interpretations are not mutually exclusive. One is that a certain time is necessary for an abnormal signal to develop. The other is that abnormal patients, because of their brain injury, have difficulty with daily living, including getting themselves to the scanner.

Using a low-field low-resolution magnet in patients with more severe injury, Levin et al. (1985) showed persistence of signal 5 years after injury in his patient. Four of our 25 patients who were scanned 1 year or later after their injury had UBOs. Wiedmann, Hadley, Wilson, Brooks, and Teasdale (1987) also showed resolution of nearly half the lesions in individual patients who had suffered more severe injuries. In both these examples, the patients were hospitalized and the scanners used were low resolution.

Just as lucency on CT is a marker for an old event, we think that signals detected late after injury will *not* resolve. But how soon after injury will these lesions appear?

CT lesions in stroke patients provide a useful analogy. Patients with ischemic infarction and dense hemiparesis all have normal CT scans right after the ictus. Scans become positive only a few days later. Depending on size of the infarct, a radiographic signature of abnormality may remain, or the scan can revert to normal. The time course is extremely variable, as any clinician knows.

TABLE 9.12. Days to HCF and MRI for injuries after March 1985.

Days to HCF		Days to MRI	
Normal MRI	Abnormal MRI	Normal MRI	Abnormal MRI
43±25	52±19 t = ns	101±45 t = 2.8	139±103 $p > .02$ $df = 15$

Note. $N = 18$.

Gomori, Grossman, and Goldberg (1985) showed that the MRI lesions after hemorrhagic infarction take 1 year to resolve. We suggest that UBOs in closed head trauma found 1 year after injury will not resolve. More experience with these patients will settle this issue.

Vector of Impact and Loss of Consciousness

Thirteen of 25 patients lost consciousness. Of these, 7 (54%) had an abnormal MRI compared to 4 of 12 patients (33%) who had normal MRIs who did not lose consciousness. That is, one is nearly twice as likely to have an abnormal MRI if unconscious, while analysis of impact region by sector indicates that one is more likely to lose consciousness with a lateral impact, particularly a left fronto-temporal one. This fact may be related to design of shoulder restraints in this population, who all had auto accidents. There were nearly equal numbers of cases of single impact versus multiple impact in groups who lost consciousness and those who did not.

For location of lesion by either HCF or MRI, the vector of force did not accurately predict the traditional coup-contracoup lesions. This theory may indicate the *magnitude of trauma* and be suitable for surface lesions found at autopsy, or for contusions and hemorrhages seen on CT scans, but not hold for subjects with shaking injuries of the brain. Strich (1961) framed the same opinion nicely:

> Because it is tedious to examine a brain histologically, pathologists have been content to study the damage visible to the naked eye—such as lacerations or coup and contre-coup lesions—which, though interesting, are often not the cause of the patient's death or even of his neurological signs.

Our point is not that one magnet is better than another. The point is that any neuropsychologist can outperform several million dollars worth of equipment and yield more valuable information that can influence the patient's treatment. Patient's are being denied treatment for want of an abnormal image.

To characterize and delineate the severity of cognitive impairment, the neuropsychological evaluation of higher cerebral function remains the examination of choice. Patients are often comforted to know that their problems are "real" even if their impairment is not always visible to the latest high-technology machinery.

Ideally, "high tech" and "old hat" should complement each other. There is a tendency for physicians to rely on "imaging" at the expense of clinical examination or functional testing. Closed head trauma (CHT) is known *not* to cause large focal lesions, which imaging techniques are best suited to detect. CHT causes diffuse axonal injury, although some regions of the inhomogenous brain tissue (Metz, McElhaney, & Ommaya, 1970; Ommaya 1968) will receive more force than others. Perhaps the UBOs are markers of these focal points of sheer-strain forces.

If one wants an image, an MR with high field strength and resolution is mandatory. In well over half of our patients *who are impaired*, we cannot demonstrate an anatomic lesion, although this may change with spectroscopy, which can measure the chemical constituents of nervous tissue. Ultimately, integrity of cognitive function depends on the integrity of individual neurons and their synaptic connections. Cognition—to the extent that it can be measured—is best done by neuropsychological means.

Return to Work

Why people of disparate psychological constitutions should categorically use the fact of a "trivial" head injury as an excuse to stop working and get on the dole makes no sense. Yet this truism persists.

Kelly (1981) showed that a delay in settlement may *increase* the risk of not returning to work. Average time from injury to settlement for his 170 subjects was 3.8 years for patients not back at work before settlement compared to 3 years for those who did return to work before settlement. Age and occupation influence the ability to return to work, with older patients and those in more dangerous occupations tending not to return.

Barth, Macciocchi, Giordani, Rimel, Jane, & Boll (1983) showed correlation of Halstead impairment index >0.4 (mild injury) with considerable difficulty in returning to work at 3 months postinjury ($R=0.41$, $p<.001$), whether or not patients with suspect employment histories were included in the analysis. Cognitive impairment was also correlated with a decline in personal care and household effectiveness ($R = 0.24$, $p<.02$).

In a study of 66 New Zealand men ages 17 to 48 who were off work 0 to 26 days (mean 4.7), Wrightson and Gronwall (1981) found that 66% were symptomatic on returning to work and that 46% could not perform as well for an additional 14 days. Leisure activities were similarly affected. At 3 months postinjury, 20% were still symptomatic at work and without compensation claims. Patients had typical symptoms. Persistence of symptoms had no correlation with age, posttraumatic amnesia, or other factors.

They point out the limitation of posttraumatic amnesia as an index for severity of injury; that return to work may be a useful index of severity but obviously does not indicate recovery; that age is an important factor, with effects seen statistically beginning at 35 years; that the uniformity of symptoms suggests general impairment rather than separate and individual defects. That symptoms are more numerous in those who return to work early suggests that precipitation of symptoms may occur when too much is asked of a reduced capacity.

Rimel, Giordani, Barth, & colleagues (1981) evaluated 424 patients 3 months after head injury. All had lost consciousness less than 20 minutes and were hospitalized less than 48 hours. Glasgow scores were 13 to 15. They found 79% had persistent headache, 59% complained of memory problems, and 34% had not returned to work. Most of 69 patients evaluated had neuropsychological impairments in attention, concentration, memory, and judgment.

Rimel et al. suggested that emotional stress caused by persistent symptoms may be significant in long-term disability, a point made earlier by Dikmen and Reitan (1977), who showed that patients with greater initial and residual neuropsychological impairment experience greater emotional distress than those with lesser injuries. There is some decline in distress over time. Lastly, Rimel et al. suggested that litigation and compensation play minimal roles, concluding that high rates of morbidity and unemployment in patients 3 months after seemingly trivial head trauma is evidence that many of them have, in fact, neuropsychological organic brain damage.

Gronwall and Wrightson (1975) indicated that the effects of concussions are cumulative, particularly regarding the rate of information processing. The cumulative effects of repeated concussion and shaking of the brain is particularly well demonstrated in boxers (Casson et al., 1982; Morrison, 1986; Ross, Cole, Thompson, & Kim, 1983). Maguire and Benson (1986) discuss retinal injury in this type of injury. Our patients with multiple head injury have shown multiple, bilateral UBOs on MRI.

Neck Injury

It is axiomatic that head and neck injuries go together. Biomechanical factors responsible for injury have been studied, but appear to be better known to safety engineers and designers of automobiles than to physicians. Much also has been learned from the drilling behavior of woodpeckers to support the rotational theory of impact brain trauma and the associated neck factors (May, Fuster, Haber, & Hirschman, 1979).

The incorrect general impression is that neck injuries are either minor (whiplash) or catastrophic (quadriplegia). Yet fatal injury following whiplash without direct head contact is documented (Ommaya & Yarnell, 1969). The subdural and subarachnoid surface hemorrhages in brain and spinal cord in monkeys with whiplash severe enough to cause concussion could be the source of neck stiffness, reflex myodystonia, and increased intracranial pressure (Yarnell & Ommaya, 1969). Jennett (1975) emphasizes that "fatal brain damage can occur without a fracture of the skull or any blemish on the scalp."

Whiplash was recognized in World War II when pilots of catapult take-off craft had to be discharged from service because of intractable neck pain and occasional concussion! The solution was to extend the seat back to support the head (MacNab, 1964, 1975; Ommaya, personal communication).

All injuries to the neck are the result of tensile, shear, and compressive strains resulting from a combination of overbending, axial compression and rotational loads. Ommaya (1984) showed that experimental tearing of the anterior longitudinal ligament and separation of the disc from the vertebra are always associated with anterior neck muscle injury and could never be demonstrated by conventional x-ray.

Our experience is consonant with that of others who have shown a wide range of serious problems following the shaking injury of whiplash, but who have documented a small number of patients from the point of view of their own specialty. These findings include subdural hemorrhage in adults (Ommaya & Yarnell, 1969) and children (Zimmerman, Bilaniuk, Bruce, et al., 1978); foveal splinters and macular whisps (Daily, 1979); retinal hemorrhages (Carter & McCormick, 1983); neurotransmitter deregulation and orthostasis (Baron et al., 1979); vocal cord paralysis (Helliwell, Robertson, Todd, & Lobb, 1984); hearing loss and vertigo (Berman & Fredrickson, 1978; Griffiths, 1979; Healy, 1982; Hinoki, 1984); endolymphatic fistulae (Fitzgerald, 1984); and a dissociated amnesia similar to transient global amnesia (Nielsen, 1959).

In this retrospective group, we did not pay sufficient attention to injury of the anterior neck structures, which are always involved when there is a hyperextension injury, as is most often the case in automobile accidents. Also, patients in this retrospective series were usually referred beyond the acute phase, when the anterior neck symptoms had resolved. Now, when patients are being referred soon after their injury, we note change in voice, painful swallowing, pain on palpation of the sternal insertion of the sternocleidomastoid muscle and longissimus colles, and impaction of the nasal septum. Otolaryngological evaluation, which includes fiberoptic laryngoscopy, can detect vocal cord paralysis due to stretch injury of the recurrent laryngeal nerve, retropharyngeal hematomas, and impaction headaches. Impaction headaches disappear with cocainization of the nasal septum. Nosebleed at the time of impact is pathognomonic of nasal fracture and should prompt an investigation of this additional peripheral cause of post-traumatic headache. These types of physical findings should be taken as evidence of blunt trauma in future studies.

Conclusions

Our message is not new. Shaking the human body does cause brain injuries. Yet decades of prejudice emphasizing compensation neurosis and malingering as characteristic of patients with closed head injuries, particularly those not rushed to hospital *in extremis*, continues. Their plight is stereotyped and devalued by no more scientific authority than *ex cathedra* pronouncements that appeal to common sense (Read, 1981).

Why are derangements of higher cognitive function and behavior not more readily apparent? Culpability is probably not due to negligence or omission, but rather the historical development of cognitive neuroscience. Its broad interdisciplinary basis needs no emphasis, but the fact that its study is not routine in neurology, neurosurgery, psychiatry, or clinical psychology training programs does.

Acquisition of neuropsychological expertise is self-elected, the methodology somewhat alien to the clinical neurosciences, and nowhere does the adage that one finds what he or she is looking for more readily apply.

Weinstein and Wells (1981) illustrate the point well in their case of a 24-year-old man, misdiagnosed for 6 years, during which he was subjected to four psychiatric hospitalizations and 6 months in jail after numerous encounters with the police. He was unable to finish college or a tour in the Navy. Twice, neuropsychological testing pointed to organic disease but his behavior was not acknowledged as such. Physicians without a special interest in higher cognitive functions fail to recognize cognitive or personality changes due to acquired brain pathology.

This background should help illuminate why assumptions, which have no scientific basis, that closed head injuries have no cognitive-behavioral sequelae are perpetuated. Assumptions based on common sense can be wrong, however. Kelly and Smith (1981) refuted four common myths that "everybody knows" and are "obvious" about postconcussion syndrome in a prospective study of 170 patients, namely: 1) symptoms of concussion do not occur in patients who have no prospect for compensation, 2) the severity of symptoms is inversely related to the severity of injury, 3) symptoms never develop in white-collar managerial or professional workers, and 4) no one ever recovers and returns to work before settlement. Those who take the time to look will find that such patients manifest a wide variety of objective findings commensurate with injury to the central and peripheral nervous systems. Voltaire was more strident: The greater the ignorance the greater the dogma.

But it is not totally a question of ignorance that explains this professional bias. Kelly (1981) and Kelly and Smith (1981) suggested that organic "symptoms may be neurotically prolonged because of failure of the medical profession to recognize" them. Patient resentment is common, understandable, and "compounded when they meet disbelief from the medical profession and lawyers, a refusal to treat their symptoms, and a vague hint of moral disapproval."

The basis for the pervasive disbelief among medical practitioners is partly historical. Physician training emphasizes intervention at end-stage disease. In the 17th and 18th centuries, the art of physical diagnosis – the systematic categorization of symptoms and signs – reached its peak and became a science when it was correlated with Virchow's new cellular pathology. The clinicopathological exercise was born. Thus, physicians have a strong bias of expectation toward gross disease and its outward physical manifestation. That cognitive symptoms should be entirely relegated to "psychological factors" is no surprise.

With the advent of technology, starting with Laenec's stethoscope and currently represented by the MR scanner, scientists have developed technology to probe physiological function and structure. The gradual introduction of the x-ray machine and the cardiogram into hospitals in the 1920s and 1930s was followed by an explosion in laboratory analysis and instrumentation. The historical paradigm grew for physicians to order "tests" if the physical exam did not lead to diagnosis. As a good word in a living language, "diagnosis" stopped meaning "through knowledge" and came to stand for "through machines." Indeed, the faith in technology became so strong that "test results" became the final arbiter in clinical medicine, supplanting clinical and cognitive skills, even judgment. Negative tests came to mean that nothing was wrong.

There is still no test for cognitive function, at least machine tests comparable to EKGs, x-rays, including CT scans, and blood chemistry analyzers. It is difficult for people to consider engaging another human being in a stylized series of situations as a "test," but this is exactly what neuropsychological assessment is. This kind of interaction, using paper and pencil and other tools of the trade like pegboards and finger tappers, is no different than the neurological exam with its reflex hammers and hat pins.

Acknowledgment. This work was supported in part by the Medlantic Research Foundation (formerly the Research Foundation of the Washington Hospital Center).

References

Adams, J.H., Graham, D.I., Murray, L.S., et al. (1982). Diffuse axonal injury due to nonmissile head injury to humans: An analysis of 45 cases. *Annals of Neurology, 12,* 557–563.

American Psychiatric Association. (1980). *Diagnostic and statistical manual of mental disorders* (3rd ed.). Washington, DC.

Armaly, M. (1969). Ocular pressure and visual fields: A ten year follow up. *Archives of Ophthalmology, 81,* 25–40.

Baron, J.B., Tangapregassom, M.J., Ushio, N., et al. (1979). Neurotransmitters disregulation related to the orthostatic postural activity disorders in cases of post concussional syndrome after head or whiplash injuries. *International Journal of Neurology, 13,* 237–249.

Barth, J.T., Macciocchi, S.N., Giordani, B., Rimel, R., Jane, J.A., & Boll, T.J.: (1983). Neuropsychological sequelae of minor head injury. *Neurosurgery, 13,* 529–533.

Benna, P., Bergamasco, B., Bianco, C., Gilli, C., Ferrero, P., & Pimessi, L. (1982). Brainstem and auditory evoked potentials in postconcussion syndrome. *Italian Journal of Neurological Science, 4,* 281–287.

Bennett, H.S., & French, J.H. (1980). Elevated intracranial pressure in whiplash shaken infant syndrome detected with normal computerized tomography. *Clinical Pediatrics, 19,* 633–634.

Berman, J.M., & Fredrickson, J.M. (1978). Vertigo after head injury—a five year follow up. *Otolaryngology, 7*(3), 237–245.

Carter, J.E., & McCormick, A.Q. (1983). Whiplash shaking syndrome: Retinal hemorrhages and computerized axial tomography of the brain. *Child Abuse and Neglect 7*(3), 279–286.

Casson, I.R., Sham, R.A.J., Campbell, E.A., et al. (1982). Neurological and CT evaluation of knocked-out boxers. *Journal of Neurology, Neurosurgery and Psychiatry, 45,* 170–174.

Daily, J. (1979). Whiplash injury as one cause of the foveolar splinter and macular whisps. *Archives of Ophthalmology, 97,* 360.
Dikmen, S., & Reitan, R.M. (1977). Emotional sequelae of head injury. *Annals of Neurology, 2,* 492–494.
Fitzgerald, D.C. (1984). Endolymphatic fistula. *JAMA, (Journal of the American Medical Association), 252,* 1407.
Gennarelli, T.A., Thibault, L.E., Adams, J.H., et al. (1982). Diffuse axonal injury and traumatic coma in the primate. *Annals of Neurology, 12,* 564–574.
Gerard, G., & Weisberg, L.A. (1986). MRI periventricular lesions in adults. *Neurology, 36,* 998–1001.
Gomori, J.M., Grossman, R.I., & Goldberg, H.I. (1985). Intracranial hematomas: Imaging by high-field MR. *Radiology, 157,* 87–93.
Griffiths, M.V. (1979). The incidence of auditory and vestibular concussion following minor head injury. *Journal of Laryngology and Otology, 93,* 253–265.
Gronwall, D., & Wrightson, P. (1975). Cumulative effect of concussion. *Lancet, November 22,* 995–997.
Healy, G.B. (1982). Current concepts in otolaryngology: Hearing loss and vertigo secondary to head injury. *New England Journal of Medicine, 306,* 1029–1031.
Helliwell, M., Robertson, J.C., Todd, G.B., & Lobb, M. (1984). Bilateral vocal cord paralysis due to whiplash injury. *British Medical Journal, 288,* 1876–1877.
Hershey, L.A., Modic, M.T., Greenough, G., & Jaffe, D.F. (1987). Magnetic resonance imaging in vascular dementia. *Neurology, 37,* 29–36.
Hinoki, M. (1984). Vertigo due to whiplash injury: A neurootological approach. *Acta Otolaryngologica (Suppl.) (Stockholm), 419,* 9–29.
Holbourn, A.H.S. (1943). Mechanics of head injury. *Lancet, 2,* 438–441.
Jennett, B. (1975). *Epilepsy after non-missile head injuries* (2nd ed., pp. 5–8). London: Heinemann.
Kelly, R.E. (1981). The post-traumatic syndrome. *Journal of the Royal Society of Medicine, 74,* 242–245.
Kelly, R.E., & Smith, B.N. (1981). Post-traumatic syndrome: Another myth discredited. *Journal of the Royal Society of Medicine, 74,* 275–277.
Levin, H.S., Benton, A.L., & Grossman, R.G. (1982). *Neurobehavioral consequences of closed head injury.* New York: Oxford University Press.
Levin, H.S., Handel, S.F., Goldmann, A.M., et al. (1985). Magnetic resonance imaging after "diffuse" nonmissile head injury. *Archives of Neurology, 42,* 963–968.
Levin, H.S., Meyers, C.A., Grossman, R.G., & Sarwar, M. (1981). Ventricular enlargement after closed head injury. *Archives of Neurology, 38,* 623–628.
Maguire, J.I., & Benson, W.E. (1986). Retinal injury and detachment in boxers. *JAMA (Journal of the American Medical Association), 255,* 2451–2453.
May, P.R., Fuster, J.M., Haber, J., & Hirschman, A. (1979). Woodpecker drilling behavior: An endorsement of the rotational theory of impact brain injury. *Archives of Neurology, 36,* 370–373.
MacNab, I. (1964). Acceleration Injuries to the Cervical Spine. *Journal of Bone & Joint Surgery 46A: 1797*–1799.
MacNab, I. (1975). Acceleration Extension Injuries to the Cervical Spine. Chapter 10 in *The Spine.* Ed. Rothman, R.R. & Simeone, F.A., W.B. Saunders.
Metz, H., McElhaney, J., & Ommaya, A.K. (1970). A comparison of the elasticity of live, dead and fixed brain tissue. *Journal of Biomechanics, 3,* 453–458.

Miller, N.R., (1982). in Walsh & Hoyt (Ed.), *Clinical neuroophthalmology* (4th ed., vol. 1, pp. 153–159). Baltimore: Williams & Wilkins.

Morrison, R.G. (1986). Medical and public health aspects of boxing. *JAMA (Journal of the American Medical Association) 255*, 2475–2480.

National Head Injury Foundation, Inc. (1986, June). Annual report. 18A Vernon Street, Framingham MA, 01701.

Nielsen, J.M. (1959). Whiplash injury with amnesia for life experiences. *Bulletin of the Los Angeles Neurological Societies, 23*(4), 27–29.

Ommaya, A.K. (1968). The mechanical properties of tissues of the nervous system. *Journal of Biomechanics, 1*, 127–138.

Ommaya, A.K. (1981). Mechanisms of cerebral concussion, contusions and the physiopathology of head injury. In J. Youmans (Ed.), Neurological surgery. Philadelphia: Saunders.

Ommaya, A.K. (1984). The neck: Classification, physiology and clinical outcome of injuries to the neck in motor vehicle accidents. In *Biomechanics of impact trauma*. B. Aldeman & A. Chapon (Eds.), Amsterdam: Elsevier.

Ommaya, A.K., Hirsch, A.E., & Martinex, J. (1966, November). The role of "whiplash" in cerebral concussion. *Proceedings of the 10th Stapp Car Crash Conference* (pp. 197–203). New York: Society of Automotive Engineers.

Ommaya, A.K., & Yarnell, P. (1969). Subdural hematoma after whiplash injury. *Lancet, 2*, 237–239.

Oppenheimer, D.R. (1968). Microscopic lesions in the brain following head injury. *Journal of Neurology, Neurosurgery and Psychiatry, 31*, 299–306.

Patten, B.M. (1968). How much blood makes the cerebrospinal fluid bloody? *JAMA (Journal of the American Medical Association), 206*, 278.

Prigatano, G.P., Stahl, M.L., Orr, W.C., & Zeiner, H.K. (1982). Sleep and dreaming disturbances in closed head injury patients. *Journal of Neurology, Neurosurgery and Psychiatry, 45*, 78–80.

Read, M.R. (1981). Post traumatic psychiatric manifestations and neuropsychiatrists (editorial). *Journal of Clinical Psychiatry, 43*, 3.

Rimel, R.W., Giordani, B., Barth, J.T., et al. (1981). Disability caused by minor head injury. *Neurosurgery, 9*, 221–228.

Rock, W.J., Drance, S.M., & Morgan, R.W. (1973). Visual field screening in glaucoma: An evaluation of the Armaly technique for screening visual fields. *Archives of Ophthalmology, 89*, 287–290.

Ron, S., Algom, D., Hary, D., Cohen, M. (1980). Time-related changes in the distribution of sleep stages in brain injured patients. *Electroencephalography and Clinical Neurophysiology, 48*, 432–441.

Rowe, M.J., & Carlson, C. (1980). Brainstem auditory evoked potentials in postconcussion dizziness. *Archives of Neurology, 37*, 679–683.

Ross, R.J., Cole, M., Thompson, J.S., & Kim, K.H. (1983). Boxers—computed tomography, EEG, and neurological evaluation. *JAMA (Journal of the American Medical Association), 249*, 211–213.

Scott, W.R., New, P.F., & Davis, K.R. (1974). Computerized axial tomography of intracerebral and intraventricular hemorrhage. *Radiology, 112*, 73–80.

Strich, S.J. (1956). Diffuse degeneration of the cerebral white matter in severe dementia following head injury. *Journal of Neurology, Neurosurgery and Psychiatry, 19*, 163–185.

Strich, S.J. (1961). Shearing of nerve fibers as a cause of brain damage due to head injury. A pathological study of twenty cases. *Lancet, 2,* 443–448.
Strich, S.J. (1970). Lesions in the cerebral hemispheres after blunt head injury. In S. Sevit & H.B. Stoner (Eds.), The pathology of trauma (pp. 116–171). London: BMA House.
Stuss, D.T., Ely, P., Hugenholtz, H., Richard, M.T., LaRochelle, S., Poinier, C.A., Bell, I. (1985). Subtle neuropsychological deficits in patients with good recovery after closed head injury. *Neurosurgery, 17,* 41–47.
Travell, J. (1967). Mechanical headache. *Headache 7*(1), 23–29.
Travell, J. (1976). Myofascial trigger points: Clinical view. In J.J. Bonica et al. (Eds.), *Advances in pain research and therapy* (Vol. 1, pp. 919-926). New York: Raven Press.
Travell, J., & Simmons, D.G. (1983). *Myofascial pain and dysfunction: The trigger point manual.* Baltimore: Williams & Wilkins.
Wall, M., & George, D. (1987). Visual loss in pseudotumor cerebri. *Archives of Neurology, 44,* 170–175.
Walsh, F.B. (1966). The pathological clinical correlations: 1. Indirect trauma to the optic nerve and chiasm. 2. Certain cerebral involvements associated with affected blood supply. *Investigative Ophthalmology, xx* (Oct.), 433–439.
Ward, J., & Jennings, E. (1973). *Introduction to linear models.* Englewood Cliffs, NJ: Prentice-Hall.
Weinstein, G.S., & Wells, C.E. (1981). Case studies in neuropsychiatry: Post-traumatic psychiatric dysfunction, diagnosis and treatment. *Journal of Clinical Psychiatry, 42,* 120–122.
Weiss, H.D., Stern, B.J., & Goldberg, J. (1984). Chronic migraine after minor head trauma. *109th Annual Meeting of the American Neurological Association*, Baltimore.
Wiedmann, K.D., Hadley, D.M., Wilson, J.T.L., Brooks, D.N., & Teasdale, G.M. (1987). Early and late magnetic resonance imaging of head injured patients as a predictor of neuropsychological outcome. *Journal of Clinical Experimental Neuropsychology 9*(1),29.
Wiggins, W.S., Moody, D.M., Toole, J.F., et al. (1978). Clinical and computerized tomographic study of hypertensive intracerebral hemorrhage. *Archives of Neurology, 35,* 832–833.
Wrightson, P., & Gronwall, D. (1981). Time off work and symptoms after minor head injury. *Injury (British Journal of Accident Surgery), 12*(6), 445–454.
Yarnell, P., & Ommaya, A.K. (1969). Experimental cerebral concussion in the rhesus monkey. *Bulletin of the New York Academy of Medicine, 45,* 39–45.
Zimmerman, R.A., Bilaniuk, L.T., Bruce, D., et al. (1978). Interhemispheric acute subdural hematoma: A computerized tomographic manifestation of child abuse by shaking. *Neuroradiology, 16,* 39–40.

Appendix 9.A. Head Injury Information Questionnaire

Exact and specific detail about the nature of your injury is very important in helping the doctor evaluate your injury. Please take the time to consider some of these specific questions.

Name ______________________ Age _____ Right or Left Handed _____

Highest grade you finished in school? ________________ What type of work do or did you do?: ____________ If Federal Employee, what GS level? ____

. . . .

1) Date of accident ____ Type Of Injury:
   - ☐ Auto (D P M S SB)
   - ☐ Happened at Work
   - ☐ Sports Injury (describe)
   - ☐ Fall/Something fell on my head
   - ☐ Attacked by someone

2) Is this your <u>first</u> accidental head or neck injury? If not, describe date of other(s) and whether you have <u>completely recovered</u> or have any lingering injury because of that.

3) Did you lose consciousness (black out, pass out)? For how long?

4) Did you hit your head? Steering wheel, windshield, or the back of your head hit the headrest?

5) If you did <u>not</u> lose consciousness did any of the following occur? Circle Yes answers.

   Saw stars   Confused   Threw up/Nauseated   Had a bad headache
   Dizzy   Lost my hearing   Vision funny

6) <u>Check</u> any of the following problems you have and <u>circle</u> its severity;

	Mild									Severe
☐ Headaches	1	2	3	4	5	6	7	8	9	10
☐ Memory/concentration	1	2	3	4	5	6	7	8	9	10
☐ Dizziness	1	2	3	4	5	6	7	8	9	10
☐ Neck/back pain	1	2	3	4	5	6	7	8	9	10
☐ Short temper/irritable	1	2	3	4	5	6	7	8	9	10
☐ Sensitive to light/noise	1	2	3	4	5	6	7	8	9	10
☐ Blurred vision	1	2	3	4	5	6	7	8	9	10
☐ Sleep disturbance	1	2	3	4	5	6	7	8	9	10
☐ Anxiety or depression	1	2	3	4	5	6	7	8	9	10
☐ Fatigue/tired	1	2	3	4	5	6	7	8	9	10

   ☐ Irregular menses/sex difficulties   ☐ Pain/numbness in arm or leg
   ☐ Hearing/ringins in ears

7) What other doctors are you seeing for your accident? ________________
   ____

8) What medicines are you taking? ________________________________

9) Who is your regular doctor? ______________________________

10) What medical conditions do you have? What medicine do you take for it? ______________________________

____

Note. The purpose this form is to help obtain details of the mechanics of injury and bring out information that the patient may think is "not important." It forces patients to reconstruct the events of their accident and the sequence of their symptoms. It is filled out during registration for their first consultation, before they see the doctor. The 10-point rating scale of severity was not included in the current retrospective study. Copyright 1987, Capitol Neurology.

10
Activation of Semantic Relations in Alzheimer's and Huntington's Disease

STAN SMITH, NELSON BUTTERS, and ERIC GRANHOLM

Recent studies have demonstrated that the memory disorders of patients with cortical (e.g., Alzheimer's disease) and subcortical (e.g., Huntington's disease) dementias involve different processing deficits. For example, whereas patients with dementia of the Alzheimer type (DAT) have unusual difficulty storing new information and are highly sensitive to proactive interference, patients with Huntington's disease (HD) are deficient in the initiation of retrieval strategies for searching short- and long-term memory (Butters, Granholm, Salmon, Grant, & Wolfe, in press). Although it is often stated that the organization of semantic memory may be altered in both cortical and, to a lesser degree, subcortical dementias (e.g., Cummings & Benson, 1984), few investigators have attempted to elucidate and compare the exact nature of these changes. In the present chapter, we review some recent investigations that focus on this issue and demonstrate that the deterioration of semantic memory in DAT and HD is markedly different.

In the most dominant theory of semantic representation (Collins & Loftus, 1975; Collins & Quillian, 1967), semantic memory is represented as a network of conceptual nodes. Each concept is linked to other concepts and their lexical representations by a variety of relationships (e.g., category membership, functional association), such that activation of one node representing a given concept automatically activates other related nodes in the network. Those nodes representing more highly associated concepts are more strongly activated than those representing less highly associated concepts. This differential activation, though transient, is maintained over a period of time and can have a facilitative effect on lexical access, as has been demonstrated by numerous priming studies (Loftus, 1973; McKoon & Ratcliffe, 1979; Meyer & Schvanaveldt, 1971).

Evaluations of language abilities in patients with Alzheimer's disease (Irigaray, 1973; Schwartz, Marin, & Saffran, 1979; Whitaker, 1976; Appell, Kertesz and Fisman, 1972) are consistent with the notion that DAT involves a disruption in this system of spreading activation among nodes. The word-finding difficulty in the earlier stages of DAT progresses to a fairly pronounced anomia in the middle and later stages of the disease. In its more advanced stages, DAT often mimics transcortical sensory and Wernicke's aphasias, both of which involve a severe loss of comprehension as well as, frequently, semantically "empty" speech production (Goodglass & Kaplan, 1972).

Further evidence from language assessments demonstrates impaired confrontation naming in patients with DAT (Bayles & Tomoeda, 1983), as well as a compromised ability to find the semantic similarity between lexical items (Miller, 1973). In addition, DAT patients are impaired in their ability to use semantic information to facilitate episodic memory (Corkin, 1982; Granholm & Butters, in press; Martin, Brouwers, Cox, & Fedio, 1987). For example, in a study by Granholm and Butters (in press), patients with DAT were unable to exploit semantic relations between associated word pairs to facilitate verbal recall. Finally, DAT patients are impaired in their ability to generate members of a category (Butters, Granholm, et al., 1987; Weingartner et al., 1981), even though letter fluency may be relatively preserved in the early stages of DAT (Butters, Granholm, et al., 1987).

The above findings have led a number of investigators (Bayles, 1982; Martin & Fedio, 1983; Schwartz et al., 1979) to suggest that DAT involves a breakdown in the structure and usage of semantic knowledge. Such a deterioration could reflect a disruption in the system of cortical activation that represents semantic memory. This proposal is consistent with neuropathological evidence that DAT is characterized by widespread damage to cortical brain areas, including the entorhinal region and temporoparietal association cortices (Hyman, Van Hoesen, Damasio, & Barnes, 1984; Terry & Davies, 1980; Whitehouse et al., 1982).

Despite the problems that DAT patients have with semantic processing, orthographic and phonological (as well as grammatical) processing abilities appear to remain relatively intact through the early and middle stages of the disease. In fact, orthophonemic processing may be preserved even in advanced stages of DAT, as is dramatically demonstrated in a case reported by Schwartz et al. (1979). These investigators described a profoundly demented patient who could correctly read aloud a wide range of words having inconsistent or exceptional spelling-sound relations (leopard, shoe, flood, tortoise, etc.), even when she was not able to match the written or spoken word to the appropriate object, or even to determine whether the word denoted an animal or nonliving thing.

In contrast with DAT, the dementia of HD is believed to largely spare language abilities, particularly semantic representation, at least during the early and middle stages of the disease (Butters, Sax, Montgomery, & Tarlow, 1978; Josiassen, Curry, & Mancall, 1983; Josiassen, Curry, Roemer, DeBease, & Mancall, 1982). Although HD involves deficits in memory, problem solving, visuoperceptive processing, and spatial and arithmetical reasoning (Brouwers, Cox, Martin, Chase, & Fedio, 1984; Butters, 1984; Butters, Albert, & Sax 1979; Caine, Hunt, Weingartner, & Ebert, 1978; Fedio et al., 1979), most of the HD patient's language difficulties are believed to be linked to a dysarthria that worsens as the disease progresses. This apparent sparing of language is rather striking in light of a number of investigations (Cappa, Cavallotti, Guidotti, Papagno, & Vignolo, 1983; Damasio, Damasio, Rizzo, Varney, & Gersh, 1982; Naeser et al., 1982;

Sterzi & Vallar, 1978; Wallesch et al., 1983) that have demonstrated that left unilateral lesions of the basal ganglia involved in HD (e.g., caudate nuclei, putamen) may result in aphasia or quasi-aphasic language deficits.

Although investigators agree that language is largely spared in moderately demented HD patients, several recent studies (Butters, Wolfe, Granholm, & Martone, 1986; Josiassen et al., 1982; Mildworf & Albert, 1978) have reported impaired performance among HD patients on tasks that involve lexical access or that require knowledge about specific semantic relations between lexical items. Such tasks include the Boston Naming Test and Body Parts Test (Mildworf & Albert, 1978) from the Boston Diagnostic Aphasia Examination (Goodglass & Kaplan, 1972), the Comprehension and Similarities subtests of the Wechsler Adult Intelligence Scale–Revised (WAIS-R) (Josiassen et al., 1982), and tests of verbal fluency (Butters et al., 1986). Similar deficits on category and word fluency tests, and in the production of synonyms and antonyms, have also been demonstrated in patients with left unilateral lesions of the basal ganglia (Wallesch et al., 1983).

The above findings suggest that, despite the absence of frank aphasia, there may be some deterioration of the lexicosemantic representational system in HD. However, the above-cited language deficits in HD are usually attributed to general performance factors (i.e., excess processing demands). Butters et al. (1986), for example, have suggested that impaired performance of early HD patients on tests of verbal fluency may result from a difficulty in initiating and maintaining a systematic search of semantic memory. Similarly, tests like the Similarities subtest from the WAIS-R may be attributed to an impaired ability to perform operations on acquired knowledge (Brandt & Butters, 1986).

More recently, a similar line of reasoning has been used to argue that the DAT patient's apparent loss of semantic representation may be explained in terms of excess processing demands. For example, Nebes, Martin, and Horn (1984) proposed that impaired semantic processing in DAT may be attributed to attentional deficits (Corkin, 1982; Miller, 1973). This explanation is most applicable to those tasks that require patients to make conscious decisions about the semantic features of stimuli, to organize items according to their semantic relationships, or to actively search their memories for specified semantic information.

In an attempt to minimize demands on active working memory, Nebes et al. (1984) employed a verbal priming paradigm that assessed the intactness of semantic networks in patients with mild DAT. Naming latencies to target words were measured under two conditions: 1) when the word was preceded by a semantic associate (e.g., doctor-nurse), and 2) when it was preceded by an unrelated word (e.g., shoe-nurse). In this paradigm, any decrease in the amount of processing time from the unrelated to the related condition reflects facilitation produced by spreading activation between concepts in the semantic network. Because priming is largely automatic (Hasher & Zacks, 1979; Posner & Snyder, 1975), it places little processing load on working memory. Hence, if semantic representation is preserved in DAT, Alzheimer patients should benefit as much as do normal intact subjects from semantic priming. Nebes et al.'s results were consistent with this expectation. Although DAT required significantly more time to pronounce tachistoscopically presented words than did intact controls, the amount of facilitation produced by semantic primes was equal for both groups.

A limitation to the generalizability of the above finding involves Nebes et al.'s exclusive use of strong semantic associates. Less highly associated word pairs might produce little or no priming effects in patients with DAT. A further restriction involves the interval between presentation of primes and target words. In Nebes et al.'s study, target items were always presented *immediately* following the disappearance of primes. This lack of delay conditions might mask evidence that activation of semantic relations may be more transient in DAT patients than in normal processors, regardless of whether such activation is elicited by automatic or attentional processes.

In a more recent investigation, Nebes, Boller, and Holland (1986) evaluated mildly demented patients with DAT on three tasks that assessed the effect of semantic context on lexical access. On a sentence priming task, DAT patients and intact control subjects showed comparable facilitative effects of congruous semantic contexts. However, DAT patients were impaired in their ability to *generate* appropriate last words for sentences, except when highly constraining semantic contexts were available. Notably, an *inhibitory* effect of *incongruous* semantic contexts on DAT patients' response latencies for the sentence priming test was attributed to a conscious, conceptually driven response strategy. The existence of such a strategy would suggest that DAT patients are able to access semantic representations in some situations that involve effortful processing. Finally, on a category decision task, the dominance (i.e., degree of association) of word pairs affected response times of DAT patients as much as those of intact control subjects. However, a positive response bias of DAT patients on this task obscures potential conclusions regarding the preservation of semantic representation in DAT.

The above findings suggest that the extent to which semantic representation appears to be preserved in dementia is highly task dependent. That is, the degree to which demented patients are impaired on verbal performance tasks may depend on a number of factors in addition to demands on active working memory. Hence, an understanding of the nature of changes that occur in semantic representation with the progression of dementia may require an evaluation of demented patients' semantic processing under a *variety* of conditions.

Two recently completed investigations from our laboratory have focused on the organization of semantic memory in DAT and HD. The first of these studies (Smith, Butters, White, Lyon, & Granholm, in press) evaluated HD patients' performance on a brief battery of language tests and on a semantic priming task. The second (Salmon, Shimamura, Butters, & Smith, in press) analyzes DAT and HD patients' performance on both lexical and semantic priming tests. The remainder of this chapter deals with these studies' findings and their theoretical implications regarding the nature of semantic representation in dementia.

Lexicosemantic Processing in HD

The investigation of Smith et al. (in press) yielded two kinds of evidence regarding a possible degeneration in the organization of semantic representation in HD. The first originated from an analysis of HD patients' performance on a short battery of language tests, which included tests of confrontation naming, category and letter fluency, and vocabulary. The second form of evidence emanated from an experiment that employed a free-association paradigm in which semantic relations between stimulus and target words were either primed or not primed. In addition, the strength and type of relation between stimulus and target words were varied systematically in two ways: First, half of the target words were strongly associated with their corresponding stimulus items, while the other half were only moderately related. This type of manipulation has also been used with amnesic patients (Gardner, Boller, Moreines, & Butters, 1973). Second, half of the stimulus-target pairs bore a category-exemplar relationship (e.g., animal-dog), while the other half were related functionally, that is, had complementary roles in a function-action sequence (e.g., soup-spoon). Since both free association and priming are primarily automatic (Hasher & Zacks, 1979; Posner & Snyder, 1975), they do not require active manipulation of knowledge or a systematic search of semantic memory. Hence, processing demands were minimized in this investigation.

Thirty-three subjects participated in the study: 21 patients with Huntington's disease and 12 neurologically intact, normal control subjects. The HD patients had been diagnosed by a senior staff neurologist on the basis of a positive family history and the presence of choreiform movements. The patients were divided into mildly demented (MI-HD) and moderately demented (MO-HD) groups. Group membership was determined by the patient's score on a recent administration of the Dementia Rating Scale (DRS) (Mattis, 1976). Patients scoring above 123 (maximum score = 144) were included in the MI-HD group (N = 10) and the remaining patients formed the MO-HD group (N = 11). The 12 normal controls (mean DRS = 141.3) were recruited from fraternal and religious organizations in the community. Respondents with a history of alcoholism, drug abuse, learning disabilities, or serious neurological or psychiatric disorders were excluded.

Table 10.1 shows the mean age, years of education, and DRS scores for the three subject groups. Analysis of variance indicated no significant differences between groups in age or education. There were, however, significant differences in DRS scores between intact controls and MI-HD patients, between intact control subjects and MO-HD patients, and between MI-HD and MO-HD patients. Shoulson's (1981) Functional Disability Scale, which rates HD patients on a 5-point scale (1 = minimal disability; 5 = maximum disability), was used to judge the stage of the illness. The mean stages for the MI-HD and MO-HD patient groups were 2.5 and 2.7, respectively. Although all of the patients in Stages 3 and 4 were dysarthric to some degree, all were sufficiently articulate to participate in the study.

TABLE 10.1. Demographic and psychometric characteristics of the three subject groups.

Group	Age	Years of education	DRS score
Normal control	56.1	13.0	141.3
(*N*=12)	(10.0)	(1.7)	(2.5)
Mild HD	51.2	12.2	130.9
(*N*=10)	(15.8)	(1.6)	(5.6)
Moderate HD	54.6	12.8	113.0
(*N*=11)	(17.4)	(2.5)	(7.2)

Note. Numbers represent the mean; numbers in parentheses represent standard deviation.

Battery of Language Tests

The language assessment included tests of letter fluency (FAS) (Benton, 1968), a test of category fluency from the Boston Diagnostic Aphasia Examination (Goodglass & Kaplan, 1972), the Boston Naming Test (Kaplan, Goodglass, & Weintraub, 1983), and the WAIS-R vocabulary subtest (Wechsler, 1981). For the letter fluency test, subjects were read the letters *F*, *A*, and *S* successively and asked to produce as many words as they could think of beginning with the given letter. Similarly, for the category fluency test, subjects were asked to produce as many different animal names as possible. For the Boston Naming Test, subjects were shown a series of pictorially depicted objects and asked to name them. Scores were assigned on the basis of the number of correct spontaneous and cued responses. Finally, for the Vocabulary subtest from the WAIS-R, subjects were presented with a series of 35 words, one at a time, and asked to provide definitions for the words. Each definition was given a score (0, 1, 2) based on standardized preestablished criteria (Wechsler, 1981).

The results of the language tests are shown in Table 10.2. Group comparisons showed that on the letter fluency (FAS) test both the mild HD and moderate HD groups performed significantly worse than did age-matched intact controls. In addition, performance of MO-HD patients was significantly worse than that of MI-HD patients. A similar pattern was found for the category fluency test. Both MI-HD and MO-HD patients named significantly fewer animals than did control subjects, and the MO-HD patients performed significantly worse than the MI-HD patients. This result replicated previous findings (Butters et al., 1986) that HD patients' impairments on tests of verbal fluency are evident quite early in the disease process. It should be noted that HD patients' impaired performance on tests of verbal fluency cannot be attributed to the patients' dysarthria. The HD patients who participated in this study were only mildly dysarthric, and all of their responses were generated in the first 35 to 40 seconds of the allotted 60 seconds. If the impaired verbal fluency of HD patients were due to dysarthria, the distribution of responses would likely have been equal throughout the 60-second period.

TABLE 10.2. Measures of language function.

Group	Letter fluency (FAS)	Category fluency (animals)	Boston Naming Test	WAIS-R Vocabulary[a]
Normal control ($N=12$)	45.8[b] (17.1)	19.4[c] (4.0)	56.3[c] (2.4)	12.6 (1.7)
Mild HD ($N=10$)	23.5 (8.6)	11.8 (2.7)	52.4 (5.3)	9.0[d] (2.0)
Moderate HD ($N=11$)	13.3 (6.4)	8.1 (3.1)	41.4 (9.4)	7.3 (1.7)

Note. Numbers represent the mean; numbers in parentheses represent standard deviation.
[a] Scaled scores.
[b] $N=11$.
[c] $N=10$.
[d] $N=9$.

On the Boston Naming Test, both groups of HD patients performed significantly more poorly than did the intact control subjects, and the MO-HD patients named significantly fewer items than did the MI-HD patients. This finding provided further evidence, along with results of previous studies (Bayles & Tomoeda, 1983; Mildworf & Albert, 1978), that HD patients are mildly impaired in confrontation naming. A similar pattern of results was evident from analysis of the groups' performances on the WAIS-R Vocabulary subtest. Scaled scores of both the MI-HD and MO-HD groups were significantly lower than those of intact control subjects. In addition, scaled scores of MO-HD patients were lower than those of MI-HD patients, although this difference just approached statistical significance.

The overall results of the language tests are consistent with the notion that HD patients are impaired on certain tasks that involve lexical access, or that require knowledge of specific semantic properties of words (Butters et al., 1986; Josiassen et al., 1982). Although these data seem to suggest that HD may involve a breakdown in the organization of lexical-semantic representation, it is not possible to rule out the possible influence of general performance factors (e.g., active retrieval processes). Even a confrontation naming task requires an active search of semantic memory, and a test like the WAIS-R Vocabulary subtest requires an active manipulation of acquired knowledge. Since the semantic priming paradigm involved far less processing demands, it provided a better index of the organization of semantic memory in HD.

SEMANTIC PRIMING

In order to generate functionally related word pairs (e.g., soup-spoon), each of 24 stimulus words from the Minnesota Word Association Norms (Jenkins, 1970) was paired with a strongly associated (ranks 1–3) and a moderately associated (ranks 8–11) response item. Similarly, to create categorically related word pairs (e.g., bird-robin), each of 24 category superordinates from the Battig and

Montague (1969) category norms was paired with a strongly associated (ranks 1–3) and a moderately associated (ranks 8–11) exemplar. Finally, six unrelated word pairs were created to control for the possibility that subjects would respond with target words on the free-association task, not because an existing semantic association had been primed, but simply because the two words had been presented together.

The priming test was administered in three identical blocks, each composed of a rating and a free-association task. On the rating task, subjects were asked to rate 12 visually presented word pairs on a scale ranging from 1 (not related) to 5 (strongly related). Studies conducted within a levels-of-processing framework (Craik & Lockhart, 1972; Craik & Tulving, 1975) have shown that this type of manipulation facilitates the maintenance of activation of semantic information in normal individuals. Each group of 12 word pairs (4 categorical, 4 functional, 2 unrelated, and 2 filler) was presented in the same order to each subject twice in succession. Of the category-exemplar and functional pairs, half of each type were strongly associated, while the other half were moderately associated. A comparison of means and standard deviations of rating scores indicated that groups did not differ with respect to the way they approached the task.

Immediately following the rating task, subjects were shown the first words of categorical, functional, and unrelated pairs presented during the rating task and asked to free associate to them (i.e., "Say the first word that comes to mind"). In addition, to establish nonprimed hit rates, the first words from eight strongly and moderately associated categorical and functional pairs that had not appeared in the rating task were presented. Use of stimulus words for primed and nonprimed conditions was counterbalanced across subjects.

In assessing the organization of semantic representation in HD patients, the most pertinent results from this experiment involved group comparisons on hit rates for the *primed* condition of the free-association task. (It should be noted that the groups did not differ with respect to general nonprimed response biases.) First, all three subject groups (intact control subjects, MI-HD patients, and MO-HD patients) showed positive priming effects regardless of the strength of association or type of relation between word pairs. Since target hits for unrelated pairs were rare and isolated, it is not likely that these effects resulted from a conscious recall strategy. More importantly, collapsed across all other variables, intact subjects, MI-HD patients, and MO-HD patients primed equally well (see Figure 10.1). In processing terms, there were no overall group differences in the degree to which enhanced activation of connections between nodes was maintained from the priming task to the free-association task.

The above finding, alone, would seem to indicate that semantic representation remains intact throughout the mild-to-moderate stages of HD. However, although the type of relationship (i.e., functional, categorical) between words did not prove to be significant for any of the subject groups, group differences in the effect of association strength (i.e., strong, moderate) on subjects' hit rates suggest that HD may result in subtle changes in the organization of semantic activation. Specifically, there was a trend toward reduction in the magnitude of strength

FIGURE 10.1. Overall primed hit rates for each of the three subject groups. The dotted line represents the mean hit rate for nonprimed words. NC = normal controls; MI-HD = mildly demented patients with Huntington's disease; MO-HD = moderately demented patients with Huntington's disease.

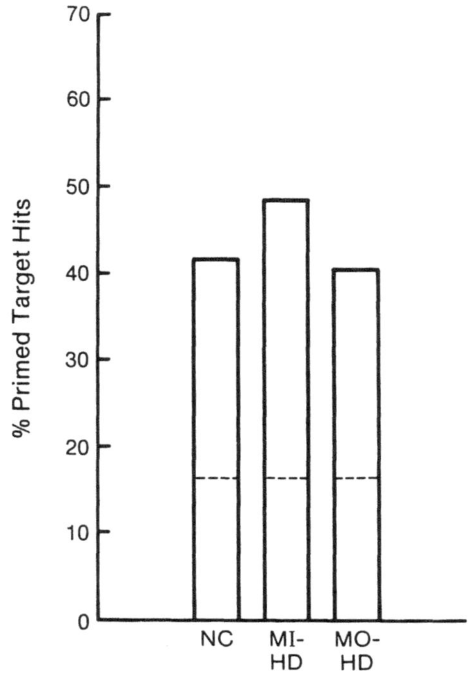

effects from intact control subjects, to MI-HD subjects, to MO-HD subjects. Figure 10.2 shows hit rates for target items from strongly associated pairs and moderately associated pairs for each of the three subject groups. For intact subjects, there was a difference of 37% between hit rates for target items from strongly associated pairs and those from moderately associated pairs. This difference was 30% for the MI-HD group, and for the MO-HD group it was only 16%.

The reported reduction in magnitude of strength effects is due not only to an apparent tendency among HD patients to show *decreased* priming effects for *strongly* associated pairs with the progression of the disease, but also to an apparent tendency for HD patients to show *larger* priming effects, relative to intact subjects, for *moderately* associated pairs. As can be seen in Figure 10.2, there was a reduction in the MO-HD group, relative to intact and MI-HD subjects, in hit rates for strongly associated pairs. Normal control subjects, MI-HD patients, and MO-HD patients had hit rates of 60%, 63%, and 48%, respectively, for this condition. However, there was also a difference between groups in hit rates for moderately associated pairs, for which normal subjects were lower (23%) than either the MI-HD group (33%) or the MO-HD group (32%). Post-hoc comparisons indicated that these differences represented an *overall* decline, across the three subject groups (intact controls, MI-HD, and MO-HD) in the degree to which associative strengths of word pairs affected subjects' hit rates.

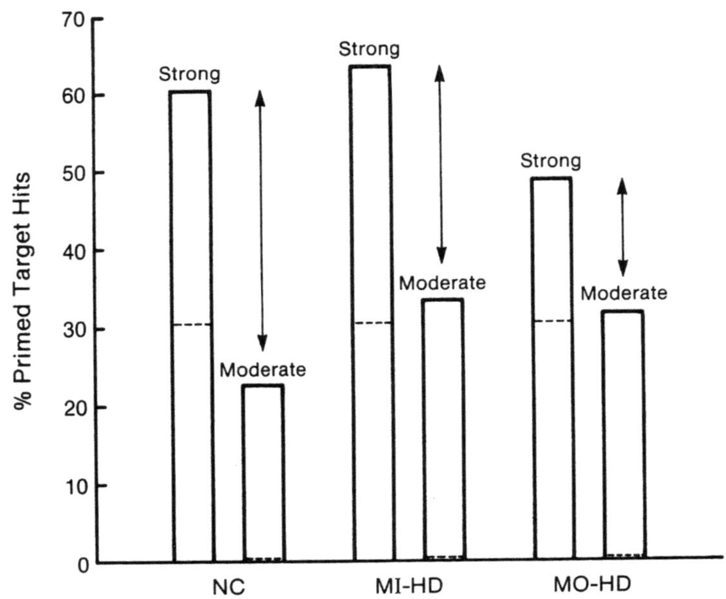

FIGURE 10.2. Primed hit rates for strongly and moderately associated word pairs for each subject group. Dotted lines represent hit rates for nonprimed words. NC = normal controls; MI-HD = mildly demented patients with Huntington's disease; MO-HD = moderately demented patients with Huntington's disease.

This finding, along with the results of the language tests, provides evidence that HD involves some breakdown in the organization of lexicosemantic representation. Specifically, although HD patients showed no impairment in their ability to prime per se, there was a progressive decline among HD patients in the degree to which association strengths of word pairs affected priming of semantic relations. This change represents a qualitative difference between subjects in the way activation of semantic relations is initiated and maintained over a period of time. Although these results do not support the view that HD involves an actual *loss* of representation of concepts in semantic networks, they are consistent with the notion that the dementia of HD involves a deterioration in the system of *activation* of concepts and relations in a network.

Lexical and Semantic Priming in DAT

Salmon et al.'s (in press) study evaluated DAT and HD patients' performance on two kinds of priming tasks: The first was a lexical priming (i.e., stem completion) task in which subjects are exposed to a list of words (e.g., *motel, abstain*) and then asked simply to say the first word that comes to mind in response to orthophonemic cues (i.e., three-letter stems, such as *mot, abs*). The second experiment made use of the semantic priming paradigm employed by Smith et al. in the first study reviewed in this paper. As in the prior study, a free-association task was preceded by a rating task that specifically, though implicitly, elicits activation of semantic relations between word pairs. Again, the strength and type of relation between stimulus and target words were varied.

Like the semantic priming study by Nebes et al. (1984), both the stem-completion and free-association experiments made use of automatic processing paradigms in order to minimize processing loads. However, an important difference between these experiments and the one reported by Nebes et al. involved the elapsed time between priming and testing phases. That is, Nebes et al. presented target words to subjects immediately following presentation of stimulus words, whereas in Salmon et al.'s experiments, priming effects depended on the *maintenance* of activation across a period of several minutes.

Stem Completion

Fifty-five subjects participated in the stem-completion part of this study: 13 patients with DAT were matched for age and education with 13 nonneurologically impaired control subjects. In addition, 8 patients with HD were matched with 8 intact control subjects. Finally, 7 patients with alcoholic Korsakoff's syndrome (KS) were matched with 6 alcoholic controls.

For DAT subjects, a diagnosis of probable DAT was made by a senior staff neurologist according to criteria developed by the National Institute of Neurological and Communicative Disorders and Stroke (NINCDS) and the Alzheimer's Disease and Related Disorders Association (ADRDA) (McCann et al., 1984). All DAT patients were mildly to moderately demented, with a score of at least 102 out of a possible 144 points on the Dementia Rating Scale (DRS) (Mattis, 1976). For HD patients, the same diagnostic criteria used in Smith et al.'s (in press) study were again employed. The 7 KS patients had an extensive history of alcoholism and malnutrition prior to an acute onset of Wernicke's encephalopathy. Although they were severely amnesic (both anterograde and retrograde), the KS patients were relatively intact in terms of other cognitive functions. In all cases, the KS patients' intelligence quotient was at least 20 points higher than their memory quotient. The 6 alcoholics were current or former participants in alcohol treatment programs in San Diego County. The mean age, years of education, and the DRS scores of the three patient groups and their respective control groups are shown in Table 10.3.

The stem-completion task was administered as follows: Each subject was shown 10 words (e.g., *motel, abstain*), each of which was printed on a separate 3 × 5-inch card, and asked to rate how much they liked each word on a 5-point scale (1 = like extremely, 5 = dislike extremely). In order to reduce primacy and recency effects, five additional filler words were presented—three at the beginning of the list and two at the end. This rating task was repeated with the same words presented in the same order. Following the rating task, subjects were shown 20 three-letter stems (e.g., *mot, abs*) and asked to complete each stem

TABLE 10.3. Mean age, years of education, and Dementia Rating Scale scores of the three patient and control groups in the stem-completion experiment.

	DAT (N = 13)	DAT CON (N = 13)	HD (N = 8)	HD CON (N = 8)	KS (N = 7)	KS CON (N = 6)
Age	71.2 (7.5)	66.5 (5.5)	48.8 (10.5)	49.4 (8.2)	53.6 (9.2)	50.3 (6.2)
ED	12.4 (2.4)	14.0 (2.3)	13.1 (2.0)	13.5 (2.1)	11.0 (1.5)	12.5 (1.8)
DRS	116.6 (10.8)	139.5[a] (2.5)	121.8 (10.8)	142.0[b] (1.6)	128.3 (8.8)	138.7 (4.0)

Note. ED = years of education; DRS = Dementia Rating Scale; CON = control group; DAT = dementia of the Alzheimer type; HD = Huntington's disease; KS = Korsakoff's syndrome. Standard deviations are presented in parentheses.
[a] N=12.
[b] N=7.

"with the first word that comes to mind." Of the 20 stems, 10 could be completed using words that had appeared in the rating task. The other 10 were used to assess baseline (nonprimed) hit rates, and were used as target stems for other subjects. There were at least 10 possible words that could be used to complete the stem, one of which had been presented in the rating task. The entire rating task/stem-completion procedure was then repeated using 10 different target words.

Figure 10.3 shows primed and nonprimed hit rates on stem-completion for each of the patient and matched control groups. Subject groups did not differ with respect to *nonprimed* target hit rates, indicating that none of the patient groups was impaired in the ability to perform the basic task of completing three-letter stems with words. However, hit rates for *primed* targets were significantly worse for DAT and HD patients than for matched intact control subjects. In addition, the primed stem-completion performance of DAT patients was significantly worse than that of either of the other two patient groups. As anticipated on the basis of a previous report (Shimamura, Salmon, Squire, & Butters, 1987), KS patients showed normal priming on this task.

The finding that HD patients have a mild deficit on stem-completion priming seems to conflict with a previous report (Shimamura et al., 1987) of intact performance in this patient population. This difference may be at least partly attributed to elevated priming scores obtained by control subjects in this study, relative to those of control subjects in Shimamura et al.'s study. This seems especially likely in view of the fact that priming scores for HD patients were comparable across experiments in the two studies (this experiment: completion = 44.3%, baseline = 9.4%; Shimamura et al.'s experiment: completion = 41.3%, baseline = 10%).

In contrast to the HD patients, the DAT patients' impairments on stem-completion priming were unequivocal. Although DAT and HD patients had similar levels of overall dementia (as judged by DRS scores) and of deficiency on

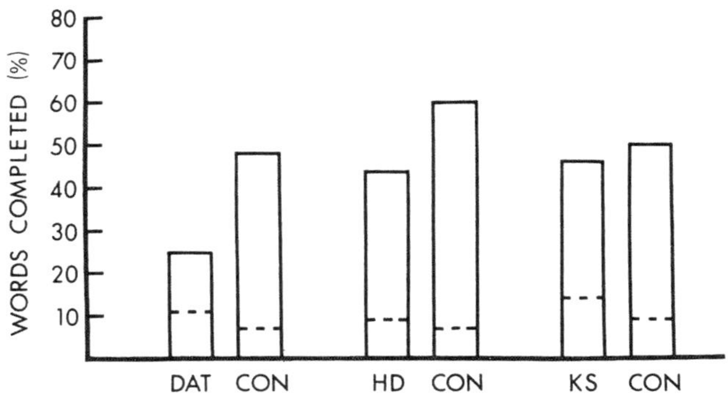

FIGURE 10.3. Percentage of target words completed for patient and matched control groups on stem-completion priming. Dotted lines represent hit rates for nonprimed words. DAT = dementia of the Alzheimer type; CON = controls; HD = Huntington's disease; KS = Korsahoff's syndrome.

verbal recall and recognition tests, the DAT patients performed significantly more poorly than did the HD patients on the stem-completion task. This priming deficit is somewhat surprising in light of the observation that orthographic and phonemic levels of representation are relatively spared in DAT (Bayles, 1982; Whitaker, 1976), an observation that is borne out by DAT patients' lack of impairment in their ability to generate words from stems. The impairment is even more striking when one considers that stem-completion priming is automatic and makes minimal processing demands on active working memory. Apparently, automaticity alone is not a sufficient condition for normal processing in patients with DAT.

One possible explanation for the DAT patients' severe impairment is that stem-completion priming depends on the activation of *semantic* representations of lexical items. This proposal is consistent with findings of studies conducted within a *levels-of-processing* framework that show that, for normal processors, maintenance of semantically encoded material in memory is superior to that of phonemically encoded material (Craik & Lockhart, 1972; Craik & Tulving, 1975). In processing terms, the maintenance of activation of a lexical representation may depend on the activation of a corresponding network of concepts and relations in semantic memory. Accordingly, the failure of DAT patients to show priming effects in the stem-completion experiment might reflect organizational changes in semantic representation or even an actual shrinkage of semantic networks (Bayles & Tomoeda, 1983; Martin et al., 1987). An alternative explanation for the DAT patients' deficits on the stem-completion task assumes that this failure reflects an inability to *spontaneously* use semantic criteria for encoding lexical material, even though semantic networks remain intact. Thus, a procedure that specifically elicits activation of semantic relations may result in normal priming effects for patients with DAT. This question was further explored in the semantic priming study reported in the following section.

TABLE 10.4. Mean age, years of education, and Dementia Rating Scale scores of the patient and control groups in the second semantic priming experiment.

	DAT (N = 9)	ENC (N = 9)	HD (N = 10)	MNC (N = 10)
Age	71.4 (5.9)	71.4 (5.3)	51.9 (15.8)	49.9 (10.6)
ED	13.0 (2.6)	13.0 (2.8)	13.3 (2.0)	13.1 (1.7)
DRS	118.5 (11.1)	138.6 (3.2)	113.1 (7.6)	141.6 (2.1)

Note. ED = years of education; DRS = Dementia Rating Scale; CON = control group; DAT = dementia of the Alzheimer type; HD = Huntington's disease; ENC = elderly normal controls; MNC = middle-age normal controls. Standard deviations are presented in parentheses.

SEMANTIC PRIMING

Nine patients with DAT and 10 patients with HD participated in this experiment, along with 9 intact elderly control subjects matched to DAT patients for age and education, and 10 middle-age control subjects similarly matched to the HD group. The criteria for selection of HD and DAT subjects, as well as for intact normal control subjects, were identical to those reported for the stem-completion experiment. Table 10.4 shows the mean age, years of education, and DRS score for each subject group. The DRS scores of DAT (mean = 118.5) and HD (mean = 113.5) groups were significantly lower than those of their respective control groups (mean DRS scores for elderly and middle-age control subjects were 138.6 and 141.6, respectively). However, the DRS scores of DAT patients and HD patients were not significantly different.

Materials and administration procedures for the semantic priming test were the same as those reported for the study on semantic priming in HD discussed in the previous section of this chapter (Smith et al., in press). It is important to note that DAT patients, HD patients, and intact control subjects did not differ in the way they approached the rating task, since means and standard deviations of rating scores for each of the four subject groups did not differ significantly. In addition, there were no significant differences between subject groups in *nonprimed* hit rates on the free-association task, for which all subject groups showed a significant effect of association strength. For the *primed* condition of the free-association task, target hits from previously presented *unrelated* pairs were extremely rare and isolated, indicating that subjects in all groups treated the task as one of free association, rather than adopting a conscious recall strategy.

Figure 10.4 shows the percentage of *primed* target hits for each subject group. Patients with DAT had a significantly lower hit rate than any of the other subject

FIGURE 10.4. Overall primed hit rates for each subject group in the second semantic priming experiment. Dotted lines represent hit rates for nonprimed words. ENC = elderly normal controls; DAT = dementia of the Alzheimer type; MNC = middle-age normal controls; HD = Huntington's disease.

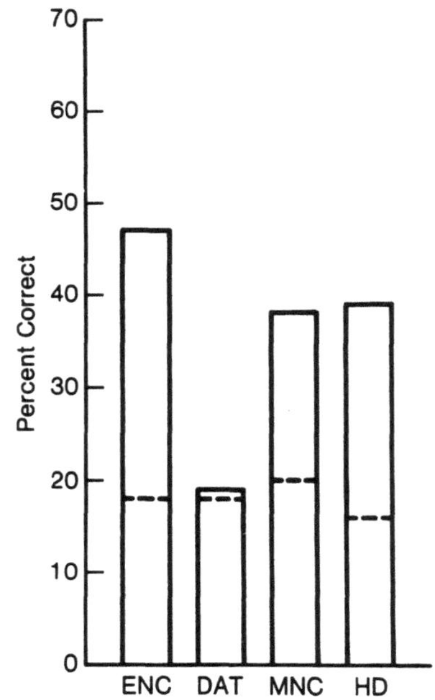

groups. In fact, DAT patients failed to exhibit any significant effect of priming whatsoever. In contrast, as in Smith et al.'s study, patients with Huntington's disease did not differ significantly from intact control subjects in their *overall* primed response rates, and evidenced a reduction in the magnitude of strength effects on primed hit rates.

Because of the automatic nature of both priming and free association (Hasher & Zacks, 1979; Posner & Snyder, 1975), the failure of DAT patients to show normal priming effects cannot be attributed to excess processing demands. Since DAT patients did not differ from normal control subjects in the nonprimed conditions of the free-association and stem-completion tasks, it is unlikely that the poor performance of patients with DAT is due to a problem with lexical access per se. Rather, the DAT patients' difficulty seems to lie in an inability to *maintain* the activation of semantic relations across a period of time (several minutes in this case).

Incorporated in a levels-of-processing framework is the empirically supported assumption that, within a given domain (e.g., semantic, phonemic), memory strength is proportional to the number of attributes and features encoded for to-be-remembered material (Craik & Tulving, 1975; Klein & Saltz, 1976). Accordingly, the failure of DAT patients to show priming effects on the free-association task is consistent with the proposal that DAT involves a breakdown in activation (or loss of representation) of attributes and features that relate and differentiate concepts in a semantic network. This interpretation is supported by the observation that DAT patients are impaired in their ability to distinguish between semantically related words within a category (Martin & Fedio, 1983; Schwartz et al., 1979; Warrington, 1975).

A related proposal has been made by Martin and his colleagues (1987), who suggest that a compromised ability to encode attributes of concepts may contribute to impaired performance of DAT patients on tests of conscious verbal recall. This is consistent with a finding of Granholm and Butters (in press) that DAT patients are unable to exploit semantic relations between words to facilitate episodic memory. However, the demands that conscious recall tasks place on processing resources prevent conclusions regarding structural changes that may occur in the semantic representational systems of DAT patients. In contrast, the present study provides substantial evidence for a breakdown of semantic representation in DAT.

General Discussion and Conclusions

The results of the studies reviewed in this paper provide evidence for contrasting semantic processing deficits in DAT and HD. First, we reviewed some evidence of a possible disorganization of semantic representation in HD. An evaluation of HD patients' performance on language tests involving lexical access or requiring knowledge of specific semantic properties of words was consistent with earlier findings (e.g., Butters et al., 1986; Josiassen et al., 1982) that there is a general performance deficit among HD patients on tests of this nature. Although these results suggest that there is a disruption of semantic representation in HD, the particular processing demands of each of the language tests in the battery (Brandt & Butters, 1986; Butters et al., 1986) reduce the certainty of this conclusion.

Less equivocal evidence for a breakdown in the organization of semantic representation in HD was provided by an analysis of HD patients' performance on a semantic priming test in which processing demands were minimized. The pattern of performance displayed by HD patients on this test represents substantial evidence for a degeneration in the system of spreading activation in semantic networks. Specifically, although HD patients showed no impairment in their ability to prime per se on either the stem-completion or semantic priming test, there was a progressive decline among HD patients in the degree to which the association strength of word pairs influenced the priming of semantic relations. Thus, HD patients and intact subjects differ in the way activation of semantic relations is initiated and maintained over a period of time.

To demonstrate how a breakdown in the organization of semantic networks can account for HD patients' pattern of performance on the semantic priming test, Smith et al. (in press) described a model that incorporates aspects of *interaction activation* (McClelland & Rumelhart, 1981; Rumelhart & McClelland, 1982). In such a model, the various connections representing relations between conceptual nodes in a semantic network have varying *resting levels* of activation. These resting levels may be influenced by a variety of factors, including frequency and recency of activation and can be elevated temporarily. In priming, for example, the resting level of activation for a particular relation or concept is temporarily elevated, such that less subsequent activation is required to activate it beyond a threshold level.

Since HD patients did not differ from intact control subjects in hit rates for *non-primed* targets, it is not likely that group differences reported for the effect of association strength stem from general *long-term* differences between HD patients and normal processors in resting levels of activation of semantic relations. Rather, group differences seem to originate from differential effects of association strength on the extent to which resting levels of activation were *temporarily* elevated and/or maintained. One possible explanation for this effect may involve group differences in the role of *inhibition* in processing.

In an interactive activation model, as a given relation is activated, there is a proportionate inhibition of competing concepts or relations. When relations between strongly related words are primed, as in the rating task of the semantic priming study, the effects are twofold: Not only are the resting levels of activation strongly elevated for these relations, but also there is a strong *inhibition* of activation for *competing* relations. This inhibition, in turn, results in a reduction of inhibition *received* from competing relations, thereby *facilitating* priming effects for strongly related word pairs. In contrast, when relations between moderately associated pairs are primed, not only is there *less elevation* of the resting level of activation of the relation, but also *less inhibition* of activation for competing relations (e.g., relations between one of the words and more strongly associated items). Therefore, primed relations between moderately associated words are more susceptible to inhibition from those competing relations, resulting in an inhibition of priming effects for moderately associated word pairs. A progressive breakdown in this system of simultaneous activation and inhibition would result in a decline in the degree to which association strengths of word pairs affects semantic priming (i.e., the pattern of performance displayed by HD patients in the studies reviewed in this chapter).

The analysis of DAT patients' performance on lexical (stem-completion) and semantic priming tasks yielded evidence of a severe semantic processing deficit. The failure of DAT patients to show normal priming effects on either of these tasks demonstrates that semantic processing in DAT is impaired even under conditions that minimize demands on processing resources. More importantly, these results also provide substantial evidence for a deterioration of semantic representation in DAT. Specifically, within a depth-of-processing framework, the impaired ability of DAT patients to *maintain* activation of semantic relations suggests that DAT involves a breakdown in the activation (or loss of representation) of attributes and features that relate and differentiate concepts in a semantic network. This interpretation is supported by the observation (Martin & Fedio, 1983; Schwartz et al., 1979; Warrington, 1975) that DAT patients are impaired in their ability to distinguish between semantically related words within a category, and is consistent with findings (Granholm & Butters, in press; Martin et al., 1987) that these patients are unable to exploit semantic relations between words to facilitate performance on conscious verbal recall tasks.

A loss of features and attributes in semantic memory can account for apparently discrepant findings regarding the intactness of semantic representation in the mild-to-moderate stages of DAT. That is, *incomplete* representations of concepts may be sufficient to provide the impression of normal processing on some tasks, while resulting in obviously impaired performance on others. For example, activation of a few central attributes of concepts may result in "normal" priming for highly related word pairs with short stimulus-onset asynchronies, as in the paradigm reported by Nebes et al. (1984). Similarly, deciding that a given lexical item belongs to a category may be accomplished by matching a few criterial features. Moreover, activation of a *reduced set* of features may explain DAT patients' difficulty in rejecting category nonexemplars (Nebes et al., 1986), which may require the activation of less central attributes of concepts. Finally, a degeneration in the activation of semantic features that relate and differentiate concepts may underlie DAT patients' impaired ability to generate members of a category (Butters, Salmon, Heindel, & Granholm, in press; Weingartner et al., 1981). This seems especially likely in light of the finding (Martin & Fedio, 1983) that DAT patients' output of semantically related items is negatively correlated with a tendency to confuse words from the same semantic category.

In conclusion, it should be noted that the results of the studies reviewed herein are consistent with Cummings and Benson's (1984) distinction regarding the relative preservation of language abilities in cortical and subcortical dementias. The apparent derangement of semantic processing in HD patients is not only much less severe than the breakdown found in DAT, but is also of a very different nature. The evidence reviewed in this paper suggests that the progression of HD may involve subtle changes in the organization of activation in semantic networks. In contrast, it appears that DAT may involve an actual *shrinkage* of semantic networks, resulting in incomplete representation of concepts and their relations in semantic memory.

Acknowledgments. The research reported in this manuscript was supported by funds from the Medical Research Service of the Veterans Administration, NIA Grant AG05131 to the University of California at San Diego, and by NIA Fellowship, AG05378 to Stan Smith.

References

Appell, J., Kertesz, A., & Fisman, M. (1972). A study of language functioning in Alzheimer patients. *Brain and Language, 7*, 73–91.

Battig, W.F., & Montague, W.E. (1969). Category norms for verbal items in fifty-six categories: A replication and extension of the Connecticut Category Norms. *Journal of Experimental Psychology Monographs, 80*(3), 1–45.

Bayles, K.A. (1982). Language functions in senile dementia. *Brain and Language, 16*, 260–280.

Bayles, K., & Tomoeda, C. (1983). Confrontation naming impairment in dementia. *Brain and Language, 19*, 98–114.
Benton, A.L. (1968). Differential behavioral effects in frontal lobe disease. *Neuropsychologia, 6*, 53–60.
Brandt, J., & Butters, N. (1986). The neuropsychology of Huntington's disease. *Trends in Neurosciences, 9*, 118–120.
Brouwers, P., Cox, C., Martin, A., Chase, T., & Fedio, P. (1984). Differential perceptual-spatial impairment in Huntington's and Alzheimer's dementia. *Archives of Neurology, 41*, 1073–1076.
Butters, N. (1984). The clinical aspects of memory disorders: Contributions from experimental studies of amnesia and dementia. *Journal of Clinical and Experimental Neuropsychology, 7*, 181–210.
Butters, N., Albert, M.S., & Sax, D. (1979). Investigations of the memory disorders of patients with Huntington's disease. In T. Chase, N. Wechsler, & A. Barbeau (Eds.), *Advances in neurology: Vol. 23. Huntington's disease*, (pp. 203–214). New York: Raven Press.
Butters, N., Granholm, E., Salmon, D., Grant, I., & Wolfe, J. (1987). Episodic and semantic memory: A comparison of amnesic and demented patients. *Journal of Clinical and Experimental Neuropsychology, 9*, 480–497.
Butters, N., Salmon, D., Heindel, B., & Granholm, E. (in press). Episodic, semantic and procedural memory: Some comparisons of Alzheimer's and Huntington's disease patients. In R. Terry (Ed.), *Aging and the Brain*. New York: Raven Press.
Butters, N., Sax, D., Montgomery, K., & Tarlow, S. (1978). Comparison of the neuropsychological deficits associated with early and advanced Huntington's disease. *Archives of Neurology, 35*, 585–589.
Butters, N., Wolfe, J., Granholm, E., & Martone, M. (1986). An assessment of verbal recall, recognition, and fluency abilities in patients with Huntington's disease. *Cortex, 86*, 11–32.
Caine, E., Hunt, R., Weingartner, H., & Ebert, M. (1978). Huntington's dementia: Clinical and neuropsychological features. *Archives of General Psychiatry, 35*, 377–384.
Cappa, S.F., Cavallotti, G., Guidotti, M., Papagno, C., & Vignolo, L.A. (1983). Subcortical aphasia: Two clinical CT-scan correlation studies. *Cortex, 19*, 227–241.
Collins, A.M., & Loftus, E.F. (1975). A spreading-activation theory of semantic processing. *Psychological Review, 82*, 407–428.
Collins, M., & Quillian, M. (1967). Retrieval time from semantic memory. *Journal of Verbal Learning and Verbal Behavior, 8*, 240–247.
Corkin, S. (1982). Some relationships between global amnesias and the memory impairments of Alzheimer's disease. In S. Corkin et al. (Eds.), *Aging: Vol 19. Alzheimer's disease: A report of progress in Research* (pp. 149–164). New York: Raven Press.
Craik, F.I.M., & Lockhart, R.A. (1972). Levels of processing: A framework for memory research. *Journal of Verbal Learning and Verbal Behavior, 11*, 671–684.
Craik, F.I.M., & Tulving, E. (1975). Depth of processing and retention of words in episodic memory. *Journal of Experimental Psychology: General, 104*, 268–294.
Cummings, J.L., & Benson, F. (1984). Subcortical dementia: Review of an emerging concept. *Archives of Neurology, 39*, 115–120.
Damasio, A.R., Damasio, H., Rizzo, M., Varney, M., & Gersh, F. (1982). Aphasia with nonhemorrhagic lesions in the basal ganglia and internal capsule. *Archives of Neurology, 39*, 115–120.

Fedio, P., Cox, C., Neophytides, A., Canal-Frederick, G., & Chase, T. (1979). Neuropsychological profile of Huntington's disease: Patients and those at risk. In T. Chase & A. Barbeau (Eds.), *Advances in neurology: Vol. 23. Huntington's disease*, (pp. 239–256). New York: Raven Press.

Gardner, H., Boller, F., Moreines, J., & Butters, N. (1973). Retrieving information from Korsakoff patients: Effects of categorical cues and reference to the task. *Cortex, 9*, 165–175.

Goodglass, H., & Kaplan, E. (1972). *The assessment of aphasia and related disorders*. Philadelphia: Lea & Febiger.

Granholm, E., & Butters, N. (in press). Associative encoding and retrieval in Alzheimer's and Huntington's disease. *Brain and Cognition*.

Hasher, L., & Zacks, R.T. (1979). Automatic and effortful processes in memory. *Journal of Experimental Psychology: General, 108*, 356–388.

Hyman, B.T., Van Hoesen, G.W., Damasio, A.R., & Barnes, C.L. (1984). Alzheimer's disease: Cell-specific pathology isolates the hippocampal formation. *Science, 225*, 1168–1170.

Irigaray, L. (1973). *Le language des dements*. The Hague: Mouton.

Jenkins, J.J. (1970). The 1952 Minnesota word association norms. In L. Postman & G. Keppel (Eds.), *Norms of word association*, (pp. 1–38). New York: Academic Press.

Josiassen, R., Curry, L., & Mancall, E. (1983). Development of neuropsychological deficits in Huntington's disease. *Archives of Neurology, 40*, 791–796.

Josiassen, R., Curry, L., Roemer, R., DeBease, C., & Mancall, M.L. (1982). Patterns of intellectual deficit in Huntington's disease. *Journal of Clinical Neuropsychology, 4*, 173–183.

Kaplan, E., Goodglass, H., & Weintraub, S. (1983). *Boston Naming Test*. Philadelphia: Lea & Febiger.

Klein, K., & Saltz, E. (1976). Specifying the mechanisms in a levels-of-processing approach to memory. *Journal of Experimental Psychology: Human Learning and Memory, 2*, 671–679.

Loftus, E.F. (1973). Activation of semantic memory. *American Journal of Psychology, 86*, 331–337.

Martin, A., Brouwers, P., Cox, C., & Fedio, P. (1985). On the nature of the verbal memory deficit in Alzheimer's disease. *Brain and Language, 25*, 323–341.

Martin, A., & Fedio, P. (1983). Word production and comprehension in Alzheimer's disease: The breakdown of semantic knowledge. *Brain and Language, 19*, 124–141.

Mattis, S. (1976). Mental Status Examination for organic mental syndrome in the elderly patient. In L. Bellack & T.B. Karasu (Eds.), *Geriatric psychiatry*, (pp. 77–121). New York: Grune & Stratton.

McCann, G., Drachman, D., Folstein, M., Katzman, R., Price, D., & Stadlam, E.M. (1984). Clinical diagnosis of Alzheimer's disease: Report of the NINCDS-ADRDA Work Group under the auspices of Department of Health and Human Services Task Force on Alzheimer's disease. *Neurology, 34*, 939–944.

McClelland, J., & Rumelhart, D. (1981). An interactive activation model of context effects in letter perception: Part 1. An account of the basic findings. *Psychological Review, 88*, 375–402.

McKoon, G., & Ratcliffe, R. (1979). Priming in episodic and semantic memory. *Journal of Verbal Learning and Verbal Behavior, 18*, 463–480.

Meyer, D., & Schvanaveldt, R. (1971). Facilitation in recognizing pairs of words: Evidence of dependence between retrieval operations. *Journal of Experimental Psychology, 90*, 227–234.

Mildworf, B., & Albert, M. (1978). *Cognitive function in elderly patients*. Masters thesis, Hebrew University.

Miller, E. (1973). Short- and long-term memory in presenile dementia (Alzheimer's disease). *Psychological Medicine, 3*, 221–224.

Naeser, M., Alexander, M.P., Helm-Estabrooks, N., Levine, H., Laughlin, S.A., & Geschwind, N. (1982). Aphasia with predominantly subcortical lesion sites. *Archives of Neurology, 39*, 2–12.

Nebes, R.D., Boller, F., & Holland, A. (1986). Use of semantic context by patients with Alzheimer's disease. *Psychology and Aging, 1*, 261–269.

Nebes, R.D., Martin, D.C., & Horn, L.C. (1984). Sparing of semantic memory in Alzheimer's disease. *Journal of Abnormal Psychology, 93*, 321–330.

Posner, M.I., & Snyder, C.R. (1975). Attention and cognitive control. In. R.L. Solso (Ed.), *Information and cognition*, (pp. 55–85). Hillsdale, NJ: Erlbaum.

Rumelhart, D., & McClelland, J. (1982). An interactive activation model of context effects in letter perception: Part 2. The contextual enhancement effect and some tests and extensions of the model. *Psychological Review, 89*, 60–94.

Salmon, D.P., Shimamura, A.P., Butters, N., & Smith, S. (in press). Lexical and semantic processing in patients with Alzheimer's disease. *Journal of Clinical and Experimental Neuropsychology.*

Schwartz, M., Marin, O., & Saffran, E. (1979). Dissociation of the language functions in dementia: A case study. *Brain and Language, 7*, 277–306.

Shimamura, A.P., Salmon, D.P., Squire, L.R., & Butters, N. (1987). Memory dysfunction and word priming in dementia and amnesia. *Behavioral Neuroscience, 101*, 347–351.

Shoulson, I. (1981). Huntington's disease: Functional capacities in patients treated with neuroleptic and antidepressant drugs. *Neurology, 31*, 1333–1335.

Smith, S., Butters, N., White, R., Lyon, L., & Granholm, E. (in press). Priming semantic relations in patients with Huntington's disease. *Brain and Language.*

Sterzi, R., & Vallar, G. (1978). Frontal lobe syndrome as a disconnection syndrome: Report of a case. *Acta Neurologica, 33*, 419–425.

Terry, R.D., & Davies, P. (1980). Dementia of the Alzheimer type. *Annual Review of Neuroscience, 3*, 77–95.

Wallesch, C., Kornhuber, H., Brunner, R., Kunz, T., Hollerbach, B., & Sugert, G. (1983). Lesions of the basal ganglia, thalamus, and deep white matter: Differential effects on language functions. *Brain and Language, 20*, 286–304.

Warrington, E.K. (1975). The selective impairment of semantic memory. *Quarterly Journal of Experimental Psychology, 27*, 635–657.

Wechsler, D. (1981). *Wechsler Adult Intelligence Scale—Revised manual*. New York: Harcourt Brace Jovanovich.

Weingartner, H., Kaye, W., Smallberg, S., Ebert, M., Gillin, J., & Sitaram, N. (1981). Memory failures in progressive, idiopathic dementia. *Journal of Abnormal Psychology, 90*, 187–196.

Whitaker, H. (1976). A case of isolation of the language function. In H. Whitaker & H.A. Whitaker (Eds.), *Studies in neurolinguistics (Vol. 2)*, (pp. 1–58). New York: Academic Press.

Whitehouse, P.J., Price, D.L., Struble, R.J., Clark, A.W., Coyle, J.T., & DeLong, M.R. (1982). Alzheimer's disease and senile dementia: Loss of neurons in the basal forebrain. *Science, 215*, 1237–1239.

Author Index

Subject Index

MIX
Papier aus verantwortungsvollen Quellen
Paper from responsible sources
FSC® C105338

If you have any concerns about our products,
you can contact us on
ProductSafety@springernature.com

In case Publisher is established outside the EU,
the EU authorized representative is:
Springer Nature Customer Service Center GmbH
Europaplatz 3, 69115 Heidelberg, Germany

Printed by Libri Plureos GmbH
in Hamburg, Germany